Routledge Revivals

The Hygiene of Mind

The
Hygiene of Mind

by

T. S. Clouston

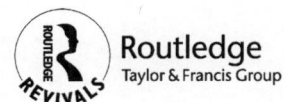
Routledge
Taylor & Francis Group

First published in 1906 by Methuen & Co.

This edition first published in 2019 by Routledge
2 Park Square, Milton Park, Abingdon, Oxon, OX14 4RN
and by Routledge
52 Vanderbilt Avenue, New York, NY 10017, USA

Routledge is an imprint of the Taylor & Francis Group, an informa business

© 1906 by Taylor and Francis

Publisher's Note
The publisher has gone to great lengths to ensure the quality of this reprint but points out that some imperfections in the original copies may be apparent.

Disclaimer
The publisher has made every effort to trace copyright holders and welcomes correspondence from those they have been unable to contact.

A Library of Congress record exists under ISBN:

ISBN 13: 978-0-367-25351-6 (hbk)
ISBN 13: 978-0-367-25365-3 (pbk)
ISBN 13: 978-0-429-28740-4 (ebk)

THE HYGIENE OF MIND

THE

HYGIENE OF MIND

BY

T. S. CLOUSTON, M.D., F.R.S.E.

LECTURER ON MENTAL DISEASES IN THE UNIVERSITY OF EDINBURGH
PHYSICIAN-SUPERINTENDENT OF THE ROYAL EDINBURGH ASYLUM
VICE-PRESIDENT OF THE ROYAL COLLEGE OF PHYSICIANS, EDINBURGH
AUTHOR OF "THE NEUROSES OF DEVELOPMENT"
"CLINICAL LECTURES ON MENTAL DISEASES," ETC.

WITH TEN ILLUSTRATIONS

METHUEN & CO.
36 ESSEX STREET W. C.

First Published in 1906

PREFACE

H OW Science can benefit Life is the greatest practical problem of modern civilisation. It is now being solved in a thousand ways. Whether this treatise on *The Hygiene of Mind* will in the least aid in its solution remains to be seen. Health is now in the air. How the mind of man can be strengthened, widened, and made a more efficient instrument through the application of modern scientific and physiological knowledge is a question of intense interest. I well know how presumptuous a thing it will seem to some persons to suggest that modern Science may succeed in doing what all the great philosophers, moralists, and religious teachers of the past have been trying to do for six thousand years. The justification of that suggestion is that evolution, physiology, psychology, and modern preventive medicine have now placed knowledge at our disposal which none of those great men of old had access to. If the scientific view that Mind has been evolved, like all else in the world, through the long ages of the past and has slowly reached its present stage through fixed laws is true, then it assuredly follows that it may still further grow and reach stages it has not yet attained through the operation of the same laws. The exclusively metaphysical view of Mind has so taken possession of the world that it will die hard. The wisdom and experience of the ages, with their axioms, rules, and assumptions as to how Mind should be educated and treated must, in this later time, at least receive a scientific interpretation in so far as they are true. No one can look into the problems treated of in this book and the literature of the subject without being deeply impressed by the way in which modern scientific conclusions about health of body and mind have often been anticipated by the wise men of the pre-scientific era. It is not generally realised that a necessity is laid on modern Science to bring morals, conduct, and even religion, under fixed laws and to harmonise them with the reign of law everywhere apparent in the universe. It is now a universally accepted fact that the body is capable of improvement by the application of hygienic rules, and that thereby the life of man and his happiness are bettered. It is also proved by physiology that mental action is absolutely co-related with brain action, and it therefore does not admit of doubt that the mind may also be bettered through brain and bodily hygiene. To put into popular language some of the known facts thus far ascertained and to extend the conclusions from those facts in regard to mental betterment through physiological, psychological, and medical means is the object of this book. Its aim is practical, and by that standard only it should be judged. The chief excuses for its many faults and omissions must be the novelty and the difficulties of the subject, the imperfection of our knowledge and the incomplete equipment of the author.

TABLE OF CONTENTS

CONTENTS

The most difficult study in Nature—Chemical processes—Physical processes—Vital processes and mental processes all associated—Reflex action is easily conceivable, not so consciousness and organisation, a chasm with no bottom—Consciousness and mind conditioned by brain processes—The nerve-cell and the muscle—Relations of cell to blood—Anabolism and Katabolism—Mind-cell stimuli—Stimuli from senses, from action of internal organs—Registration of stimuli—Printing on the brain—The phonograph—Laura Bridgman and Helen Keller—Brain and mental attributes and faculties and how they work and are related.

Necessity to Energise : Implies continuous repair, adjustment, and regulation of stimuli—All the brain cells do not act at the same time—Presentation and Representation.

Sleep : Brain repair—Dreaming.

Reactiveness : Different results of the same and of different stimuli in different brains—Range of man's reactiveness the greatest in Nature to influences and stimuli from within and without—Disturbed brain reactiveness from disease.

Brain and Mental Resistiveness : Importance—Defence against ever-present enemies—Microbes—Hygiene largely consists in strengthening Nature's defences—Alcohol, opium, &c., and resistiveness—Examples of broken-down resistiveness—Sound "health" and resistiveness.

Brain and Mental Solidarity : "Whether one member suffers, all the members suffer with it."

The Hierarchy in the Brain : Nerve centres and faculties higher and lower in grade—A regiment—Inhibitory centres—Colonel-in-chief—Innate differences in different persons and races—Limits to all faculties and powers—Do not approach those limits—Hereditary weaknesses.

Brain and Mental Habit : Physiological doctrine and universality of habit in all vital processes.

Habit and Inhibition : Brain fibre connections formed in child go with repeated action—Habit and Memory.

The metaphysical mental faculties, instincts, appetites, vitalities and organic necessities, and their relation—Consciousness—Feeling—Emotion—Idealism— Reasoning—Volition—Inhibition—Power of attention—Representation—Imagination—Association of ideas—Moral faculties—Religious instincts—Memory—Love of Life—Reproductive instinct—Gregarious and

CHAPTER VI

CONTENTS

CHAPTER XI

CHAPTER XIII

A 2

CONTENTS

CHAPTER XIV

Hygiene of manhood and womanhood not so important as that of adolescence—Psychologically and physiologically, functions and faculties mature—Masculine and feminine characteristics complete—Heredity no longer an advancing process—No longer a shadow coming out of the darkness—Full age implies work and stress—This healthy and natural—Enjoyment must not be excluded—The questions are, Are there weak points ? What are they ?—" Know thyself "—Fair health and average luck go to most—Greater responsibility of full age—Altruism a great hygienic duty—Selection of occupation—Use of the " preventive doctor "—Keep reasonably fat—An axiom for all serious people— A reasonable mental gymnastic possible for most men—Look at natural objects—Conscientiousness—A blend of St. Paul and Marcus Aurelius recommended—Solidarity of brain—The minor virtues—"Moderation in all things"—The bore, the critic, and the egotist are psychologically "unfit"—Mental and moral health and capacity cannot be precisely measured—Strychnine tonic *v.* a good dinner—Head work v. Routine mechanical work—Principles of hygiene for the two different—Equally good hygiene to think or to walk in different cases—The loss and wastage of human brain power through the neglect of hygiene—Pitt, Burns, Robert Louis Stevenson, Keats, Alexander the Great, Charles the Fifth—A medical reading of history and biography needed.

Mental Hygiene of Womanhood : Many special considerations of sex and duties—Her nervous organisation—Necessary repressions in her life—Child-bearing and nursing and their mental risks—A working man's wife and her hardships—The risks of the unmarried woman—Woman not so hungry as man—More subject to neurasthenia—Better times in recent years—Sex rivalry preposterous—The ideal woman—Different pictures— Woman undergoing evolution faster than man which makes her position more trying—Certain qualities she must have, modesty, &c., &c.—Marriage—Its psychology yet to be written from the point of view of modern science—Many pictures—The married state undergoing evolution—The greatest by far of all social institutions—Different theories of the married life at different times—The scientific theory—Large assortment of qualities needed—Some risks always—Love *v.* Passion—Love fused into a helpful comradeship—Nature provides the best hygiene of the married state—A mutual admiration society of two—Exceptions to rules—Innumerable love marriages turned out failures—Royal marriages—A woman with children takes a lot to make her unhappy—Only three-fourths of the marriages ideal—What is to

CHAPTER XVI

Modern medicine and psychology much concerned with sex
questions—Science cannot accept ignorance on any subject,
however dangerous it may appear—A sexless world a joyless
world—Emotion, art, poetry, &c., mixed up with it—Religion
and sex—National decadence largely connected with wrong sex
views and practices—All degenerate nations sexually corrupt
—Riches and luxury—St. Paul's view—A key to individual
happiness and national longevity—Wrong practices fatal to
emotional and moral perfection—The physiological law as to
the commencement of sex exercise—Developmental nutrition
must have ended before reproduction begun—Mental results of
disobedience—Impairment of manliness and modesty—Less
capacity for work—Nervous excitement—Morbid attention to
reproduction—Waste of precious energy—Nature will exact her
penalty—Tainted hues given to innocent subjects—Social and
family intercourse poisoned—Ideal of womanhood should be
founded on that of mother and sister—Unnatural practices not
inevitable and not harmless—*Obsta principiis*, the essential thing
—Control is best established by diverting attention and energy
to other subjects—Transform the energy into work and
thinking—Muscular exercise—Bathing—Foods commonly too
stimulating—Work, Nature's antidote—Self-denial strengthens

CHAPTER XVII

CONTENTS

LIST OF ILLUSTRATIONS

THE HYGIENE OF MIND

CHAPTER I

THE HYGIENE OF MIND—THE PROBLEM

HEALTH Science, or "preventive medicine," arose in the latter half of the nineteenth century. It has done wonders in its fifty years of existence in saving life, improving health, increasing happiness, and educating public opinion in regard to hygiene. A lowered death-rate only expresses a small part of what has been accomplished. The sufferings of the living have been decreased to an incalculable degree, and the race of the future is to be a better one than that of the past. The *mens sana* was always associated with the *corpus sanum*, but of old, and indeed up to very recent times, the sound mind was always held to be " in " the sound body rather than "of" it. The views of the physiologist, the psychologist, and the doctor have changed on that point. They now absolutely refuse to admit the possibility of a healthy mind in an unsound body, or at all events in an unsound brain, just as the electricians would refuse to admit that a steady electric current could be produced by an imperfect dynamo. No doubt an unsound mind and an unsound brain may appear to co-exist with what popularly would be called "good bodily health," but that is a misapprehension. Whatever Mental Hygiene is it cannot be dissociated from soundness of brain. The solidarity of brain and mind is an axiom of modern medicine. A man may have a sound heart with a bad liver, but he cannot have an unsound heart and a good circulation. To preserve health and to prevent disease are the objects of the great modern science and art of preventive medicine. Hygiene is the short term to express this science and art. Unsoundness, inefficiency, or weakness of mind may have to do with factors which ordinary preventive medicine has hitherto only touched lightly. Such factors are modes of education, social customs, human feelings, passions, morals, and religion. The man who writes about preventive medicine in the ordinary sense must know something of physics, chemistry, physiology, medicine, bacteriology, and laboratory work. The man who writes about Mental Hygiene must, in addition, have a special acquaintance with brain structure and function, and must take into special account mental evolution, heredity, psychology, ethics, education, sociology, and the religious instincts. It implies also a special study of mental disease and derangements and the modes of dealing with them. Perhaps even more than a study of fully developed mental disease, it needs a knowledge of those innumerable mental eccentricities, stupidities, lethargies, impracticabilities, losses of control, obsessions, impulses, asocialisms, perversions of feeling, morbid laziness, and all such mental and moral abnormalities as fall short of actual insanity. It therefore requires special qualifications. Who is sufficient for these things? I certainly do not feel myself to be so. Our data for an entirely satisfactory treatise on Mental Hygiene do not at present exist. Our knowledge is, as yet, immature in regard to many of the sciences on which such a treatise must be based. Thoroughly to know the human brain and how it works would imply a comprehension of the very highest, most difficult, and most complicated facts in organic nature. Its mechanism and its energies are as yet only in process of being studied. It is the driving wheel of human history, the apex of the vast evolutional pyramid of life whose basis consists of the swarming millions of microbes in which life began. Such perfect knowledge would imply a going back for millions of years of life. The human brain is not only the apex but the evident aim of the whole evolutional process. To ask if it is of importance that every means should be used to keep this marvellous organ healthy and efficient for its mental work would indeed be a cynical inquiry. The only possible objection to any attempt made to treat of the hygiene of mind is that the problem is as yet too difficult for the full application of the methods of modern science. The conditions which would absolutely ensure mental and brain health are infinitely complicated and are as yet largely impossible of attainment. It may be said that an organ whose essence and purpose is to respond and react to every force in nature—many persons would say to supernatural influences as well—must be so subtle in its working as to defy most of the ordinary hygienic measures at present known to us. The prescriptions of the modern preventive physician would be too simple to effect the end in view. Yet it is certain that we do now know enough to enable us to strengthen mental life and prevent mental failure and deterioration to a large extent.

If he would apply his knowledge to the lives of men, the mental hygienist must, in the first place, assume that man is a " bit of nature," and that the brain and its highest function of mind work through natural laws as sure and invariable as the law of gravitation. Our ignorance or incomplete knowledge of many of those laws should not be held as an excuse for complete inaction. Some good should certainly come out of every practical attempt to work the brain on right lines, to point out the causes of brain and mind failures, and to anticipate some of the effects of evil heredity, bad environments, and disease. Nearly all attempts to explain the causes of human ill-health and to lay down rules for its prevention and cure have been at first met with popular neglect and even derision. The laws and conditions of health, mental and bodily, are but faintly realised by the mass of mankind It will not credit that health rests on law. Ignorance commonly sits in the scorner's chair. Human nature is never so selfish as when, feeling itself happy and in good health, it sees efforts to prevent disease which it does not understand or sympathise with. This human nature weakness we often see exhibited in our popular literature and newspapers when health subjects are treated of. Microbes are commonly enough used to point a jest, and precautions against disease are frequently treated as if they were only suitable for amusing hypochondriacs and fools. No doubt to a certain extent the pendulum sometimes swings to the other side, a blind credulity taking the place of a blind scepticism. The sensational triumphs of modern surgery, which Lister has brought about by a study of the microbic enemies of mankind, the good effects of anti-serums and the abolition of malaria by killing mosquitoes are often looked on as miraculous tales of the supernatural rather than as the result of scientific study. The former sceptics are often inclined to believe every improved wonder of healing chronicled by the ubiquitous reporter and to swallow any nostrum that the quack or the enthusiast recommends. In no department of medicine have quackery, duplicity, and unreasoning credulousness found so sure a field as where the mental action of the brain is disturbed. The history of the occult arts, of mesmerism, of " faith healing," and of " Christian science " abound in illustrations of human credulity. Rational Mental Hygiene must rest solely on a sound physiological conception of the true relation of the brain and mind to each other and to the rest of the human organism. It must suspect all hygienic or other procedure that leaves the brain out of account. It must be distrustful of all conclusions that rest only on subjective experience, not backed by objective facts capable of proof. Reliable evidence is difficult to obtain. Fact and fancy are often so inextricably mixed up in the human mind, and are so difficult to disentangle that it is no wonder the one is taken for the other. A really scientific and reasoning state of mind usually needs so much training to acquire that it is necessarily rare. Human imagination is so active and subtle and needs so little basis of fact that it riots in the obscure and the wonderful. Medicine requires so much intellectual clearness and honesty in its study and in its practice that it is not surprising that its history is full of fallacies and immature generalisations. Mental Hygiene must assume as its basis that mind, in its every faculty and exhibition, implies and requires accompanying brain action. Whether we have to deal with reasoning or emotion, memory or will, appetite, passion, or instinct, whether exhibited in normal or abnormal forms—for every one of them brain activity is the essential basis. Consciousness itself, partial or entire, can never otherwise exist, in this world at least. " No brain, no mind " must be an unquestioned axiom to the student and practitioner of Mental Hygiene. All this is so contrary to a certain uneducated human instinct and appears to be so at variance with certain metaphysical and religious assumptions as to the entity and essential independence of mind, personality, and soul, that it is no wonder the scientific view has great difficulty in being popularly realised.

A treatise on Mental Hygiene might be written by the religious teacher, the moralist, the sociologist, the educationalist or the parent, each from his own point of view. From each of these we might learn much, but the modern physiologist or physician would almost certainly have to refuse to accept or to modify many of their conclusions, as not being founded on scientific data. This would not be the result of any mere "materialistic" assumption. The scepticism of a physicist who refused to accept generalisations that were founded on the study of energy alone without relation to its sources, its transformations, or its necessary relation to matter, would be perfectly justified by scientific methods. Such a man would believe in heat as the source of energy, but he would also believe that it had, as the necessary condition of its existence, a relation to the molecular or electric changes in matter. For this he would only receive approbation from his fellow-scientists, and the public would probably accept his conclusions unquestioningly. They would accept the fact that he knew about this branch of science, and was able to judge and decide on questions relating to it. They would not set up any opinion of their own in regard to it. They would not invent such a nickname for him as "materialist." The physiologist believes in the transcendental qualities and special attributes of mind as firmly as does the metaphysician. He knows that it stands apart from and above all other energies. He may even agree with Spencer that its special connection with organisation is "unthinkable," but he also knows that Lord Kelvin, the greatest living physicist, says the same thing about the precise nature of the connection of heat, light, and electricity with matter as Spencer does in regard to mind and organisation. It is sufficient as a scientific fact in both cases that the connection is absolute, that it follows fixed laws which can be studied by the methods of modern science.

The evolution of mind can be traced in living beings from the earthworm up through the lower to the higher animals and then at last to its highest exhibition in man. Science sees no break in the chain. The facts relating to sensation, the prelude of mind, having as its material instrument a specialised organic tissue, the nervous system, the fact that mind arose in its first simple beginnings out of sensation, that it becomes connected in its earliest stages with muscular movements, and that mind, sensation, and movement slowly, in the evolutionary process, became integrated and enlarged from a lower to a higher stage as the nervous system becomes specialised and more highly developed—such facts are just as surely proved as any physical phenomena. They are the basis of physiology, of medicine, and of the hygiene of mind. The further study of nerve and mind gives the great hope of health and happiness and even of still further evolution for the human species. Its practical importance to the future of mankind becomes thus incalculable. No study of physics and no mechanical invention can approach it in importance.

The practical and the true view of a science of Mental Hygiene may therefore be thus shortly stated. The study of the physiological processes of the body, so far as these affect the mental functions of the brain, must be its basis. All the organs of the body, so far as they have special relation to the brain, must also be taken into account. The more we know of bodily processes, be they nutritive or dynamical, the more we study the organism, the surer will be our conclusions. The brain must be assumed to be not only the most important organ in the body, but its essential organ, for the sake of which all else exists. It is, in fact, the microcosm of the whole organism, its centre and its master. It receives help from every other organ, but it also largely controls the working

of each.   By its mental action alone it can hurry the
heart's beat or slow its pace ; it can make the skin shrivel
or flush, it can quicken or stop the digestion, it can stop or
change the character of all the secretions, it can arrest
or improve the general nutrition of the body. Every organ
and every vital process is represented in the structure
of the brain by special "centres" and groups of cells that
have a direct relation with such organs and processes, and
through which they are controlled. This fact of itself
gives the widest range to the study of Mental Hygiene.
To do the brain good, to accentuate its mental action,
to avoid influences that would hurt it, is the aim of our
science.   That implies not only a knowledge of the brain
but of the functions and work of all the other organs
which are, as it were, its satellites. Their diseases and
weaknesses must be taken into account in its hygiene.
Its own special mechanism and its own marvellous
working, whose difficulties of investigation have hitherto,
in many respects, defied the patience and ingenious
researches of multitudes of the keenest investigators, must
be taken into account, so far as they are known. The
conditions and the substances that conduce to its vigorous
nutrition and to its healthy action must be attended to,
while the things that impede and injure its proper working
must be avoided. How it grows and how its functions are
slowly perfected during the perilous years of childhood,
youth and adolescence, from birth to the age of twenty-five,
and what the enemies of that marvellous developmental
process are, must be ascertained and taken into account.
How hereditary influences act for good or evil, during the
developmental period, forms a most important, but as yet
a very obscure, study relating to our problem. Can such
heredity, if evil, be antagonised or counteracted ? if good,
can it be helped ? are questions of the last importance to
the mental hygienist. There is reason to suppose that

the effects of heredity towards strength and weakness are exhibited in the brain more than in any other organ. The special diseases and disorders that affect the growing brain need to be known and fought against. The onset of the reproductive period of life and all that it implies, bodily, mentally, and morally, for health, pleasure, and work, form momentous problems for the individual and the race. The mind and brain management of this period of life, if we knew how to carry it out successfully, might alter the fate of millions of men and women. How educational methods, religious influences, moral sanctions, the right control of passions, the scientific forming of the growing mind may be carried out, has to be inquired into. Dr. Ballantyne would no doubt say that the intra-uterine or pre-natal period of brain life needs some care and attention. Certainly the mental condition of the pregnant woman is notoriously, in many cases, apt to be peculiar and unstable, requiring hygienic and medical attention. The middle period of life, between the ages of twenty-five and forty-five, with its efforts, its worries, its responsibilities and work, is subject to many upsets, preventable and un-preventable. Brain strength and efficiency make all the difference between success and failure, between productive citizenship and dependence, between good and bad father-hood and motherhood, between the ability to provide good and bad conditions of up-bringing for children. The period of decadence, retrogression, and old age, between forty-five and death, is one when, specially in its later stages, the brain cells are undergoing gradual shrinkage, and consequently the power of energy is diminishing and the joys of life are lessening in intensity. During this period there is, in many cases, a special necessity for such hygienic measures as tend to make the process of mental decay gradual and quiet instead of taking on an abnormal and explosive energy which the brain cannot safely tolerate. The waning nerve power needs to be used up with discretion. The diminished recuperative energy of this period must also be taken into account. A happy and comfortable old age is quite possible ; indeed, it seems to be becoming the rule rather than the exception among our comfortably-off classes, and stands in very sharp contrast to the unhappy and irritable old age which is neither a comfort to itself nor to others.

Among the most practical of all the questions in Mental Hygiene are the two following : By what means can we detect the preludes and beginnings of brain and mental abnormality and exhaustion ? Can we adopt any measures in those early stages for the counteraction and eradication of such abnormalities? To answer those, and so to help humanity in its need, implies a knowledge of the whole facts of brain development and of the laws which regulate that development. The beginnings of evil are always the most difficult to detect. Advanced evils are easy enough to diagnose. A bad brain and mental habit, if not corrected early, becomes evident enough after it has been thoroughly established. Looking to the variety of human nature and the normal range which is seen in every family and every community of men it is by no means easy to say definitely when the road which leads to abnormality has been entered. It is desirable to avoid false alarms or such undue introspection and self-centredness as would lead to hypochondria. Slight and commencing danger must neither be underrated nor overrated. *Obsta principiis* is, however, the most valuable motto in all effectual Mental Hygiene.

Few evils can be effectually counteracted except their causes are ascertained. Now the possible causes of mental and brain ill-health are legion. Heredity in every degree, bad education in many forms, and evil environments of innumerable sorts go towards its causation. Causes that will act on one brain and constitution unfavourably may have no effect on another. Nay, it is well known that a cause of weakness in one person will be a cause of strength in another. One young man mixes much with society and his mind is brightened and stimulated ; another does the same and his mental power is dissipated, while his attention is withdrawn permanently from serious study One young woman takes to athletics with her brothers and develops the strength of her womanhood ; another does the same and becomes a disagreeable tomboy. If we could clearly ascertain first what are the general causes of mental ill-being and inefficiency, and could then find out how those causes individually and in conjunction act on the multiform kinds of human constitutions, we should have solved half the problem of Mental Hygiene.

Some mental qualities are of so much more importance than others for a successful and happy life that one branch of Mental Hygiene consists in studying where strength lies and where weakness is exhibited in every individual child. The faculties are developed, as we shall see, in a definite order. Speech, sensitiveness, conscience, sex feelings, the religious instincts, may all appear either too soon or too late in a child where the brain is abnormal and the heredity is not good. The natural order of development is departed from in any individual to his very great danger. The faculties and powers are developed in relation to each other and in relation to the needs of life and of the whole organism in a normal child. This order and this relationship need, therefore, to be known before we can detect that anything is amiss. It would seem to be the object of some systems of education and upbringing to interfere with Nature's methods and to fight against her beneficent laws.

I have by no means thus exhausted the scope and

objects of Mental Hygiene, but have merely taken prominent illustrations of its work and aims.   Sound and strong mind is unquestionably the greatest asset of mankind. There is, unfortunately, a general feeling of fatality in the public mind about it.   It is now admitted that the bodily health and condition of a nation may be improved, but it is assumed most wrongly that its mental state and strength is a fixed quantity that cannot be altered.   To rouse discontent and promote inquiry on the subject would be a great gain.   It would lead to knowledge and to effort.   The problem would be assumed to be soluble. The first stage of progress would thus be reached.

CHAPTER II

THE MIND MACHINERY IN THE BRAIN

MENTAL energy of all kinds, mind in every shape, needs a mechanism through which it can manifest itself, in this world at least. That mechanism is found in perfection in the human brain and is of extraordinary complication and delicacy. The brain may be said to have four chief functions. The first is that of motion. It presides over and stimulates all the voluntary muscular movements of the body, regulating their force and co-ordinating in their working the different groups of muscles needed to perform them. The muscles of the legs and arms and body do not move on their own initiative, they need nerve currents from the brain to set them going. The apparatus for this in the brain is necessarily in close relationship to the sensory and mental apparatus. Mind and muscular movement have the closest connection with each other, acting and reacting on each other. The second brain capacity is that which gives the power of feeling or sensation. Different organs and tissues of the body have this power of feeling in very different degrees. Some, like the skin of the face and fingers, have it in great intensity ; others, like the hair and nails and cartilages, have no feeling at all. The mechanism through which it arises is also closely allied to the mechanism of the mind. All mind was slowly evolved out of sensation, looking to the evolution of the lowly animal life of millions of years ago, up to man. Sensation is closely related to motion, there being a form of movement called reflex, where an impression being made on a sensory nerve a muscular movement results therefrom, without any will being exercised or mental action of any kind. Sensation is specialised in the organs of the senses, the eye, the ear, the smell, the taste, and the muscular sense. Those have the closest of all the sensory relations to mind. Without them mind could not be developed at all, and their deficiency or disease always affects it adversely. The third great function of the brain is that of nutrition ; through this its own nourishment and that of the rest of the body is regulated. Every bodily organ or tissue has an innate power of extracting nourishment from the blood, altering its chemical constitution, and building it up as part of itself, but this nutritive process needs regulation by the brain, without which it would be irregular and unrelational. As part of this great nutritive process the brain regulates the distribution of blood by the arteries and capillaries. Those blood-carrying tubes are made larger or smaller by nervous impulses from the brain and the nerve centres. Much or little blood is thus supplied to the bodily organs. How mind affects this function is well seen in blushing, when the whole of the blood capillaries in the face are suddenly enlarged. The general tone of the walls of the blood-vessels is steadily kept up from the brain. We can give certain medicines which act on the brain and increase this tone, so improving the nutrition of the body. The fourth function of the brain, its highest and most important, is that of mental action. The largest part of the human brain, the most delicate and the most complicated portion, is devoted to this all-important function. All these functions of the brain are connected with each other in the most definite way. One without the other would be imperfect.

Working, as they do, harmoniously together, they form by far the most perfect mechanism known in nature.

The actual physical machinery that does the work of the brain consists of cells, fibres, blood-vessels, drainage apparatus, and a connective substance which holds these

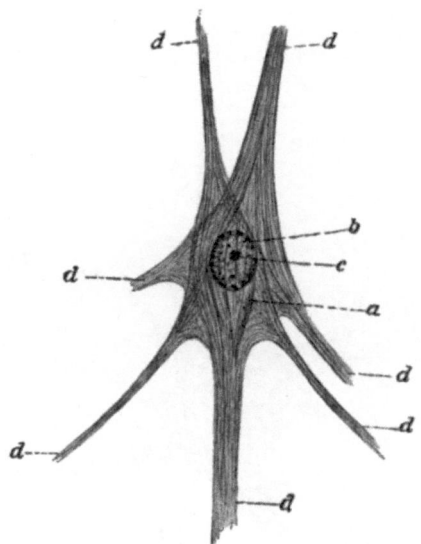

FIG. I.—A NORMAL BRAIN CELL OF
LARGE SIZE.

a. Body of cell with innumerable minute fibres passing through it. *b.* Its nucleus. *c.* Its nucleolus. *d.* The outgoing and incoming fibres through which it is related to other cells, to the spinal cord, and to the nerves of the body.

all together in their proper places and prevents them being displaced or injured by such physical shocks as are implied in walking, jumping, or coming in contact with hard substances. The cells are the most important and the most wonderful of these. They have each an exquisite internal structure which it has taken fifty years of

hard and ingenious work by physiologists to discover, and
we do not know it fully yet (see fig. 1).   The brain has to
be first hardened by chemical agents and sliced into the
thinnest shreds, stained with different coloured pigments

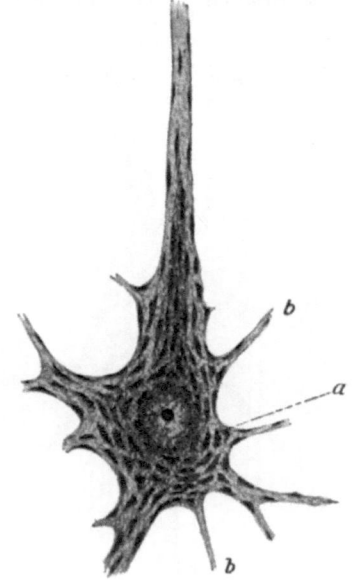

FIG. 2.—A LARGE BRAIN CELL PREPARED BY A
DIFFERENT PROCESS—THE "NISSL METHOD"—
FROM THE ONE SHOWN IN FIG. I.

There are many methods of such preparation and
staining, each bringing out the different parts
and characteristics of the cell.   This one shows
the cell full of material for potential work,
"chromatic granules," such as a young man or
woman in good health and after rest and sleep
should have.   a. Chromatic granules.   b. Outgoing and incoming fibres.

and then examined by microscopes magnifying a thousand diameters to see the internal structure of the cell.
Each cell has the power of taking up from the blood
and storing within it the nerve substance for its proper

nourishment. A nerve cell, after rest and sleep, can be seen to contain this substance (see fig. 2). An empty nerve cell, after a hard day's work or thinking, or in certain states of exhaustion and disease, can be seen to have much less of this nutritive pabulum (see fig. 3). Every

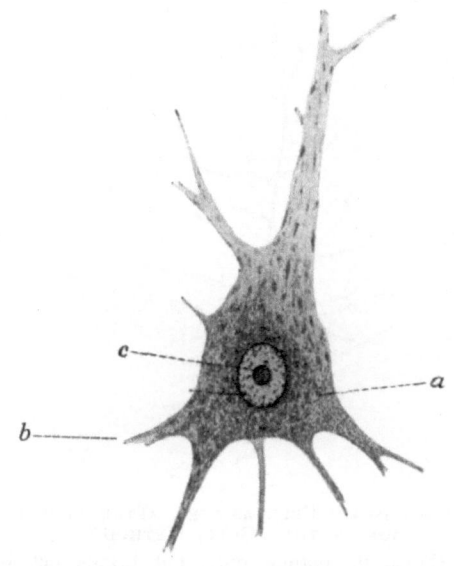

FIG. 3.—A LARGE BRAIN CELL PREPARED BY THE SAME METHOD AS FIG. 2,

Showing that the material for potential work, "chromatic granules," exists in very small quantity. This diminution of chromatic material is found after exhaustive conditions and great overwork. *a.* Pale chromatic granules. *b.* Outgoing and incoming fibres. *c.* Nucleus.

cell has connected with it and forming a part of it, like the legs of a spider, a series of minute fibres or processes (see fig. 4). Some of those are for the purpose of communicating with the other cells near it, while one main process of each large cell passes right out of the brain to the spinal

c

cord and the other parts of the body (fig. 4 *c*). The nearest analogy to the working of a nerve cell is a small electric battery.   This has first to be supplied with chemicals. Those are gradually used up through the transformation of

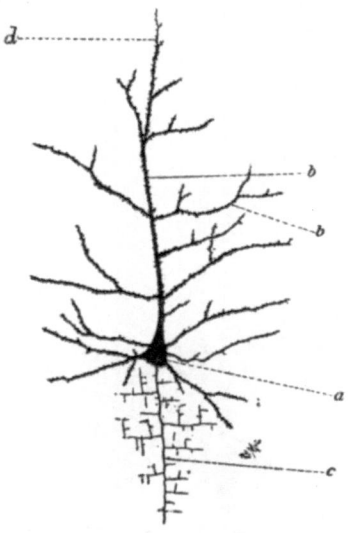

FIG. 4.—A BRAIN CELL AS SEEN AFTER PREPARA-
TION BY THE "GOLGI METHOD."

This shows its outline only, but brings out its
branches—"dendrites"—and "axis cylinder," or
the fibre that passes down from the cell into the
spinal cord and nerves of the body, so enabling
the cell to transmit its energy to the most distant parts of the body. The branches are seen
to be covered with innumerable small knob-like
projections, the "gemmules." *a*. The cell. *b*. Its
branches or dendrites.   *c*. The "axis cylinder"
and its processes. *d*. The "gemmules."

potential into active energy, and so the electric force is generated. The electric current so created is then trans- mitted through the copper wires that are attached to the battery. The cell, through its internal action, evolves nerve force and sends it out through its attached fibres as the battery evolves electricity and sends it out. Mind may be regarded as the highest form of nerve force. It is not " created " in the brain but it is absolutely conditioned by that organ. These cells do not work each for itself and by itself, they are associated together in groups of hundreds or thousands, as the case may be (see fig. 5), those groups doing the combined work of the brain. Different groups have different kinds of work assigned to them. Some have motion, some have sensation, some have nutrition, and some have mind, while many forms of mind, *e.g.*, inhibition, has special tracts of brain to carry it on. Every group, while it does its own work, is related to and combined with others, influencing them and being influenced for the purpose of producing a harmonious effect. The impressions conveyed to each from the body and the outer world beyond the body leave a fixed registration. This process is one of the many brain marvels which we are yet quite unable fully to understand. But it is just as certain that the impressions received from the skin and from the eye and from the ear and from the taste and smell are imprinted on those cells and laid up there as it is that the types leave an imprint of the letters and words on the pages of a printed book. Those printed impressions upon the cells can be revived and seen and heard by the mental consciousness, just as a printed book can be opened and seen and read by its owner. There is this difference, amongst others, between the two—that no book has so many words and ideas contained within it as one human brain has, let us say, at the age of forty. As we have the power of opening a book and reading its contents, so every human being can revive the sights and the sounds and the sensations he has previously experienced.

Those brain cells are of very different sizes. It is one of the largest of them that is represented in the picture (fig. 1). The number of them is absolutely inconceivable. I asked my friend, Dr. Ford Robertson, who devotes his whole life to the study of the brain, to compute the average

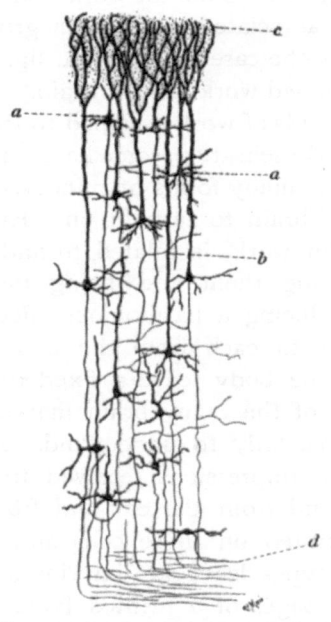

FIG. 5.—THIS SHOWS HOW THE CELLS ARE ASSOCI-
ATED TOGETHER IN GROUPS IN THE BRAIN, EACH
CELL MEMBER OF THE GROUP WORKING WITH
THE OTHERS. ("GOLGI METHOD" OF PREPA-
RATION.)

a. Cells.   *b.* Branches ("dendrites").   *c.* Method in
which the branches are associated at the surface
of the brain, enabling all the other groups to
receive impressions from this group.   *d.* The
"axis cylinders" passing from the cells through
the brain, forming part of its "white substance,"
and then down to the spinal cord and to every
sensitive and muscular part of the body.

number of cells in a human brain. He estimates that they reach the astounding figure of three thousand millions. No human mind, it is said, can take in the idea of a million units. It is not wonderful, therefore, that we have difficulty in even imagining the mechanism and the working of a human brain. If all the telegraph batteries in the world with all their communicating wires were thrown together and worked in relationship to each other, it would be a mechanism not to compare with the human brain in complexity and number of individual units. A man with great thinking power has far more cells than a stupid man, and an idiot has few and badly formed cells (fig. 6 c).

The fibres connected with those brain cells connect every unit and every group with each other and also connect them all with every organ and part of the human body. If a toe or a finger is touched, at once the brain feels it through the sensory cell and the impression is then instantaneously analysed by the mental cells as to whether it is a touch, or heat or cold. The spinal cord is a prolongation of the brain down the spine and has functions of its own, all relating to motion and sensation, but it has no direct relationship to mind. The brain cells that subserve mental action form the greater part of the mass of the brain convolutions, and they mostly lie outside of and above the other cells. Those cells are not perfect in their form and structure and connection till long after birth. At birth the cells are small (see fig. 6 b). Each then contains only a little "protoplasm," and its fibres of connection with other cells are few and imperfect compared with the fully developed brain. On the process of their slow and gradual development and the formation of the connections of cell with cell and groups of cells with groups of cells by means of new strands of fibres depend the development of the mental processes of thought, feeling, and will. During this most subtle and marvellous growth of the mind machinery, the influences of right or wrong environment and conditions are all important for good or evil. It is then that a scientific Mental Hygiene should come in to avert evil and help right development in certain cases.

The brain requires and has an enormous blood supply. The large arteries come into the brain from different points, and at their base are connected in a circle, so that if one is accidentally blocked there are others to take its place. When those arteries split up and become

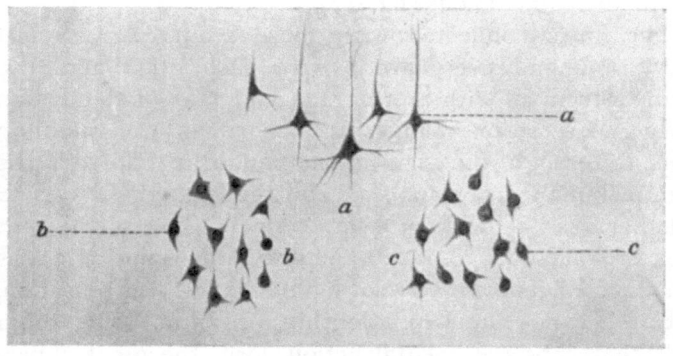

FIG. 6.—THREE GROUPS OF BRAIN CELLS.

One (a) showing the normal appearance of the cells in a grown man or woman ; the next (b) showing their undeveloped state in a newly-born child, with normal nucleus but small cell contents and few short processes ; and the third (c) showing the cells arrested in their development in an idiot of 20, those being in much the same state as in the newly-born child. The brain cells have not grown and the mind has not developed.

"arterioles" they spread out in all directions round and through the brain. When the arterioles split up and become capillaries those pass to the cells in innumerable directions. Each cell has a capillary near enough to enable it to absorb from the blood the nourishment that it needs (see fig. 7 b). As showing the great importance of the cells, they are found to have five or six times as many capillaries in every square inch as the fibres. This means that they use up that proportion of the blood. It is perfectly clear from this alone that the cells are there to produce the chief energies of the organ, while the fibres merely conduct that energy from one place to another, just as in telegraphy the battery evolves the electricity and needs constant renewing

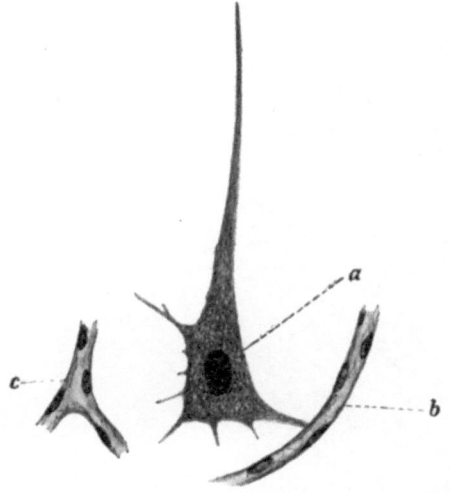

FIG. 7.—SHOWS HOW A BRAIN CELL GETS ITS SUPPLY OF BLOOD FROM A CAPILLARY BLOOD-VESSEL LYING IN CONTACT WITH OR VERY NEAR IT.

a. Cell. *b*. Its capillary blood tube. *c*. Another capillary. The brain cells need for their proper mental working a very large supply of pure blood. This is how they get it.

while the copper wire merely sends it on to another place and needs little care. The capillaries of the brain are not only more numerous but they are smaller in size and their walls are thinner than those of any other tissue. This means that the chemical and physical processes through which the nourishing part of the blood passes from the vessels into the cells need to be done more quickly than anywhere else. The demand for blood in abundance is more urgent than elsewhere.

The packing and supporting tissue of the brain, called the "neuroglia," consists of small cells quite different

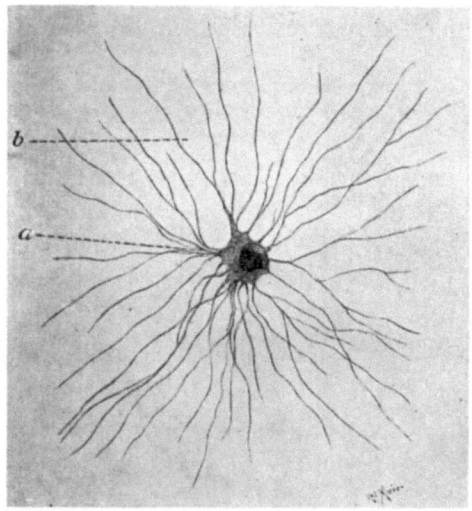

FIG. 8.—A CELL OF THE PACKING AND BINDING MATERIAL OF THE BRAIN, THE "NEUROGLIA."

By means of those innumerable fine fibrils which are fixed to the blood-vessels a strong network is formed for the cells where they lie free from the risks of injury. Those fibrils act as guy-ropes to the capillaries and small vessels. A strong framework is thus given to the brain.

in appearance from the brain cells, each sending out innumerable fibres of the most extraordinary fineness (fig. 8). Each cell in this way has multitudes of supporters. The capillaries, too, are held in their proper places by those guy-ropes. As everybody knows, the brain is encased and protected outside by a strong, bony envelope, the skull. No other organ has such a complete protection.

The brain has also an elaborate drainage system through which its waste products are instantly removed. If they are not taken away thoroughly, the cells are poisoned and act more slowly. The mental processes then become slow, confused, and distorted.

Mental Hygiene must take account of the working of every part and constituent of this most delicate and intricate mechanism. Derangement in any part of it, will derange or diminish mental force. Non-development will arrest mind growth. Improper blood will alter mind, imperfect drainage will confuse mind, and mechanical shocks will kill mind.

CHAPTER III

HOW THE BRAIN MECHANISM WORKS IN REGARD TO MIND

THE mode of working, or the physiology of the brain, is probably the most difficult study in all nature. It includes chemical processes, physical processes, vital processes, and mental processes of astounding complexity. Scientists do not, as yet, pretend to have solved one-tenth of the mysteries of brain-working. The human mind is quite capable of conceiving how an impression made on a nerve of the skin can be transmitted through a sensory nerve up to the brain, and when that stimulus reaches the brain cells that they may be set into action and transmit another kind of stimulus down through a motor nerve to a muscle so that we have "reflex" movements resulting therefrom. The analogy of pressing a button and so turning on an electric current to move a lever in a mechanism and setting wheels in motion enables us to understand in some degree this nerve process; but when we try to imagine what takes place when the impression is consciously *felt* in the brain we fail to understand it through any analogy with any other known process. We realise that we have entered a region of knowledge entirely different from chemistry, physics, or physiology. The leap from those sciences to mind and consciousness is one over a chasm with, as yet, no bottom.

Spencer's gradation hypothesis from molecular action to sensation and then to mental working was but a shot in the dark. We only know that mental action is evolved and conditioned in all sorts of ways by physical agencies acting on the organ of mind. But let us first look at what rouses muscular movement. The cells of the brain which preside over it originate and regulate the force which causes the muscles to move, just as an electric car moves quickly or slowly according to the strength of the current. All cells require constant recharging with the source of the energy that they are so constantly giving out. This means that there are in each of them two processes going on. The one is that of taking from the blood the source of such energy, converting this into nerve material, which, as we have seen, is laid up in the cell (fig. 2.) The coal has to be made on the spot and stored handy for use. Each cell is, in short, a powerful chemical factory. We call this process that of *anabolism*, or building up. The second process, that of *katabolism*, is that of using the material thus laid up in the cells. If one thinks for a moment how we use this motor force we see how subtle must be its action. We want to lift a pin, and the cells send down a very minute amount of stimulus indeed to the finger muscles. We want to lift a hundredweight, and a perfect flood of the same energy is sent down to the arms. We want to play the piano, and there are hundreds of cell groups that must send out regulated stimuli to the scores of muscles that are to be employed and co-ordinated.

Mind-cell Stimuli.—A primary fact to be recognised about those cells which are the vehicle of mind is this— they undergo almost all their development during child-hood from stimuli coming from without the brain. When a child is born its brain is absolutely mindless. The cells have infinite possibilities and potentialities. What sets them going on their marvellous course of future action ?

It is undoubtedly the impressions and stimuli which they are constantly receiving from the eyes, the ears, the touch, the taste, and the smell.   There is another series of constant impressions from within the body, but outside of the brain, that are thus reaching the cells from the senses, and those are from the muscles.   In addition to those the working of the heart and lungs and the other organs are all felt by and stimulate the brain cells.   In addition, each cell and each group of cells is laying up not only the nourishment—the coal supplies of which we have spoken— but it is constantly registering through a subtle series of molecular changes the stimuli of which I have spoken. The colour and qualities of objects and their nearness or distance, the different kinds of sounds and tones are all printed on the brain as on a book.   The processes of subjective thought, apart from sense impressions, are also registered.   This process is all the time helping to develop the actual physical structure of the cells of the growing brain.   The writing is there, and by a more wonderful process still than anything we have yet contemplated it can be read and brought before consciousness at any time during the whole of the rest of life.   This constitutes the process of memory, without which no intelligence could be developed and no process of imagination could take place.   Every kind of mental activity and every kind of feeling needs and uses up the brain energy of the cells.   To think, we need plenty of healthy blood supplied to the cells.   To make that healthy blood we need abundance of fresh air supplied to the lungs and a vigorous heart to pump it up to the brain.   When we think or feel it can be demonstrated that the brain becomes redder and more full of blood than when we are not thinking or feeling, and when we cease to feel or think actively or are fatigued it is pale.   To think and feel properly should mean to act rightly as a physiological corollary. Brain cells must be ever vigorous in action, and this vigour can only be attained through the many years of steady stimulation from the senses and through the power of memory to recall the impressions of those stimuli. The phonograph offers a distant analogy of some of the brain processes. We first have the voice and its modulation into words. We then need the electric wire to convey the energy. We then need the phonographic plate—that is, the brain cell—to receive the impression through its appropriate mechanism. We then have those plates put aside for future use. They require to be arranged and assorted so that each may be got at when needed, and when so needed they are put again into active use. What piles of phonographic plates lie assorted in every human brain! No one can think of this process which I have tried so imperfectly to describe without saying to himself, " How enormous must be the importance of having those processes and their machinery rightly provided for and properly attended to ! " Two of the most instructive studies in mental development through sensory and mental stimuli are to be found in the biographies of Laura Bridgman and Helen Keller. Both girls lost the senses of hearing and sight and the faculty of speech early in life. They both from this cause remained for years in a condition of virtual idiocy through brain arrestment. The only sense available for their development was that of touch. By a marvellous process of teaching, devised in the case of Bridgman by Dr. Howe, of Boston, touch was made to take the place of the other lost senses, and they both became intelligent members of society. They were restored to the enjoyment of intellect, emotion, imagination, inhibition, morals, and the social contact of their fellows. They both reached a high degree of happiness. They both attained keenly intellectual and emotional lives. Their stories are the romance of Mental Hygiene.

Brain and Mental Attributes and Faculties.—I shall now shortly describe some of the fundamental brain attributes that are relevant to Mental Hygiene. One of the most important of these is what may be called the *necessity to energise*—that is to say, the brain cells generally and the mental mechanism particularly is of such a nature and constitution that it cannot absolutely rest—at least during waking hours. There is a necessity for them to act in some way, and this action necessarily produces mental action. No doubt they may act slowly or with great rapidity. The engine may go at five miles an hour or it may be pushed to go at a hundred, but go it must—it cannot stand still. Different brains have different capacities of energising, both in regard to speed and force. This continuous action implies continuous repair. There must be a delicate adjustment between what I have referred to as the anabolic or reparatory force and the katabolic or dynamical output. Blood is needed, air is needed, and the right kinds of stimuli are needed. If wrong or improper stimuli are applied the energising will be perverted or too continuously active in regard to its sensory and emotional qualities. Mental cells have only limited periods during which the highest kind of activity can persist. Few men can feel intense joy or sorrow or suffer intense pain for very long without a dulling process setting in. That means that the cells are exhausted and the brain is ceasing to be able to feel keenly. It may be asked, "Do all those millions of cells act at once?" It is certain that they do not. Nature has provided, in the first place, probably fifty times the number of cells that are required for the brain's activity at one time. The different groups of cells have different functions, and those groups are put in action according to the faculty or function that is in action. When a man is thinking over the memory of past events and scenes in his life one group of cells is called into action; when he is devising plans for the future another group. When those memories are called up before consciousness we call it *representation;* when the original pictures are actually seen by the eye or heard by the ear and reach consciousness we call it *presentation.* During presentation the record is made in the brain. This takes a little time. If the time of presentation is too short an imperfect record is made. If the same presentation is made again and again it deepens the record. This is ever to be kept in mind by the mental hygienist. Repeat and deepen the presentation of all good and pleasant things and thoughts. Representation is a fainter process than presentation, but its vividness differs enormously in different people.

Trying to remember a bit of scenery or a face, many people have the power of what is called "visualising," that is, they actually see before them the object that they had previously seen. When a man feels, a different set of cells are put into action. When a man wills, another still different set of cells are employed. When any of those mental operations are accompanied by muscular movements, there is, as it were, a projection downwards of stimuli to the motor centres. The brain looks within as well as without, and records its own thoughts and feelings just as it registers the impressions of outward objects. The subjective and the objective are not different in the essential conditions of their registration and remembrance. It is the same brain process through which both are accomplished.

Sleep.—The process of repair and the complete physiological rest which the brain cells absolutely need, are provided for by the marvellous brain function of sleep. What precisely happens and what causes the cessation of consciousness, the suspension of thinking and feeling and the stoppage of muscular action in sleep is not accurately known, but it is known that activity of the brain cells is then chiefly confined to absorbing their proper nourishment from the blood and so laying up a stock of energy for use during the waking hours. This needs less blood and less oxygen than katabolic activity, for the brain is then pale. We know that the mental powers are not absolutely suspended at all times during sleep. The process of dreaming, that close analogue to delirium and insanity, shows that there is then a kind of automatic and disordered mental activity. The pictures that have been laid up come out casually in grotesque groups and unrelated sequences. The phonographic plates are taken out at random. No Mental Hygiene that does not take account of the sleep process can be a complete one.

Brain and Mental Reactiveness.—There is an all-pervading and most subtle quality of the brain which may be called its *reactiveness*, which distinguishes it, at least, in degree and kind from all other organs. What is meant by brain reactiveness is that when stimuli are applied of various kinds they rouse energy, mental or otherwise, corresponding in kind and degree to the stimulation applied. It sympathises, as it were, with favourable forces that impinge on it, and it antagonises others that are unfavourable. Plants react to light, air, heat, moisture, and soil only. The lower kinds of animals, such as fish or frogs, react to a few more environments than plants, and the higher animals react to many more than such cold-blooded creatures. In man's brain there is a reactiveness to almost every force and stimulus in nature. No doubt some of the means of communication with the outer world, chiefly the organs of sense, are not so acute in man as those of some of the higher animals. We do not smell like the dog, nor do we see like the eagle. It is doubtful if we possess some of the sense capacities of birds and certain wild animals as to weather, atmosphere, and orientation.   But the range and the effects of all our sense impressions taken together are infinitely larger and more subtle than those of the highest animal.   The range of an animal's reaction to its sense impressions is mostly limited to food, sex, and self-preservation.   Our sense impressions, on the contrary, have the power of calling up memory images of vast extent, of rousing imagination, of stimulating thought, and of powerfully acting on volition. The chief sources of human brain reactions are light, sound, colour, smell, taste, touch, air, heat, cold, electricity, music, harmony, the beautiful, the terrible, the sublime, and our fellow-men in life or in their books.   Brain reaction also results from impressions and stimuli from within the body and the brain itself.   The subtle but continuous influences on brain and mental action of the healthy or unhealthy working of the skin, the lungs, the heart, and stomach, are causing continuous reactions.   The influences of sex and reproduction are specially powerful and affect morality or immorality, action or inaction, affection or hatred. The effect of want of food on human brains has often been to stir up revolutions.   It was not ideas only that caused the French Revolution.   The starvation and the bodily miseries of the common people powerfully contributed to it and affected its character.   The quality of the blood has the power of producing reactions of all sorts in the brain cells which it is nourishing.   Brain reaction, if excessive, may take the form of loss of self-control, delirium, or insanity.   In mental disease, the reactiveness of the brain so affected is often completely altered, so that heat and cold may produce no effects, hunger may not stimulate efforts to get food, and sex no impulses to satisfy its cravings.   The sight of those nearest and dearest may not produce happiness or any effect whatever ; or the re- actions in such cases may be completely perverted from their normal conditions, so that in the instances quoted

D

the presence of those nearest and dearest to a patient may simply aggravate the morbid pain. But it would need a treatise to exhaust what could be said on this all-important brain and mental quality.

Brain and Mental Resistiveness.—Another brain and mental quality of great importance in Mental Hygiene is what may be called *resistiveness.* This means that a brain with a high degree of this quality will not suffer from such injurious stimuli and environments as would destroy one with a low degree of this quality. A high degree of this quality, together with the possession of surplus energy—and often it is the possession of such energy that gives resistiveness—forms a strong brain that lives long. It is now known to modern science that life of every sort, and human life particularly, is surrounded by innumerable microscopic living enemies to its existence. On the power of defence against those enemies, its health and its existence depend. The chief of those enemies to life and health are swarms of microbes which we constantly breathe in the air and swallow in our food. Nature has provided a most elaborate process for our defence against them. The blood contains millions of microscopic particles called "leucocytes," whose purpose is to swallow and antagonise such enemies. The harmful microbes produce the toxin, or poison; the guardian leucocytes at once produce the anti-toxin, or antidote. The latest studies in mental medicine show that probably many mental diseases and many conditions of mental disturbance, short of actual insanity, such as lethargy, irritability, inability for work, and depression are of microbic origin. Part of the work of hygiene, bodily and mental, is, according to modern science, to strengthen nature's vital defences and so increase this resistiveness. Many symptoms of disease, which are themselves often put down as actual disease, such as inflammation, cough and fever, are nature's processes of resisting disease and death. To be able to resist the early symptoms of depression and painful emotion, excitement, and loss of control, would be to avert attacks of mental disturbance in many cases. Looked at from the ethical point of view, conduct might thereby be improved, immorality might be avoided, and sweetness and light let into our lives. But for such resistiveness many of our race would become so unhappy that they would die, and our slum population would become so fierce that they certainly would steal and murder more than they do. Many of our social customs are so inharmonious with healthy life, and many of the things we use are so destructive to resistiveness that it is no wonder our people suffer so largely from ill-health, mental and bodily. Of all the articles largely used by mankind, probably alcohol in excess, as we shall see, has the power of diminishing resistiveness to disease to a greater degree than anything else used by our modern urban populations.[1] But regarding that and the effects of other such agents as tobacco, opium, tea, and other poisons from without or from within, I shall have more to say in detail afterwards. Take the following example of the way in which mental and moral resistiveness may be broken down. A strong man of high principle became ill, and a relative who was his nurse put such pressure on him that he made a will, leaving her all his money, and so doing gross injustice to his other relatives equally nearly connected with him, and of whom he was equally fond. The moment this cause of the breaking down of his resistive power was removed he altered his will and did justice to his relations. " Lead us not into temptation " is another way of putting " Increase our mental resistiveness." Normal resistiveness usually goes

[1] [Alcohol has lately been shown to paralyse the guardian leucocytes of the blood : *cf.* Prof. Metchaikoff's Harben Lectures, 1906. *Editor s Note.*]

with sound health, vigorous muscular power, and exercise in the fresh air. A man in this condition will resist the effects of cold, of pain or injury, and, if hurt, will heal more quickly than a man in a lower condition of health, in addition to being able to resist mental evil influences. When a man or a woman is said to " break down " it is usually a case of diminished brain resistiveness. This quality is closely related to will power and moral capacity.

We doctors meet with curious examples of brain resistiveness produced by disease against certain drugs. I have known many cases of acute mental disease who could take and be the better for poisonous doses of sedatives and sleep-producing medicines, while the strongest purgatives will sometimes not act on their bowels nor the most active sudorifics produce perspiration in them.

Brain and Mental Solidarity.—The brain, though composed of many parts and centres, representing many functions, has at the same time a *solidarity*, or oneness of function, which must always be taken into account by the mental hygienist. No single function can be overdone, and no one part can be injured or suffer disease without every part suffering more or less in consequence. " And whether one member suffer all the members suffer with it," is good physiology and correct psychology. Exhaustion of one function always weakens the others more or less. Mosso has clearly proved that fatigue of mind, through mental exertion, diminishes the power of walking and writing somewhat ; while excessive muscular exercise is incompatible with the best thinking or the highest volition. Solidarity and localisation both exist in the brain, but not in a complete form. One conditions the other.

The Hierarchy in the Brain.—The various portions of the brain which represent different functions and capacities, the different nerve centres and the different mental powers and faculties are related to each other as higher or lower according to their importance. There is, in fact, a hierarchy in the brain, each part of which has a different authority. It is made up like a regiment with the colonel, major, captain and the rank and file, as Hughlings Jackson puts it. Certain portions of the brain exist, not, as it were, to do special work of their own, but to stimulate or to inhibit the work of other centres. Those " inhibitory centres " of muscular movement, of nutrition, and of nerve action represent the mental and the moral qualities of control, such qualities being of the highest rank in the hierarchy. Mental inhibition is the colonel-in-chief of the brain hierarchy. There is a power of high import-ance in Mental Hygiene, and that is the action of mind on mind. I do not mean that this can take place except through the brain, the senses, or the corporeal presence of the person who so acts and is acted on. As yet there is no scientific proof of the mental action of one person on another who is at a distance, the so-called " telepathy " or pure transmitted will power without any bodily presence. But that one human being acts on and influences others for good or evil through the exercise of mind force, sympathy, antipathy, and will power is an unquestioned fact in psychology.

Differences in Brain.—There are enormous innate dif-ferences between the brain and mental power of different individuals. To compare the lower sort of savages with the man of genius in a civilised country is to compare things that have almost nothing in common—at least when looked at superficially. The power of a superior brain in force, in intensity, subtlety of action, in acquisition and pro-ductiveness is often a hundred times that of the average man. Taking one faculty—that of memory—there have been many instances of such prodigious power in this faculty, that it seems miraculous when compared with that of ordinary men. This innate difference of different human brains is a thing to be taken into account by the hygienist.   It would be a perfectly futile and useless task to attempt to make one brain like another.   Unfortunately many modern educational theorists seem to go on the principle that every boy could be made into a Darwin or a Parr if only pains enough were taken with him. Every human brain has from the beginning, through heredity and innate capacity, fixed limits of power in all directions, beyond which no efforts, no teaching, and no favourable environment will make it any stronger or more powerful.   Fifty years of exercise will not make the blacksmith's arm stronger than it is after the first year of exercise.   It may be laid down as an axiom in Mental Hygiene that it is far better not to approach the limits of power of any part of the brain than to push exertion up to those limits.   Nature generally provides much reserve power in every organ, more than is needed for everyday use.   She is prodigal of capacity in a healthy organism, but one is never sure where the weak points may come in.   Especially we are often ignorant of the transmitted weaknesses by heredity until it is too late.   It is doubtful if any child is born in a civilised country without some inherited brain and mental weaknesses of some sort or in some degree.   There are many cases where, through a certain precociousness of development, a child seems to have certain faculties in great strength but where the brain basis of those faculties seems to give out early, and in reality they show themselves weak instead of strong in the long run.   I have known a child with an extraordinary memory at eight who at fifteen could scarcely remember anything at all. To push education or acquirement, mental or muscular, beyond the capacities originally provided by nature is to do certain harm.

Brain and Mental Habit.—It is one of the innate

qualities of every tissue and every organ in the body that when any vital action is done, any vital process gone through, it is easier to do it the second time, and the continuous exercise of it makes its performance more and more easy. This fact is of enormous importance in Mind Hygiene. The combination of action of one group of brain cells with another group becomes easier every time it is done. This physiological *doctrine of habit* especially applies to the working of the muscles and of the brain. During the developmental period of the brain up to twenty-five this is especially provided for, and is of especial importance. There are habits of movement, habits of sensation, habits of nutrition, and habits of mind, all depending on the same law. Every one knows that the movements needed to play the piano are at first difficult and tiresome, but that by constant practice a habit is formed so that those movements become automatic, needing no thinking, and involving no mental fatigue. Robert Houdin in early life, by constant practice, could keep four balls in the air at once, and he could do this while reading a book ; thirty years after he could only keep up three. Go higher in brain functions, and take an example from its most important function of all—that of inhibition. A child, at first, tries to grasp anything that is bright or sweet. When control is frequently exercised and taught it becomes quite easy for it to refrain from taking any object, however tempting. To think out a simple mathematical problem is to most people hard at first, but the brain habit of exercising the judgment in this particular way is soon strengthened, so that it becomes quite easy. There are, of course, limits to habit acquisition, but without it the brain would be a most inefficient organ. If everything we did and thought were as difficult as the first time we practised it, mankind could have made no progress from the lowest savagery ; indeed, it is very questionable if

man could have lived in the world at all. Habit acquisition
is closely allied to memory when both are looked at
physiologically. It may, in fact, be called a brain memory.
Different mental and muscular centres form associations
by constant use together, and those associations remain
as a permanent mechanism in the organ. To avoid bad
brain combinations is specially important. In the young
child it has been proved scientifically by Fechner that
new strands of fibres are formed continually and new
connections made between different groups of cells, as
the new mental processes go on from the simple to the
complex. Develop and encourage right brain-cell connections and action is the hygienist's rule, " form good habits "
is the immemorial motto of the parent, the teacher, and
the moralist : they are the same thing put differently.

*Mental Faculties, Instincts, Appetites, Vitalities, and
Organic Necessities.*—It is only necessary here to refer to
the metaphysical assortments of purely mental action,
otherwise called mental faculties. Standing as the basis and
conjunction of them all is consciousness, or the *ego*. The
metaphysician holds the mind to be one and indivisible.
This is so far true psychologically and physiologically.
The innate solidarity of action of the whole brain, of which
I have spoken, is its physiological correlative. Then come
feeling, perception and emotion, ideation and judgment,
volition and inhibition, power of attention, representation
and imagination, association of ideas, the moral faculties,
the religious instincts, and, lastly, that faculty which
renders them all possible—memory. Next comes that
faculty which chiefly ties together body and mind in mankind, viz., speech. Then we have the instincts which
provide for the life and the continuance of the
species, viz., love of life and desire to reproduce, the
instinctive love and care of offspring being closely
related to the latter. The gregarious and social instincts

form an essential part of the life, and of the evolution of man and of the higher animals. The appetites for food and drink, and air and light, combine bodily and mental aspects. It may be said that every tissue and every organ hungers for appropriate nourishment as an organic and vital necessity. If any one of them does not receive such nourishment, there is produced and revealed to consciousness what may be called an organic unhappiness and craving. There is not one of those faculties and instincts that does not need to be taken into account, more or less, in any system of Mental Hygiene.

Speech.—The study of no faculty of the brain is more interesting or more important than that of speech. It is an attribute of man alone, though there are in the lower animals sounds and gestures which are its humble representatives. Speech implies muscular movements, motor nerves, the sense of hearing, and the exercise of the mental volition. Most students of mind, even those who do not base their conclusions on physiology, have concluded that the existence of speech is of such essential importance in the evolution of mind that no abstract ideas could have been attained without it. Thinking without speech would be of the most primitive and simple kind. In its higher development in the best brains of civilised mankind, it is able to give outward expression to the most abstract ideas and the intensest feelings of man. Looking at its physiological and anatomical basis the large groups of nerve cells, which form the "speech centres," are localised in the left side of the brain. When these are destroyed by disease or accident in any man he ceases to be able to express himself in articulate, appropriate speech, and becomes " aphasic." When such disease is extensive, and affects the centres of hearing and sight, the patient not only cannot speak, but he does not understand the import of words spoken by others, nor of words seen in the pages of a printed book. He cannot write, and he does not understand writing. The speech groups of cells are connected above by their fibres with the higher mind centres, and below with the motor centres of the tongue, the mouth, and the throat. When we consider that there may be laid up in the molecular constitution of those cells thousands of symbols or words, and that through those words the centres have to express the intensest human feeling or the most subtle human knowledge, we can in that way realise the marvellous delicacy and scope of this piece of machinery. When we also consider that in the newly born child speech does not exist, and that its machinery is in an absolutely nascent condition, that during its slow development in the growing child speech may take on any form, from the rude phonation of the barbarian to the intricate inflection of the Chinese language, with its 43,000 characters, there is evidently scope for scientific processes of speech-teaching and speech hygiene. The mind centres express themselves in purely physical ways through speech, and the speech centres react in purely physical ways on the feelings and the ideas of the mind centres. Speech, in its making, is the most wonderful combination of mind action and muscular action to be found in nature. It is an easy thing to allow any child to speak harshly, carelessly, and unintelligibly. It is not a difficult task to teach the intelligent brain and vocal organs of a civilised child to speak in a clear, precise, and pleasurable way. Infinite attention has been paid to the vocalisation of the singer. Comparatively small efforts have been made, in a scientific way, to render the speech of the educated man and woman harmonious and fully expressive. No mind can be said to be well trained where the speaking apparatus has been neglected.

CHAPTER IV

GENERAL PRINCIPLES, ESSENTIALS, AND IDEALS OF MENTAL HYGIENE

BEFORE entering on the special applications of Mental Hygiene to the ages and conditions of life, I desire, in this Chapter, to lay down certain principles of universal application. This is necessary, in order to give a solidarity to the whole subject and to render repetitions as few as possible.

Food and Appetite.—Mental Hygiene must have, as its basis, the proper nourishment of the body and the making of good blood. The first matter to be considered, when one treats of food, is appetite. That is the mental correlative of food. The appetite is generally impaired in both mental and bodily weakness and disease. The want of appetite, or a perverted appetite, means that the processes of tissue metabolism and chemical change and waste which are going on in every organ, and, as we have seen, go on so rapidly in the brain, are disordered in some way. In a healthy organism building up and wasting are simultaneous and compensatory. Wastage is always in the process of being counteracted, and the appetite is, or ought to be, the mental signal that the organism needs more fuel. In youth, and in health and strength, the appetite for food is a periodic and recurrent sensation, which itself gives pleasure. To a certain extent it is under the control of habit, but the man or the woman or the child who is not hungry at least twice in the twenty-four hours cannot be said to be in a normal condition. Almost the first thing that a doctor asks in regard to any patient is, "How is the appetite?" and if he receives in reply that it is bad or absent, it at once suggests the questions, "What organ is not doing its duty? What vital process is incompletely performed? Are the residual chemical products of tissue waste not being properly eliminated? Are the nerve centres of nutrition doing their work? Is there any higher mental inhibition, which is arresting this primary proof of health? Is the patient mentally happy? and if not, why?" It is a mere truism to say that appetite may be completely and at once arrested by a strong mental process, especially if that is of a disagreeable kind. The appetite may be impaired either by a want of proper digestion of the food in the stomach, by an improper digestion further down in the bowels, by an imperfect elimination from the lower bowel, or by an imperfect action of some other parts of the digestive apparatus, such as the liver or pancreas. Any one or all those things have to be taken into account by the physician who wishes to restore the appetite. The appetite may also be impaired through the imperfect performance of the subtler processes of the blood formation or the nutrition of the tissues themselves. The study of the composition and quality of the blood has made great progress of recent years. The more it is studied the more complicated and the more important it is found to be to the body in general, and to the brain and mental working in particular. It consists of a nutritive fluid, in which float a large number of cells of different appearance, and with different functions. The most numerous of these, the red corpuscles, carry oxygen to the tissues of the various organs of the body, without which they cannot work, it being especially necessary to the brain activity. When those corpuscles lessen in number we have the condition called anæmia, or bloodlessness, which is a common accompaniment of many forms of brain disorders and of mental disturbances. When there is an infection of the system through injurious microbes, the leucocytes become enormously increased for the purpose of fighting and destroying these microbes. There are certain forms of mental disorder where this increase of leucocytes, called " leucocytosis," is a very important symptom. The blood ought to be carefully examined in all conditions where there is mental languor, irritability, or marked excitement.

Air.—An abundant supply of pure air to the brain, through the blood, is essential to its working. The lassitude of the occupants of an overcrowded church, the inattention of the scholars in an ill-ventilated school, the irritability, the headaches, the feeling of organic discomfort of the persons who live in ill-aired rooms, are all danger signals and cries for more oxygen by the brain.

Other Needs.—There are certain other physical essentials to mental health. Light, colour, heat, muscular exercise, housing, right employment, mental and bodily, are all of the greatest importance. As we have seen, the brain registers every impression made on it from within or without. If the impressions are those of discomfort, gloom, darkness, and ugliness, those things being inharmonious to the constitution and working of the brain do harm and tend to set up a bad habit, which we should stop as soon as possible. The sight of the sea smiling in the sunshine is, for instance, a healing agency and nerve tonic of the most powerful kind. Many persons run down in nervous health, and convalescents from all diseases find nothing so healing as such agencies. To live in a gloomy house, with dull, ugly wall-papers, and no sunshine entering into the living-rooms, may produce in their inhabitants want of appetite, bad nutrition, and mental depression. All those agencies, therefore, enter into Mental Hygiene.   To make the environment favourable, tonic and bracing should be the first consideration.   Reduce organic discomfort, produce organic pleasure.   Take a large and physiological view of the brain and mind condition in every case.

Strengthen the Defences.—I have spoken of the brain quality of resistiveness.   To fortifiy this is an essential condition of keeping the brain and mind strong and in good working order.   To strengthen all the defences, is indeed one of the most important considerations in our science.

Education in a General Sense.—I shall treat of education in the technical sense when I come to speak of childhood and youth, but, taking education in its larger sense, as comprising all the influences which affect the mind and body of a child, it is incalculably important as a hygienic measure.   The mother, in the early stages of her child's life, through her natural instincts, cannot help realising very fully that the baby has a body as well as a mind.   The technical educationalist is very apt indeed to forget this. In a certain sense, the amount that a child learns during its first years before ever it goes under the schoolmaster nearly equals all the rest of its education put together. This is essentially the formative period in the life of the brain cells.   They are shooting out their dendrites (fibres) in all directions, and what is being written on them—that is, the impressions they are receiving—may last for the lifetime.   The cells which receive the impressions of the mother's smile are thereby acquiring a source of perennial joy and health.   During the whole of the educative period the mental qualities of imitation, acquisition, attention, memory, and imagination, have to be very carefully built up on right lines and practised in right directions.   Above all, the inhibitory or controlling processes need to be judiciously strengthened and developed.   They are the physical equivalent and correlative of self-control and morality in the after-life. A right study and care of those basal attributes of mind may make all the difference to the life of the individual. The feeling and emotional function of the cells will take care of themselves. Many evolutionists tell us that the child's natural moral qualities are those of the savage and the lower animals ; that envy, selfishness, greed, cruelty, and egotism are rampant in its constitution. The modern scientist seems to have little belief in the innate goodness of the human infant. That, he says, has to be acquired, and the evil qualities have to be antagonised. The child has to pass through, as a life experience, the savage and selfish phases of its remote ancestor before evolution and natural selection strengthened the good qualities and civilised life made them possible in practice. If the theory of evolution is right, it is no wonder that the doctrine of original sin was a very essential part of ecclesiastical belief. As a Christian doctrine it is somewhat hard to believe that it is a fact which harmonises with the idea of a wise and beneficent Father of all ordering all things aright. No one, however, who has had to do with children, and studied their natures, but must admit that both the evolutionist and the Churchman have many facts to back up their theories. It is very clear that there is room for the Mental Hygienist, working on scientific and psychological lines which certainly include ethics in their scope. He has a great field before him in the early years of a child's life. It is to be remembered, however, that good qualities, as well as evil, are hereditary. Some children are angelic through heredity, and all have some of the angel as well as of the demon in them. The good and the bad are largely determined by law.

Innate Differences in Brain Capacity and Qualities.— All children have much in common, but they also show enormous differences all along the mental lines. Those differences are clearly innate, and in many cases radical. I shall presently have to refer to the investigations of the scientists and psychologists in regard to the normal order of the development of faculties and functions in the human brain.   At present I have to emphasise it as a principle in the study and practice of the Mental Hygiene of the child, that the differences, as well as the resemblances, must be studied and taken into account.   It is certain that all weak points cannot be strengthened, that the brain of the ordinary child can never be made quite like the brain of a child who is to turn out a genius ; but, on the other hand, weak points are capable of being strengthened in many cases by judicious care and effort.   Everybody has known the cases of children brought up by a judicious mother or nurse to be changed remarkably in character and conduct as the result of an almost unconscious study on that mother's part of her children's brain and mental constitution.   By working on the affections, by rewards and punishments, by gentle pressure and subtle tact and trickery, by insistence that took no discouragement—such mothers have added to the world's happiness and to human efficiency.   Especially are such difficulties as I am now speaking of to be found in families of nervous parents. I fear I must add to nervous parents many of those of marked intellectual force, and especially of keen sensibility and of intense religious instinct, though not reckoned "nervous" at all by the world at large.   The children of families in which insanity and drunkenness have been common need especial care in their education.   It seems as though, in the slow evolution of the human brain and the natural selection of the higher qualities of that organ, that the risks of failure and the need of well-directed effort become greater.   The finer the instrument, the more it seems liable to go out of tune ; and this tendency is most markedly seen in the children of families "of distinction." To have got a human brain of very high quality, and especially to have got a family each member of which has such a brain, implies a previously severe process of selection during evolution. The average and the bad had been, perhaps, unduly eliminated in the process.

Social Instincts.—The social instincts of the human being, of which I shall have much to say, are greatly important in the formative stages of the human brain. That they must be taken into account in any system of Mental Hygiene goes without saying. It is certain that their basis appears in the cells of the brain at a very early period of life. A right training of the social instincts is beyond any doubt one of the most important means of securing happiness to the individual and order to Society. It is no wonder that at the present time the science of sociology is rising to great importance. The child's or the youth's relation to others, his affection for others, and his altruistic practices, all go to the making of society, citizenship, and patriotism in the race. A man cannot be said to be healthy mentally whose social instincts are poor or perverted. When a man is becoming disordered in mind, commonly one of the very first symptoms is the diminution of his social instincts. Notoriously the insane are a-social. The social instinct is one of the highly educable parts of the constitution of a human being.

Sex Study.—The hygienic study of the relations between the sexes, and the male and the female characteristics, is one that cannot be neglected without harm. I shall afterwards have to dwell on this aspect of Mental Hygiene. Here I merely lay down the principle that this part of the study of the human brain and mind is one that may be fruitful of the highest practical results, and that it admits, to a much larger extent than has hitherto been realised, of a popular treatment, on scien-

E

tific lines, which would steer a happy mean between a too great attention and a deplorable ignorance.

The Ideals of Mental Hygiene.—Every science must have an ideal as its goal, and every effort to benefit humanity must have this before it as its chief incentive and inspiration. It does not matter much whether the ideal is attainable or not so long as it is there. The ideals of Mental Hygiene are, in the first place, a happy childhood with the brain functions and the mental faculties unfolding in their natural order. Such a brain should be receptive in the highest degree to the innumerable stimuli that are rushing into it every moment from the senses. It should be neither too sensitive nor too obtuse. Every stimulus of a natural kind should produce pleasure. The power of acquisition should be great and should need little systematic teaching. So should glee, play, nascent capacities for work, imitativeness in all directions, instinctive reverence for father and mother as the personified deities of authority, keen social faculty, exhibited chiefly in the cravings for the presence of brothers and sisters, the inhibitory faculty, absent at first, gradually but very slowly growing into a habit, love of animals, delight in sunshine. Symbolism is markedly present. All the tastes and appetites should be natural, and even the a-social barbaric instincts of selfishness with some cruelty and destructiveness should be present in only normal amount. Such should be the ideal child in mind and brain up to seven years of age.

The next stage is the school age from 7 to 15. Then comes the perfecting of the instinctive habit of co-ordinating muscles and mind together so that the hands can do what things the mind directs, and the body can exert itself without effort, with grace and with force. The educative process at school, if conducted on proper lines, should not cause real discomfort. Acquisition of all sorts, especially by the

memory, should be easy. Bad example should not make
indelible impressions. The superstructures of conscience,
duty, and religion are laid, but with no troublesome reasoning about them. Play and air are craved for as necessities.
The feeling of honour in playing games or in screening
a schoolfellow is acquired. Vague realisations come in
towards the end of the period that duty, self-restraint,
and altruism are an essential part of life.

Then comes the period of adolescence, between 15 and
25. This stage is the crux of life. The acquisitions then
made are critical in the extreme, and often final. The real
love of right, hatred of wrong, duty, conscience, religion,
become solid and effective in forming " character." Far-
away ravishing glimpses of poetic feeling, pleasurable
altruism, citizenship and patriotism, show themselves in the
earlier stages, and give direction to life at the later. The
capacity to feel pleasure reaches its greatest intensity.
The sex relations are built up on safe and natural lines,
controlled by certain instinctive natural delicacies, by
morality and religion. An ever-increasing power of
inhibition rises up during this period, until its exercise
becomes a formed habit and even a pleasure. Music,
literature, and art, imaginative works of all sorts mix
themselves up with sex feelings, so that the two help to
form the emotional nature. An abounding capacity to
work, with real joy in work, is acquired. Love between
the sexes is capable of assuming an all-dominating
influence.

Manhood and womanhood from 25 to 55 assume
strength, beauty, power of command, originality of purpose, ambition, and a larger sense of what life means.
In short, the efficient instruments of doing the world's
work are created. Fatherhood and motherhood soften
and sweeten life.

The retrogressive period of life, after 50, should mean

restfulness, philosophy, wisdom, charity, philanthropy. Strong exertion of mind or body is not craved for as in the earlier period. There should be no irritability, no senile selfishness, and a large consideration for others should be exhibited. Poetry, love tales, and sex have ceased to set the brain on fire. The brain cells are diminishing in number, lessening in size, and not capable of the same output ; but this process should be a very gradual and almost an imperceptible one. Lots of work may be done if it is done quietly. The failure of memory and activity should come slowly and give no pain. The process of dying should be calmly regarded and accepted as simply a fact of nature like the process of birth. There should be an instinctive reliance on the greater energy of the young in return for the reverence which is paid by it.

Nature is so prodigal in her gifts of resistiveness and recuperative energy, and her attempts to attain her ideals are so strong, that in some instances a man with an apparently bad heredity, a bad education, and bad environments will largely attain them. This is the great hope for the handicapped in life. Nature, though mostly red in tooth and claw, yet is ever capable of organic mercifulness. She steadily works out her two great tendencies—the one to end a bad and tainted stock, and the other to go back to the average type. The aim of Mental Hygiene, and of all hygiene, is to help the saving and to restrict the deteriorating tendency. When an instructed and philanthropic Glasgow public authority drafts off 100 scrofulous, sickly and starved children of the slums to share the home-life of Highland farms, it is found that a surprising percentage of them react to the better environments and turn out sturdy and useful men and women. Nature is not so unkindly a stepmother if we have the wit to humour her.

CHAPTER V

THE study of heredity is admittedly one of the most difficult branches of science. It has been tackled by some of our greatest modern scientists, including Darwin himself, who put forward a theory of his own. Weismann, Lamarck, and Mendel are also among its greatest exponents. To read some of the views of the writers on heredity one might almost suppose that it was entirely a theoretical matter referring to scientific doctrine. The plain, and so far intelligible, old doctrine that "like produces like" has been so obscured by theories as to the precise way in which ancestral likenesses and qualities are transmitted, that the whole subject has become unduly complicated. The first thing to be kept in mind is this—that confusion and doubt have not arisen because of any uncertainty that like always does and always will produce like under the same conditions. Biologists are all agreed that when we go down to the beginnings of life, to the unicellular organisms, each individual consisting of one cell containing its own protoplasm, and with no relationship to any other cell except by casual contact, those organisms will, under the same temperature and in the same media of air and chemical surroundings, always produce the same kind of cell. But even in those most primitive examples of life, the environment or condition cannot be always the same, and minute differences do arise which scientists call "variations." The existence of variations is at the root of the doctrine of evolution. Out of such variations and their progeny have arisen the higher forms of life, and those most fitted to live by special adaptation to their environment. Can such variations be caused by changes of environment? is one of the burning questions of science. It is now held by most biologists that in the case of those low unicellular organisms, that such variations may be caused by changes of environment, and that the variations so produced are capable of transmitting their special characters to their descendants. When the same doctrines are applied to human beings the conditions are found to be so enormously complex that it is doubtful if the laws in regard to heredity which apply to the unicellular organism are also applicable to the human organism which possesses thousands of different forms of cells attached to each other, influencing each other, and together forming a living organism, with a wonderful solidarity in its general working.

The importance of those questions to man is at once realised when we consider that on their solution depend such practical issues as the following: Are the mental faculties of man, as developed by civilisation, by morality, by religions, and by a highly complex social system, capable of being transmitted hereditarily to successive generations, or have they all to be taught from the beginning to each child? Are the effects of bad food, vitiated air, excess of alcohol, and the use of various poisons—all these being admittedly hurtful to the individual—are they capable of being transmitted to descendants and so setting up what may strictly be called a degenerative process in the race? The great controversy in regard to heredity now ranges round the following three questions. Are the effects of environment on the individual, be they good or bad, capable of hereditary transmission to descendants ? or is such transmission strictly confined to qualities, good or bad, that have been inherited from the parents ? or is there such a combination of both influences possible that inherited character chiefly, but environmental influences also in some degrees and ways, also influence descendants, and become heritable ? The extreme advocates of the non-transmissibility of any environmental effects in man are represented by Dr. Archdall Reid, whose book on the *Principles of Heredity* has lately appeared. He has the highest opinion of the study of heredity in its results, both on its students and on human life, disease, and society. He says : " It seems to me that no kind of study can be made to bear intellectual fruit of nearly such value as the study of heredity. It lies at the root of every science and every study connected with life, from botany and zoology to medicine, sociology, or pedagogy. Who knows it not knows not life except in its superficial aspects."

" He may be a student of philosophy, or a worker in biological science, but in these days, when heredity enters so much into philosophy and links together so many biological sciences, he cannot be a very effective thinker or worker."

" It furnishes a master-key to the more tremendous events of history, and it is our only hope against disasters that loom great and terrible in the near future. It goes deep down to the springs of human life and thought and conduct, and explains why some nations are inheriting the earth and the fruits thereof, while others are dying physically or mentally. The philanthropist must know something of this science, or he will grope in the dark. The statesman must know something of it, or he may labour in vain. Transcending all else in importance is the educational value of heredity.

No nation in which a knowledge of it was widespread could possibly be stupid or brutal." If there is any truth whatever in those strong opinions by Reid, then undoubtedly heredity must play a great part in Mental Hygiene, being the hygiene of the highest of all the cells—the higher brain cells. On those brain cells act the highest and the subtlest of all forms of environment, viz., those of emotion, of passion, and of beauty. No one can deny that the worst effects on the individual of certain unfavourable environments, such as bad social conditions and alcohol, are on the brain. If the securing of good environment will not only benefit the individual, which no one can deny, but will also improve posterity through the transmission of their beneficial effects, then indeed we have an argument for improved human environments which is irresistible.

All the recent scientific authors have come to the agreement that the body generally does not directly transmit environmental effects to posterity. This is done through what is in reality an infinitesimal part of, or, as the latest theorists would say, attachment to the body, the germ cells. It may be accepted that if the effects of environment are transmitted to descendants, this is done through those germ cells, just as the ancestral qualities are so transmitted. Those who argue against such transmission very naturally say that the evils of most bad environments act on the body and not on the germ cell. In what way can they then be transmissible? The latest theory of heredity is that put forward by Dr. Beard, of Edinburgh. It would be quite impossible for me to give anything like a full detail of that theory in the space at my disposal. It is so full of technical terms and implies such a profound knowledge of physiological and biological sciences that it is difficult even to lay down its principles so that they shall be popularly understood. But one may say that the leading idea of Dr. Beard's theory is that the germ cells in all the higher animals are a direct continuation of the original primal single-cell organism. He talks of those cells being so distinct from the rest of the body, even from the embryo in utero, that they only pass a part of their lives within the body. There is, in fact, a direct continuity of such germ cells, as germ cells, apart from the rest of the body from the lowest animal up to the highest, and from the first and lowest of savage men up to the highest. An enthusiastic follower of Beard—Dr. Ford Robertson—traverses Dr. Archdall Reid's position and denies his proposition that "inborn characters are known to be transmissible from parent to offspring." Dr. Robertson says : " This teaching can no longer be regarded as accurate. Offspring, as far as can at present be determined, inherit no character whatever from their parents. Offspring are merely the realisation of the developmental potentialities of converged ancestral lines of germ cells. The distinction between inborn and acquired characters has really no justification in modern scientific fact. The definition given by Dr. Reid will not bear scrutiny." Then, too, Dr. Robertson further says : " In regard to ontogenetic evolution" (that is the development of the individual), " I would add that, although there is no inheritance of parental characters, there is an inheritance of environmental influences, to which, indeed, all that is of any importance in human ontogenetic evolution is directly due. Cut out of man's environment what Professor Karl Pearson terms 'the tradition of acquired modifications,' and his ontogenetic evolution will proceed no further than that of the brute. All the acquirements of literature, art, science, social customs, etc., form an environment to which man's inherent potentialities of development are capable of responding." When original authorities and students of heredity thus disagree in the very essence of their doctrine, the intelligent lay public may well be pardoned for applying ordinary common sense to the subject, and physicians of large practical experience may be forgiven if they adhere to the generally accepted theory that a bad, ill-nourished mother and a drunken father will produce between them a bad progeny, which progeny again will, in spite of any amount of favourable environment, often produce a very doubtful stock.   As Dr. Robertson says : " Germ cells require to be nourished like other cells.   The laws which govern their nutrition cannot be different from those that govern the nutrition of the somatic cells (those of the body) which have arisen from a germ cell.   Professor Cossar Ewart, as the result of practical experiments in hereditary characters, says that the germ cells are liable to be influenced by fever and other forms of diseases that for the time being diminish the vitality of the parents."   Dr. Robertson quotes Sevatico-Estense, who mentions the case of a healthy woman married to a drunkard.   She had five weakly children, all of whom died in infancy.   By a second husband of sober habits she had two perfectly healthy children.   The connection through heredity of such brain diseases as idiocy, imbecility, and insanity, with excess of alcohol, is very strong indeed.   Dr. Reid, in opposition to this, says " that if alcohol injuriously affected the germs the effects would accumulate generation after generation till the race became extinct."   Dr. Robertson replies : " This does not in the least follow, for the contribution from other ancestral lines of germ cells may counteract the tendencies to genetic variation produced by chronic alcoholic poisoning."

One of Dr. Reid's fundamental positions is that disease agencies, poisons, and certain deleterious influences tend, by destroying the weak, the intemperate, and the vicious, to leave a remainder which has acquired an immunity against such destructive agencies.   Logically his hygienic rule would be—"Let the weak and unfit come to an end." Dr. Ford Robertson vigorously argues that disease is a cause of human evolution through destruction of the weak only in a very limited sense. He says: "Dr. Archdall Reid asserts that diseases of parents do not affect in any way, neither for good nor for evil, offspring subsequently born, at any rate through inheritance, properly so called, that 'temperance reform is impossible from the biological standpoint,' that 'temperance reformers have failed because they have entered into a contest with Nature' and that 'every scheme for the promotion of temperance which depends for success on the abolition or diminution of the alcoholic supply, is in effect a scheme for the promotion of drunkenness.' He simply shows, it seems to me, that he has wholly misunderstood the biological significance of disease." Dr. Reid says "that the craving for alcohol is an instinctive special inborn character." Dr. Robertson contests this and says that it is "a mere specific habit." Dr. Robertson's conclusions, in regard to the bad effects of alcohol, both personal and hereditary, are the following: " My study of the question forces me to the conclusion that the effects of alcoholic intemperance upon the people of this country are much more grave and far-reaching than has generally been suspected. Most people have seen with any degree of clearness only its more immediate effects. The influence it has upon the race has only been dimly suspected by a few, and they have been derided as ignorant and unscientific. The evidence of science is, I maintain, entirely on their side."

It was right that I should have quoted the opinions of those recent writers on heredity, in its more medical and practical relations, if only to show that this important subject is still in the process of investigation and that as yet there is much doubt as to whether such definite laws can be laid down in regard to its nature as would be accepted by all scientific and medical men. I shall have occasion to refer to "atavism," or the passing over several generations of undoubted hereditary characters. We are all agreed in regard to one important conclusion as to heredity, that is, the fact that hereditary defects may occur in two forms—the one is that of definite provable changes from the normal structure and functions of the human body, such as the small brain and defective mind in many forms of idiocy and epileptic affections in early life and the paralytic affections of infancy. The other is that defects may occur which are not visible in early life or provable either in bodily structure or functional process, being then only tendencies and potentialities. The latter are as real facts as the former though not at certain times in the life of the individual demonstrable. Examples of them are seen in tendencies to mental disease and liability to certain forms of paralysis in individuals who at one time seemed to be quite healthy and free from defect. Such are of the greatest interest to the hygienist because in many of them the actual defect of disease is brought out by exciting causes, which may, in many cases, be avoided or counteracted. That is one of the greatest fields that exists for the future preventive and hygienic physician. If defects of heredity were all irremediable the future of humanity would be a dark one. I have no sort of doubt, as the result of my experience of forty years of the medical study of disordered and undeveloped mind, that heredity comes in as a causal agent in a greater degree than in any other disease. I cannot doubt, therefore, that in the whole process of development of the brain cell, which is the vehicle of mind, whether in its strong points or in its weak points or in its liability to disease, heredity is the dominating factor. On a man's ancestors it mostly depends whether he is to be a fool, a genius, or a madman, or whether he is to be a success or failure in life. This is not in the least inconsistent with the fact that the brain cell and its function of mind is also more amenable to the effects of environment or education—good or bad —than any other cell in the human body. The two facts are not contradictory but complementary. They both are proofs of the high attributes of the highest bit of organized matter in Nature. They imply the profound influence heredity plays in Mental Hygiene. A bad nervous heredity means mental unresistiveness to the causes of mental weakness and ill-health. The margin of security is less. While a man who has a good heredity may with impunity take many liberties in the way he uses his brain, this is not safe if he has a bad heredity.

There are modes of upbringing, of education, and of conduct in life that should be avoided where a man is handicapped by a bad heredity. There are special precautions and attention to physiological law which would save the minds of many men with a bad heredity from passing into inefficiency and actual disease. While heredity implies a potentiality towards good or evil it commonly needs a special exciting cause or combination of causes to bring out visible effects. It is a fate which may be averted by knowledge and the practice of law. Take the excessive use of alcohol as an example—the father and mother of a boy have indulged in it before and during his life *in utero*, he has been poisoned *in embryo*, they have both acquired an uncontrollable craving for it, the boy has thereby acquired a weak constitution, probably neurotic in its character, and his development of body and mind has not been perfect. Few students of heredity would say that he had necessarily acquired the special craving for alcohol from his parents. All that is affirmed is that his power of mental inhibition would probably be weak and his defences generally below par. The reserve stock of energy and resistance which every really healthy organism possesses is weaker in him. He would not be able to withstand social temptations, and alcohol would have a quicker and worse effect on him than on his parents. He would sooner acquire a stronger craving for it than they had. But, on the other hand, if his health in childhood and youth were specially attended to, and his body and brain thereby strengthened, if his education were made a specially suitable one, if he selected an open-air occupation, if he took no alcohol, if during adolescence especially he were guarded from severe temptation, all these influences would be likely so to strengthen his mental inhibition and antagonise his heredity that he would not fall into the alcoholic condition, and might even procreate mentally healthy children. Nature's law of striving to attain her ideal would have a chance of coming in. Everything, of course, depends on the strength of the evil heredity. Any environmental influence which weakens the constitution of the parents or poisons their blood and tissues, undoubtedly in some degree unfits them for parentage. It is a safe working hypothesis, apart from any theories of heredity, to assume that bad environments, mental and bodily, on parents will have a bad and reducing influence on children. Medical instinct and experience, as well as the common sense of mankind, strongly go in support of such an inference. The scientists are equally divided in theory as to whether personal influences can become heritable. To take precautions is therefore the part of wisdom. They do good apart from any theoretical views ; their neglect may do infinite harm to unborn generations.

The following may be laid down as the chief rules of Mental Hygiene in its relation to heredity.

1. Carefully ascertain all the facts as to the hereditary

defects and tendencies, especially in regard to the brain and nervous system of ancestry and near relations, be they good or bad.

2. Face up those facts in an honest and truthful way, both to yourself and the doctor whom you consult. To conceal or to minimise them is both cowardly and foolish.

3. In forming conclusions and in laying down rules of practice always make considerable allowance for our ignorance of hereditary law, for errors, for atavism, and for Nature's two tendencies to destroy the very unfit and to hark back to the ideal.

4. You are entitled to the benefit of the doubt.

5. If there are hereditary facts endeavour carefully to estimate their strength and import. Some such facts are strong and unmistakable, others are slight and of small import.

6. Where the heredity is bad let a careful examination be made into the bodily form, functions, and mental faculties to ascertain if there are in any of them existing defects that can be seen and proved. Are the size and shape of the head normal? Are the ears, eyes, and facial features symmetrical or irregular? Are the muscular action, the gestures, and the attitudes of the body normal? Are the reactiveness and sensitiveness of the brain too high or too low? Is there any precocity or backwardness of brain and mental function? Are the moral feelings and social instincts changed? Are there any peculiarities or idiosyncrasies in the person examined? Are all the sense organs normal in action? The results of such an examination may give valuable hygienic indications.

7. Supposing there are no visible hereditary defects of form or faculty, there still may be deadly lurking tendencies to mental evils. I have seen many young persons of almost ideal physical characteristics who

became subject to attacks of nervousness or insanity that were clearly hereditary in character, or who entirely failed in aptitude for doing their work, or who became vicious from obviously psychological peculiarities, or who became weaklings or nuisances to society from brain defects.

8. It may be held as certain that bad environments, bad education, bad food, bad air, unsuitable occupation, mental shocks and stress, the effects of disease, unsuitable marriages will all bring out latent tendencies towards mental inefficiency or disease. Many of these could have been avoided or counteracted if sufficient knowledge of hereditary risks had been acquired at early enough periods in the lives of the persons affected.

9. It must be kept in mind that hereditary defects act as "weakeners of the defences," through which mankind resists disease and death. Many of the so-called bad symptoms and evil effects of disease really result from Nature's attempts to counteract and heal. Physiologists and physicians now know that we chiefly die, not from disease, but because our defences against the innumerable enemies of our lives have become weakened. "Strengthen the defences" has therefore become a prime motto of the hygienist. To over-press and to over-educate the brain of a child in whose family insanity or neurasthenia exists may be to diminish its defences and to bring on such diseases, which by other modes of education, or the want of it, might have been avoided.

10. The following are some of the general rules, by the application of which bad mental and nervous heredity may be counteracted. Feed and strengthen the body by every possible means during childhood and onwards. Do not over-stimulate, or over-educate, or over-press the brain. Retard rather than stimulate the development of its higher functions. Let them lie fallow. They

will appear in time in a stronger and healthier form for this process. Watch most carefully the periods of puberty and adolescence. Select occupations that are outdoor, routine, unexciting, and generally wholesome. Observe heedfully the moral, the social, and the religious influences to which such an individual is subjected. Avoid the risk, as far as may be, of bad example. Do not be tempted by early acquirements, quickness, and talent to think that there is, on that account, no risk of hereditary evils. Very much the contrary is often the case.

Temperament.—From the earliest times men have observed that certain bodily and certain mental characteristics are apt to go together. Observations on this point were formulated and classified in Greek times, and formed their "Doctrine of Temperaments." Hippocrates, the father of medicine, who lived 400 B.C., gave a description of the combination of mental disposition and bodily appearance in the gods and the heroes of antiquity. He applied those inferences to the medicine of the age. He and others of the fathers of medicine observed the difference between one man and another in size and shape, in colour and constitution, in modes of action and reaction, in temper and disposition, in thinking and feeling. They saw and published their observations that the diseases to which one kind of person was subject were different in many ways from those of another, and that the treatment they needed was often very different. Those differences they assorted as "Temperaments." They were certainly not correct in their details, but their principles were founded on scientific facts. Many of their temperaments had a basis in nature, and many of their generalisations are true at the present day. Very often they assigned wrong reasons and theories in explanation of the different temperaments, because neither physiology nor psychology was then sufficiently advanced for true inferences to be

F

made. They described four temperaments—the sanguine, the phlegmatic, the bilious, and the melancholic. Every human being had one of these or a combination of them. Since the times of Hippocrates and Galen, 105 distinct treatises have been written on temperament. The late Professor Laycock, of Edinburgh, was one of the greatest modern authorities on temperament. He was able to adduce the then latest physiological discoveries, the symptoms of his patients' diseases, the facts to be found in the biographies of distinguished men and women, and the looks and actions of his friends in support of his theories. No doubt he was in many ways inexact according to the latest scientific methods, and there is still much vagueness in the doctrine of temperaments. Laycock gave enormous prominence to what he called "the neurotic temperament" and diathesis, and in that he has been followed by most modern authorities. He was, in fact, the father of that great modern department of medicine now called "Neurology." No study of Mental Hygiene can now be effective without reference to this branch of medicine. Galton's *Enquiry into Human Faculty and its Development* is a laborious investigation on truly scientific lines to settle some of the cognate questions which lie at the root of the doctrine of temperaments. The general "make up" of a man, the shape of his head, the appearance of his eyes, the mobility of his features, the texture of his hair and skin, and his kind of movement, are taken into account in the conclusion that the man is of the "neurotic temperament." The nervous temperament has now taken its place instead of the melancholic of Hippocrates. The man of this temperament is in body small, shapely, tending towards a dark complexion, thin skin, with delicate features, a well-shaped head, a quick, bright, restless eye; in figure small and wiry, nervous, highly strung and sensitive, feeling pain keenly and tolerating it badly, subject to dyspepsia and insomnia. His muscles are incessantly active. He is quick in mind and body, imaginative, keen, sensitive, ever alert, fine in the grain, subtle, fond of intellectual work, not always resolute in decision because he sees there are two sides to every question, often artistic in feeling, ambitious, and with an ill-concealed contempt for fools. When run down, this man is "ill to do with." When he grows old he gets thin, dyspeptic, irritable, and often neuralgic. The diseases he is specially subject to are nervous and mental. Every other disease he suffers from is coloured and affected by his temperament. In him the brain and mind are dominant above all others. There can be no doubt that the hurry and competition of modern life in cities, with its newspapers and telegrams and little time for resting, tend towards the development of this temperament. Men who have it can make their muscles and their bodies work by an effort of will to harmful excess. They create and follow ideals. No one can travel in America and not see that this is the prevailing temperament of the city man in that country. *Punch's* gesticulating Frenchman is one type of this temperament ; Rousseau, Nelson, and Dickens were fine examples of it in its strength. This temperament has its special temptations. Alcohol and sedative drugs are two of them. He drinks, not steadily and for social reasons, but for the sake of the effect of the drink on the brain. He is apt when he takes to drink to become an uncontrollable dipsomaniac. This temperament should unquestionably be recognised and fittingly conditioned in early life by the parent and the teacher as to diet, sleep, work, fresh air, and rest. Nature's tendency to keep the nervous child thin should be overcome by specially fattening foods. A tendency to excitability in the temperament should be counteracted by lessened animal food, no alcoholic stimulants, as little tobacco as may be, and strict limits to social excitement.

The hygiene of the other temperaments relates more to body than to mind, and therefore I need say little about them here. The child of the sanguine needs repression and control. He is apt to be rheumatic and gouty and to suffer from diseases of the heart and arteries. It is often combined with some mixture of the nervous temperament. The combination makes the men who do the world's hardest and best work, who follow adventure and discovery and build up new empires. The men of the phlegmatic and bilious temperaments take to study, to routine modes of life; are thinkers, schemers, and agnostics. An excess of any temperament tends to certain definite diseases, and thus becomes what is called by Laycock a " Diathesis."

Social Instincts.—It is a truism to say that the social instincts, which are an innate part of brain life, lie at the root of the family and the community. They are met with far down in the animal scale, even below the vertebrates. Ants and bees live in communities with a complex organisation, the work of the individual being largely subserved to the advantage of the community. Among vertebrate animals, gregariousness was the first evidence of social instinct. There is said to be only one vertebrate animal where the social instinct is so absent that even the male and the female live apart. It may be said generally that gregariousness and what is implied in it have enormously increased the intelligence and the beneficent instincts of animals. It has led to all sorts of ways of subserving the love of life and efforts for its protection, which form the primary instinct of living beings. It is closely allied to the instinct of reproducing the species and providing for the wants of the young, which is the second strongest instinct. Animals which have become domesticated and associated with men acquire social instincts often in a remarkable degree. Among primitive men the limits of the social instinct seem to have been the family.

Every one beyond that was out of the pale and usually an enemy. The more civilised man has become, the more complex and the more important have his social instincts become. It may be said that any individual who is destitute of them is in a pathological condition. In many diseases the social instincts become paralysed. This finds its acme in disorders of the mind, in which a-socialism is perhaps the most distinguishing feature. The insane can seldom combine for any purpose. In many of the chronic and incurable insane there seems to be a complete paralysis of those instincts, so that the individual has ceased to have any need or desire for the presence or the society of his fellow-creatures. The vice of selfishness is intimately associated with a congenital or an acquired loss of the social instincts. The virtue of benevolence represents a transformation of this instinct into a virtue. Citizenship and patriotism represent the social instincts expanded, idealised, and applied for the happiness and life of large communities of men and women. In the healthy child the social instinct is very early and very intensely developed, so that it may become as strong a bond of union between two or more children as it is ever capable of being in after-life.

At the school age it is one of the strongest elements of life, and one of the most powerful adjuncts in the development of mind and body at that period. In adolescence it should assume, if normally developed and rightly guided, a higher tone and a loftier sphere. It should then be definitely allied with the emotions, the morals, and religion. There are very few individuals at that time of life in whom it does not require some regulation. In the female sex it may then become overmastering, and pass beyond the bounds of reason. As between two persons, or small groups of persons, it may lead to a selfish and unsocial exclusiveness of the other members of the family or community. When combined with maternal affection, it may become one of the intensest of feelings and the strongest incentive to action of any human quality.   Its existence in communities has naturally led to all sorts of useful customs, has promoted good manners, and has created much of the law and order of civilisation.   Its artificial restriction has led to caste and to class distinctions.   In the intense reactions and enthusiasms of the greatest human cataclysm of modern times, the French Revolution, the social instinct asserted itself as one of the three great watchwords of "Liberty, Equality, and Fraternity."   "Socialism" is a revival of the social instinct which at present is leading to much legislation and effort to counteract the effects of the political economy and the *laisser faire* of last century.   The earnest study of this instinct during adolescence, and its scientific culture on right lines, would do much to mould society on a happier basis, and to do away with many of the terrible difficulties of modern life in cities. It is, of course, connected in the closest way with love between the sexes, and with the amenities and joys of marriage in family life.   If the instinct is put under rational regulation in those spheres, there would be a better chance of its taking right forms in community life.   It is capable, during adolescence, of leading to intense enthusiasms and strong efforts for the bettering of the whole community.   For its management during adolescence one needs to cultivate it where it shows deficiency by providing suitable social intercourse.   At this period it is commonly so strong, however, that regulation, rather than direct encouragement, has to be practised.   Shyness does not always imply a deficient social instinct, but rather a deficient aptitude for showing it externally.   The former life of the Scottish University student sadly lacked social opportunity and encouragement.   The consequences were apt to be a lonely, self-satisfied, bookish, professional man, gawky in manner, without tact and without polish. "Iron sharpeneth iron, so a man the countenance of his friend," was forgotten in those times ; but the establishment of University Unions and Societies, as well as the efforts of the inhabitants of Scottish University towns to give the student the benefit of family and social life, are largely remedying the effects of life in lodgings, among our students. In the English Universities the fascinations of associated college life certainly led to an exaggeration of the social instincts, with its idleness, lack of academic earnestness and waste of precious time. The happy mean during adolescence between the old solitariness of the Scottish student and the social dissipation of the English University man would seem best to follow nature's laws and society's needs. In the case of the young woman, the difference is indeed exceeding great between the a-social life of the solitary school teacher or the hard student away from home, and that of the society young woman who is out at dances every day of the week. It is much worse for a young woman not to have her social instincts ministered to than for a young man. Her cravings for social amenities are stronger and her deprivation of them more hurtful. Many sorts of self-denial come natural to a young woman, and some of them do her much good ; but this is not the case with the deprivation of right social intercourse. The strain of too much of it is, however, apt to injure her and to cause nervousness, depression, and anæmia. I believe the bloodlessness so common now in our domestic servants is largely owing to their want of natural family and social life. To many adolescents with a nervous heredity or a tendency to that thinness which leads to consumption, want of proper social intercourse may certainly mean hysteria, mental disorders, neurasthenia, or even death. Many young women who take to study, to nursing, and to social work are so intense and so conscientious that they absolutely require the antidote of a certain amount of pleasant social intercourse.

Love-making. — Closely connected with the social instincts, but having in addition a far intenser emotional basis, comes love between the sexes. This is founded on as radical a quality as heredity or temperament, and is a necessary outcome of the social and reproductive instincts. Adolescence is unquestionably the time of life when this arises and often overmasters every other feeling and every duty in life, but it is confined to no period of life, especially in woman. In its greatest intensity, indeed, it may leave nothing in life, for the time being, but itself. It may absorb all the thinking, overset all the reasoning, supersede all other feelings, turn in one direction all the will power, and dominate the whole conduct. All-absorbing as it may thus appear, I believe that the love-making and the engagements to marry of adolescents, until the later part of the epoch, are essentially shallow and ephemeral. They represent the first outburst, in a spasmodic form, of a force which afterwards acquires real strength, and which is then capable of giving a real direction to the future of the world. In adolescence it lacks depth, responsibility and prevision. Few broken hearts or spoiled lives result from the love-making of early adolescence. My belief is that no young man should form an engagement to marry till his beard is grown, and that no young woman should say "yes" to a proposal of marriage until her form is womanly and her physical strength established. The falling in love and the disappointments connected therewith during early adolescence often lead to hysteria, to attacks of depression, and changes in character and conduct. In such cases there is usually hereditary nervousness or weakness of some sort. The really healthy, plump girl, and the strong, athletic young man commonly fall in love in some sort, or think they do, during early adolescence, without doing themselves much harm. As to the making of suitable marriages, with some degree of reason and prevision coming into this momentous matter, we scientists were warned off the ground and our advice scouted as utterly impracticable by the general opinion of society. There is no doubt a great deal in this view as human nature is constituted, but I am glad to think that we are not so much out of it in all cases, as is generally assumed. My experience is that nowadays science is so influencing even those "about to marry"—many of them having already fallen in love—that they listen to, and even follow, its dictates in this matter. There is now a universal opinion among d⁻ctors of experience that the elimination of mental disease, and of many forms of drunkenness and nervous weakness must chiefly depend on the suitable mating and non-mating of the young men and women of to-day and the future. I can say very definitely, as the result of my own experience, that the proposed marriages that have been given up for such reasons, and the actual marriages that have taken place as the result of health and hereditary considerations, have resulted in greater happiness and a higher self-respect than where prudence and science were thrown to the winds and impulse alone followed. "What has posterity done for me?" was the question, not of a cynic only, but of a thoughtless enemy of his kind. The man who feels no responsibility for the future of his own possible progeny, and of the race, is indeed a man wanting in the higher reason and the altruistic principle. I say, with a deep sense of responsibility and as the result of much experience, that before this, the most important step in most lives, is taken, the inquiries by each of the parties to the life contract, by their parents and their doctors, as to heredity, temperament, and health, cannot be too carefully made. I have seen examples of the wreck of life's happiness and success of the most painful kind, from the lack of such investigations. Speaking generally, the neurotic constitution should not marry the neurotic, although there is an undoubted affinity that leads directly to this. The quick temper should marry the phlegmatic, the calm should marry the impulsive, the very intellectual and æsthetic should marry the practical and common sense. But let it be understood that I am in no way advocating in the slightest degree any marriage union where no true affection exists. After all, emotion must be the dominant note in this all-important event of life. But this emotion is only a means to an end, which is the continuance of the species. I am constantly asked the question, "Should I marry, my mother being insane?" "Should I marry a girl of a family in which mental disease is very common?" A deep responsibility rests on the doctor who has to answer such questions. The laws of the hereditary transmission of disease are as yet far from being definitely settled. In no individual can we be quite sure that the children will be insane, even if one or both parents have actually suffered from that disease, far less if there is a mere hereditary tendency thereto. The law of atavism may bring it on in a man who has had four generations of apparently sound ancestors. Good environments, and favourable conditions may, as we have seen in some cases, antagonise bad heredity. Opposite temperaments in parents may result in healthy children, even if those temperaments were exaggerated pathologically. All those favourable facts we must honestly admit and bring before our prospective brides and bridegrooms who come to us for advice. Yet we must with equal honesty and sense of responsibility point out the awful prospect of increasing the direst and most hereditary disease which can afflict mankind.

CHAPTER VI

CERTAIN IMPORTANT CONSIDERATIONS RELATING TO MIND, MORALS, AND WILL THAT HAVE A DIRECT CONNECTION WITH HYGIENE OF MIND.

Mind and Morals v. Brain.—It may be said, and no doubt will be said, by many who read this book, that however strongly it may be proved, even up to the hilt, that the brain is the organ of mind, yet that mind, looked at as mind, morals as morals, apart from brain or body, form the most important view of man's life and Mental Hygiene. They will say that a motive is the chief mental and moral force and can only appeal to mind, and that man's whole life is regulated by motives, good and bad. They will say that consciousness and the ego are so instinctively regarded as the ultimate thing in man, that it is vain to go to a secondary cause, such as brain mechanism and brain working, to explain mental action and moral conduct. They will say that no matter what are the facts as to the slow evolution of mind, what we have to do with is man as he exists with his enormous and varied power of thinking, feeling, and volition. They will ask if it is not a primary instinct in all men to attach responsibility to a man's mental action as it takes practical form in conduct? They will say that it is entirely against common sense to blame a man's brain for doing wrong and not doing right. They will say that the great moralists, the great religionists, and the wise men of past ages among all highly developed peoples could not have been entirely wrong when they regarded mind alone and took no practical notice of the mind machinery in the brain. They will ask if Jesus Christ, Buddha, Mahomet, Zeno, Epictetus, and Marcus Aurelius did not know their work as great human moral teachers and reformers when they took so little notice of the connection of mind and conduct with the working of the human brain ; most of them not only taking no notice of the place of the body in relation to mind, but taking pains to say it must be "kept under," and even holding it in contempt. The supernatural aspect of all religions will be adduced as showing that the Deity acts directly on the human mind without the intervention of any physical intermediary. How else, will it be asked, could any revelation from the Almighty or any possession by the Holy Ghost or by the evil one be imagined ? They look on the views of the modern physiological psychologist and physician as being "wrong" in a moral and religious sense and call it "materialism" and "fatalism." The "spiritualist" and the "telepathist," the "theosophist," and the "Christian Science" devotees will adduce proofs abundantly satisfactory to themselves that mind can be manifested and influenced apart from brain and the senses. Above all, the moralist will ask if those doctrines do not imply such a conditioning of man's "Free Will" as to impair his responsibility to God and the law, and to degrade him from the proud position of lord of himself and of creation ? There is, no doubt, much force in those considerations, and they cannot be lightly put aside. The real reply to all those objections is that everything in man and in the world is governed by fixed laws, and the supreme duty of science is to find out what those laws are, and when ascertained to hold to them irrespective of any objections whatever. If it is the case that all modern investigations done on scientific lines and tested by scientific proofs point to the conclusion that in this world mind is only manifested through brain as its vehicle, and is absolutely conditioned in its every form and manifestation by brain action, we must accept the fact and its consequences. It does not in the least follow from this conclusion that the mental energy so conditioned by organisation does not work by laws and on lines applicable to itself. It does not follow that the mental force does not condition the working of the brain as well as being conditioned by that working. It does not imply that mind evolved from one brain cannot act on mind evolved in another brain, though this must always be done through the senses. It in no way implies that one mind cannot be developed and educated through the efforts of another mind. Even the metaphysician does not claim that the will is free in an absolute sense. When the man with the freest and the strongest will is in an apoplexy or a fever, or is under the influence of a brain poison like alcohol, it is an evident and incontestable scientific fact that his will is no longer free. Why, therefore, may not imperfections in brain organisation and working interfere with freedom of volition and conduct? To the scientist, thinking on scientific and biological lines, it does not seem an inscrutable mystery that a man and a woman between them can create ten new minds. To the man who reasons on metaphysical lines, without reference to organisation, thinking only of the *ego*, this new creation of ten minds is simply a miracle which no one can either explain or even imagine. Mind and organisation must meantime be regarded as a dualism, organisation being the factor which can be most easily got at and influenced by hygienic means. It is capable of absolute proof that improved mind results from bettered brain. We are slowly groping by study and experiment after the processes through which this can be done. We recognise also that bad brain can be bettered and developed by purely mental processes, and we are groping and experimenting in regard to that mighty problem too. The scientist is perfectly willing to accept man's responsibility in so far as it can be proved to be a fact, but he maintains that responsibility is conditioned by all sorts of agencies affecting the brain. Many of the great philosophers of old and many of its religionists fully admitted the limited responsibility of man. St. Paul, though evidently most unwilling to admit this, yet was obliged to say, " The good that I would I do not: but the evil which I would not, that I do." On any theory, however, that of the metaphysician or of the modern scientist, the brain must be held to be the organ of supreme importance in regard to mind, and there will be little practical difference of opinion as to the importance of hygienic measures in mental improvement, especially in the earlier and formative stages of life.

The ordinary instincts of the metaphysician, the religionist, the moralist, and the educationalist have as yet, no doubt, been strongly in the direction of cultivating mind and morals apart from their organ, the brain. Men naturally point to the great philosophers, the powerful moral teachers, and the great scholars, and the heroes of old who were trained, quite irrespective of any brain knowledge. They point to the average man of the present day, and say he is a fairly good specimen of humanity developed and educated under the old system. Some of them would say if a man's mind cannot develop through mental stimuli, his body taking care of itself, it cannot be worth much. The reply to this reasoning on the part of the modern scientist I have so far anticipated. The main fact is that the mind does not exist at birth because the mental part of the brain does not exist in any organised way for effective working. The mind grows as the brain grows and the quality of the mind has a direct relation to the quality and mode of working of the brain. Those objectors to the scientific view do not seem to take into account that the great nations of antiquity have nearly all lost in mental power and have either faded away or become degenerate and have lost their virile strength in modern times. Science says that she sees no reason for this except that those nations broke the laws of Nature through ignorance in the way they lived. Science has a fervid hope that by the application of her laws to the lives of mankind, no such degeneration and decay need take place. Modern science believes that many precious lives that would have done much for the world have been lost through early preventable death or bad training and through want of mental and bodily hygiene. Take, for instance, the misery of Carlyle, the suicide of Chatterton, and the early death of Keats from consumption. Mind and brain form a dualism and both require to be taken into account equally in our system of education and in our modes of life. Many bodily processes, as we have seen, can be stimulated by mental action, while it is certain that mental action can be either promoted or interfered with by unfavourable bodily conditions. Electricity can only be produced by physical agencies, but, on the other hand, when produced, it can act on matter in all sorts of ways. No one now talks of any antagonism between electricity as one of the forms of energy and the coal and the dynamo through which that energy is created and manifests itself.

The extent to which the will and the power of inhibition can control morbid mental action and promote counteractive healthy exercises of mind and body.—The want of the power of self-control is so very common a thing amongst mankind, in respect to many matters that it may be regarded as the normal condition of our species. The perfect capacity of self-control in all directions and at all times is rather the ideal state at which we aim than the real condition of any of us. The men and the women who have attained a state of inhibitory perfection have been few and far between, and even in regard to them it may be said that they would have lost their self-control if they had been exposed to sufficient temptation or irritation. But while a perfect mental inhibition may not be attainable, there is a certain amount of this power in all directions which is expected of all sane citizens. The highest aim of Mental Hygiene should be to increase the power of mental inhibition amongst all men and women. Control is the basis of all law and the cement of every social system among men and women, without which it would go to pieces. I am to speak of the gradual development of this great power in the child, the schoolboy, and the adolescent. Sufficient power of self-control should be the essence and test of sanity. The higher inhibition can perhaps be understood best by looking at its simpler exhibitions. Grown people can control by an effort of will in many cases such morbid bodily acts as coughing or vomiting. In children it is different. If you place a bright and tempting toy before a child of two years it will be instantly appropriated. Place cold water before a sane man dying of thirst and he will drink it without any power of doing otherwise. Many persons have naturally a small supply of this power or it has not been cultivated in them in youth, so that it takes a small occasion for them to lose it. Exhaustion, mental or bodily, illness or any bodily weakness has the effect on such people of paralysing their power of self-control. They will be angels or demons just as they are fresh or tired. Some persons have it in such large degree that they have the fatal power of keeping themselves at work or at dissipation till their stock of resistiveness is entirely exhausted and they completely "break down" in their power of self-control. Woe to the man who uses up too often his surplus stock of brain inhibition! In certain neurotic people there is often a loss of self-control in regard to certain acts. Dr. Johnson had to touch each lamp-post as he passed it. If he did not do so he was unhappy and went back to do this useless and irrational act. Plenty of such people " have the feeling " that they cannot answer letters, that they cannot walk, that they cannot meet their friends, &c. In certain exceptional cases, persons constituted thus, have obscure impulses towards killing, towards destructiveness, towards dishonest appropriation of property. Possibly many of those tendencies are transmitted qualities of our far-off barbaric progenitors—reversions, in fact, to an earlier stage of human evolution. As I have said, the modern authorities in physiology and psychology now believe that there are in the brain masses of cells whose duty it is to inhibit or control the action of other parts of the brain. The question is a most important one in Mental Hygiene. Can those inhibitory centres be so developed in youth and so cultivated in mature life that they can act as antagonists to what is morbid ? Can they, in fact, be used as directly curative agencies against tendencies towards foolish and hurtful impulses? If this is so, and we could cultivate this power, it would be an educational discovery the most valuable yet made by humanity. I lately saw a lady who had consulted me frequently from her youth upwards. She came of a family in which nervousness, insanity, talent, and genius had all been found. She was herself clever and artistic, and had to earn her own liveli- hood by art and teaching. She was subject to certain foolish impulses, morbid trains of thought, and even explosive action. From the beginning I saw that she had strong inhibitory power. This I encouraged her

G

to exercise and to practise constantly and especially in regard to those tendencies which I considered morbid. Along with this I impressed on her that she must look after her general health, keep herself "fit" by plenty of fresh air, exercise, amusement, and suitable social intercourse. She had done so with such admirable effect that for many years she had been able to work hard at her profession, to earn a good income, and vastly to improve in her power of controlling what was morbid in her. In an interesting conversation I had with her in our last interview she expressed herself very strongly that this had "saved" her from unhappiness, inefficiency in her work, and possibly from mental breakdown. I believe that in this opinion she was correct, and I put her down as an example of what a strong inhibitory power, properly exercised, can do for a human life. I saw a gentleman lately, occupying an important position, who told me that he had been subject at times for most of his life to a feeling of morbid shyness, to obsessions, to feelings of unworthiness and incapacity, to religious dread and to actual vicious conduct. He had a strong power of will, and he said that by exercising that vigorously he could switch his mind off into other directions when it tended to run into such morbid grooves, and that thereby he had led a moderately happy and a useful life. When I was making some excuses for his having those obsessions on account of the nervous character of his constitution, he stopped me and said, "Now, for God's sake, Doctor, don't say I can't help those things! If you do, I shall certainly go wrong. My one hope is that you should encourage me to think that through the exercise of my will power I can stop and overcome them."

Those are examples of Mental Hygiene exercised in the highest region of the brain and under considerable difficulties. I do not say that such power of inhibition belongs to every one, or can be exercised in all circumstances. On the contrary, I know that, unfortunately, tendencies towards morbid feeling, morbid thinking, and morbid acting are often accompanied by a morbid diminution in the inhibitory power as well. This antidote for their disease does not exist in some people. But the existence of such a power of inhibition as will act thus hygienically can never be known till it is tried, and the possibility of its increase and growth can never be estimated until right means have been practised. A persistent trial is really the only practical rule for all such cases. To overcome obsessions and delusional beliefs by volitional effort it is far better to make that effort in the direction of thinking of other subjects or of doing some work that has nothing to do with the obsession than to " reason it out " and make efforts of will directly in the teeth of it. Evade it rather than stand up to it, should be the rule for most cases. Turn into a side road rather than meet your enemy in the face on his line of communication. Switch your mind on to a loop line and let your foe pass by.

CHAPTER VII

THE EMOTIONS AND THEIR MUSCULAR EXPRESSION—
THE HYGIENE OF THE EMOTIONS

THE outward expression of mind is provided for by two great powers—that of speech, of which I have treated, and that of facial and eye expression. In addition, gesture comes in, but in a very secondary way. The order of development of the different emotions and passions I shall refer to. The importance of emotion, as a part of a child's life, cannot be overestimated. Darwin, in his great work on *The Expression of the Emotions*, laid a sound foundation for all subsequent work on the subject. As the different emotions arise in the child, there is, provided by Nature, a series of muscles in the face and eyes to give them outward expression. As an index of how the subjective feelings are coming into existence it is essential to study those muscles. They are a wonderful group. Each one is very small in size, but it has an enormous number of nerve fibres coming from the brain to set it in motion. There are, including those of the eye, twenty-five of them on each side of the face (Fig. 9 a). They surround the mouth, they cover part of the nose, they surround the orbit, and they exist in the brow and cheeks. Along with those, we must take into account the small muscles of the larynx, which produce sound and regulate tone. The eye also has its own muscular apparatus round it and inside it. The number and bulk of the nerves of motion which put into action and control those " mind muscles," which altogether would weigh an ounce or two, is greater and more bulky than the nerves which move the muscles

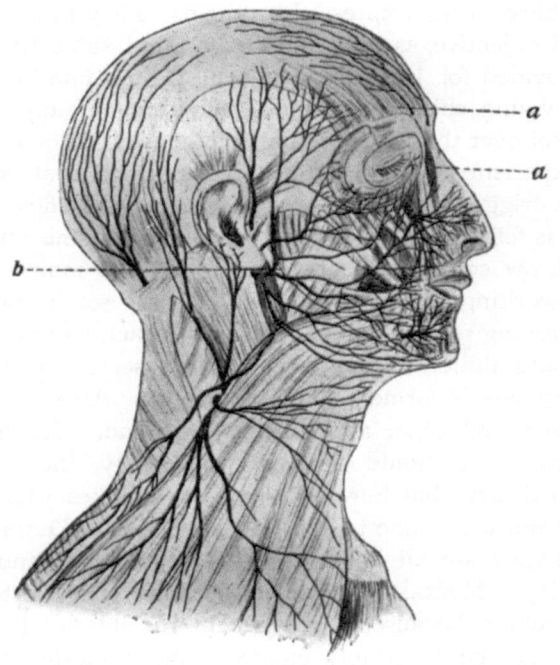

FIG. 9.—THIS SHOWS THE MUSCLES OF EXPRESSION—OF WHICH THERE ARE FIFTY—IN THE FACE AND EYE, THE "MIND MUSCLES," AND THEIR VERY ABUNDANT NERVE SUPPLY.

The muscles are shaded, the nerves are black. *a*. The muscles. *b*. The nerves.

of the arm, which would weigh several pounds. Those motor nerves of expression arise directly in the brain, are connected immediately with the mental part of the brain, and they pass from it at once to those muscles (Fig. 9 *b*).

The marvellous part of their working is that they must all work the one with the other ; in short, the power of co-ordination—a co-ordination which must be so perfect, so subtly conducted and so quick, that every tone of feeling and every passion in their every degree must be capable of being expressed by them. They form the great mind objective, as opposed to the mind subjective, which is provided for in the brain itself. Every one knows that in a young child there is no such thing as any power of control over those expressions of feeling. When a feeling is experienced by the subjective mind it is at once with "hair-trigger" velocity seen in the eye and face. When pain is felt, the muscles round the eyes and the muscles in the brow contract, the muscles round the mouth are put into working and the voice muscles are set in motion, so that crying results. The eye muscles act, so that the eye becomes duller in expression. The secretion from the tear glands is formed and pours forth. All those groups act with each other and for the same end. When a child laughs, as it should be doing frequently, those muscles again all act ; but how differently ! It takes years before those muscles come to act with perfection. During child-hood they are all being constantly exercised and put in training. Mental Hygiene is necessarily connected with their action, because, through them, the state of the child's mind can be accurately gauged. What mother does not experience one of the keenest delights of life when she sees her child's first smile ? In some children their development is arrested and they do not appear in perfection for years after the normal time. A child that at two years old cannot laugh heartily, does not weep readily, and whose face looks dull and immobile, is not in a normal condition. No one can study the facial expression of the children of the very poor and the children who are suffering from rickets and scrofula without being impressed with the deficiency in facial expression which they exhibit. They are in ill-health and need hygiene and medical care. When restored to health their muscles of mental expression gradually learn to indicate their emotions and passions. Face and eye expression becomes thus one of the chief means of diagnosing mental lack of development. In insanity the face and eye expression is also one essential means of ascertaining the mental condition. In fact, through those mind muscles largely we come to know the mental state, the intelligence, the passions, and the organic comfort or discomfort of health and disease respectively.

The muscular apparatus which I have been describing chiefly gives beauty to the face. The child that is not beautiful in some way is in a condition of retarded development of mind or body or of disease. It forms an index of how the mental centres of the brain are progressing. In idiotic and imbecile children the face has little power of expression, and the child is in most cases forbidding in appearance. Most forms of mental disease destroy beauty and attractiveness. While laying down those principles which apply in ninety-nine cases out of a hundred, there are undoubtedly a few exceptions where Nature plays a deceptive trick, and you have either bright and normal mental action with a postponement of the development and action of the face muscles, or you have an arrested, idiotic brain and some cases of insanity with much play of feature and undoubted beauty of expression. There is much scientific truth and meaning in the human craving for beauty, and admiration of it when it is seen. That craving and that admiration were not implanted in human nature for nothing. They represent the universal desire for health and, traced further back still, they represent the love of life, that primary necessity of all living things from the highest to the lowest, through which life is protected and preserved. Without such an instinctive love of beauty there can be no doubt that life would lose half its joys. In later periods of life beauty has, of course, the closest connection with the reproductive instinct.

In addition to the face muscles, however, there should be slowly developed in the child an increasing co-ordination of all the muscles of the body, so that gracefulness, harmony of movement, power to work effectively the muscles of the hands, of the arms, and of the legs, posture and gesture being thus effectively carried on. This, too, needs close observation in the development of the child. A very awkward child is an unnatural organism not uncommonly abnormal to some degree in mind. Something has gone wrong, either in its brain or spinal cord. The motor centres have not become normally co-ordinated with each other, so as to work in unison and harmony.

The Hygiene of the Emotions.—The conduct of mankind is chiefly governed by the emotions, instincts, and impulses. Spencer traces all human action to the desire for pleasure in a large and philosophical sense of that term. If this is so, then the education and the hygiene of the emotions and impulses must be of the very highest importance in the life of each individual man and woman and in the life of society. Emotion is a higher mental action than sensation, but the one commonly arises out of the other, looked at from the purely mental point of view. What emotion is has been the subject of the closest study by all students of mind. The latest theory in regard to the faculty is that of James, and it is one which lends itself to the hygienic idea more than any other. He believes, contrary to what is the old and natural way of looking at emotion, that it is not felt first by the mind, which then causes bodily changes and symptoms. " My theory," he says, " on the contrary, is that the bodily changes follow directly the perception of the exciting fact, and that our feeling of the same changes as they occur *is* the emotion. Common sense says, We lose our fortune, are sorry and weep ; we meet a bear, are frightened, and run ; we are insulted by a rival, are angry, and strike. The hypothesis here to be defended says that this order of sequence is incorrect ; that the one mental state is not immediately induced by the other, that the bodily manifestation must first be interposed between, and that the more rational statement is that we feel sorry because we cry, angry because we strike, afraid because we tremble and not that we cry, strike or tremble because we are sorry, angry, or fearful, as the case may be." He says "that every one of the bodily changes, whatsoever it be, is felt acutely or obscurely the moment it occurs." He argues very strongly in favour of this view and that it is not a materialistic view of mind at all. He says: "If our theory be true, a necessary corollary of it ought to be this—that any voluntary and cold-blooded arousal of the so-called manifestation of especial emotion should give us the emotion itself. Everybody knows how panic is increased by fright and how the giving way to the symptoms of grief or anger increase those passions themselves. In rage, it is notorious how we work ourselves up to a climax by repeated outbreaks of expression. Refuse to express the passion, and it dies. Count ten before venting your anger, and its occasion seems ridiculous. Whistling to keep up courage is no mere figure of speech. On the other hand, sit all day in a moping posture, sigh and reply to everything in a dismal voice, and your melancholy lingers. There is no more valuable precept in moral education than this—as all who have experience know—if we wish to cure undesirable emotional tendency in ourselves we must assiduously, and in the first instance cold-bloodedly, go through the *outward movements* of those contrary dispositions which we prefer to cultivate. The reward of persistency will infallibly come in the fading out of anger or depression and the advent of real cheerfulness and kindliness in their stead. Smooth the brow, brighten the eye, contract the dorsal rather than the ventral aspect of the frame and speak in a major key, pass the genial compliment and your heart must be frigid indeed if it does not gradually thaw."

Ribot says, enlarging James's illustrations : " In fear, suppress the palpitation of the heart, the hurrying breath, the trembling limbs, the widening muscles, the peculiar state of the viscera ; in anger, the heaving of the chest, the congestion of the face, the dilatation of the nostrils, the clenching of the teeth, the *staccato* voice, the impulsive tendencies ; in sorrow, get rid of tears, sighs, sobs, sorrow, anguish—what will remain ? a purely intellectual state, pale, colourless, cold. A disembodied emotion is a non-existent one." There have been many objections on the part of the psychologists and the physiologists to James's theory, but still its hygienic suggestions remain. We know that emotion, or at all events its expression, can be enormously repressed in ordinary children by teaching, persuasion, and by rewards and punishments. It is undoubtedly the aim of the English public schoolboy to repress emotion, to " take things coolly." We all know how the practice of this leads to a certain " public-school manner" in those boys. Our race has the reputation on the Continent of coolness and *sang froid* when the passions of surprise or fear would naturally exhibit themselves outwardly in other races. This, of course, implies prolonged volitional efforts and a habit thus formed. It will naturally be asked, Are such efforts possible to every child and to every grown-up man and woman ? If so, what purpose do they serve ? Are they not unnatural ? If they diminish the painful emotions do they not also tend to lessen the delights that are got out of pleasurable emotions? Take a child ; most things seem to give it pleasure, and those pleasures it learns to express by the muscular action of smiling and cooing and laughter and shouting. This is all before the will-power and self-control are developed. It is, as it were, automatic and natural. Beginning with this as our basis, this tendency to pleasure, to vivid muscular expression of emotion, are we deliberately to set ourselves by hygiene and education to exercise control over it? I say yes. Gradually acquire control over it, but not with the view of repressing or killing it out. A great principle to be observed should be, during emotional development in early life, to connect pleasurable feelings with self-control and duty. Every good deed done, every evil one repressed should receive approbation and so give pleasure, and it is right that this should happen. Nature undoubtedly implants an inner consciousness of satisfaction when good is done or self-control exercised or evil avoided. It is absolutely wrong to attempt altogether to repress this or to blame it. Far better indeed to have a little innocent boastfulness and visible self-approbation. Painful emotions should be connected in the mind with breaking Nature's laws and with immorality. Crime and badness of all sorts should be looked on, not merely as breaking human and moral law, but as going contrary to the great order of Nature under which we live. The number of the emotions, pleasurable and painful, is so great that it would be useless to attempt to go over them and ticket them with names. It is, however, undoubted that if no hygiene were exercised in regard to emotional development and its expression and action in youth, family life would be somewhat intolerable and society anything but soothing. The noisy, too demonstrative, obstreperous boy or man may be enjoying himself hugely, but he does not minister thereby to the enjoyment of others. Altruism has to come in as one of the great hygienic considerations in emotional life and its expression. It must be firmly implanted in the mind of every child that its special pleasures must not cause pain or annoyance to others. This of itself is a strong hygienic measure in regard to the expression of emotions. This principle coming in where there are many children in the family is the reason why they are so much more apt to be agreeable than where there is only one child. In schools and old-fashioned houses, as a general rule, the riotous expression of their emotions in the young is most severely handled by their teachers and elders with good enough effect, taking the system as a whole. Woman, being more emotional than man, needs, no doubt, more careful hygiene, but we would not have our women, young or old, unemotional or undemonstrative. We merely want control to the extent of the comfort and happiness of others. In modern times there is no doubt that youthful emotion is far more expressed than was allowed in family and in school life in the olden times. Possibly, a happy mean between the two methods would be the right one.

CHAPTER VIII

THE MENTAL HYGIENE OF BODILY DISEASE

THERE are few bodily diseases but what are accompanied by some mental change that is, in many cases, characteristic of and special to the condition. It is a very high condition indeed, of practical philosophy to get through ordinary work and the common troubles of life with patience, equanimity, and some degree of cheerfulness, but it implies far more than philosophy to go through a fever, an attack of bronchitis, or a severe bout of influenza without flinching in mind or becoming irritable or desponding. That needs a sound brain well trained and well treated, not being often possible even then. The common talk is that it is done through the influence of mind over body, of soul over matter. That does not quite express the truth. If the disease consists of a microbe or a poison which affects the brain especially, then no mental culture and no moral discipline will sustain a man's equanimity, for the organ of his equanimity is directly put out of gear. You might as well expect a watch with a pinch of dust among its wheels to keep time. It might be the finest instrument ever made by watchmaker, but under those circumstances it certainly will not do its work. Bodily disease is so common and so various in character that it is of enormous importance to diminish its mental effects where that is

possible.   There is a power which some men attain called
" detachment," which helps greatly in this matter.   It is,
perhaps, the highest embodiment of the Stoic philosophy
in its best period as exhibited and laid down by Marcus
Aurelius.   He says, " Efface impression, stay impulse,
quench inclination, be master of your inner self," and
again, " In the inner self and the freehold of mind, no
other may contravene.   Fire cannot touch it, nor steel, nor
tyrant, nor slander, nor any other thing, so long as it
abides poised as a sphere, self-orbed."   And again, " Pain
is either an evil for the body—and, if so, let the body state
its case—or for the soul, but the soul can maintain its own
unclouded calm and refuse to view it as evil."   Yet I have
seen the most philosophic men irritable when they had
a toothache, depressed when the liver was not working
well, irresolute when feverish, and full of delusions when
the brain was touched by the microbe of general
paralysis.   It is well known to physicians that persons
labouring under heart disease are very apt indeed to suffer
from vague fears and dreads that cannot be explained in
any other way than by the reflex effect on the mental part
of the brain when this great organ is in a condition of
disease.   The heart has always been put down as the seat
of the emotions.   It is certainly not so, but it is equally
certain that the emotions specially affect the heart's action
and that certain emotions are " felt " in the region of the
heart.   It has become part of literature to talk of " the
heart " in opposition to " the head."   There is really no
such opposition, but, on the contrary, the closest connection.   To say that a man's head is weak but that his
heart is all right, when translated into physiological
language means that a man's intellectual centres in the
brain are not strong while his emotional centres are extra
well developed and sensitive.   It is curious that the heart
should have been selected of all the internal organs as

possessing a mental function while in reality a man's mental condition depends quite as much on his stomach as his heart. The stomach, when not doing its work well, breeds all sorts of partially digested substances which act as poisons to the brain and the rest of the body. For the most part, those poisons cause vague feelings of distress, produce irritability, diminish the social instincts, and result in more or less depression of mind. Melancholy people constantly have a sinking feeling in the region of the stomach which seems to lower the whole vitality and enjoyment of life. It is an organic sense of ill-being which colours the mental life. The "precordial anxiety" of the older medical authors was really felt over the stomach and not the heart at all. The stomach and the alimentary tract, having as their function to supply the chemical substances which are absolutely necessary for the continuance of life, are naturally largely represented in the brain where the love of life, the primary instinct, resides. The stomach and the alimentary apparatus may be and are constantly disturbed from the brain, and, on the other hand, the brain is constantly upset from the stomach. Every one has experienced the fact of a keen appetite being suddenly abolished, and even of indigestion suddenly set up, by disagreeable mental emotions or distractions. On the other hand, few people but have had the experience of a perfectly happy day being suddenly made miserable by eating a bad dinner. The Mental Hygiene of the stomach is therefore obviously suggested by those considerations. Do not engage in hard mental work immediately after food, and when there is a feeling of irritability and organic distress look to the stomach and try and improve its working. I would urge in mitigation of many of the defects of this book that it has mostly been written at the end of busy days and too soon after late dinners. The liver was credited by the older medical authors such as Hippocrates, with all the depression and hypochondria that they had to treat. The "black bile"—I may say that all bile is more or less black—was put down as the cause of such complaints. It was then treated by severe doses of the purgative, hellebore. Curiously enough, one of the latest and most successful treatments for some mental complaints consists in the use of strong purgatives and antiseptics which seem to remove and counteract the poisons generated in the alimentary tract.

It is well known that the different kinds of fevers and infectious diseases produce different mental effects. The delirium of typhoid fever is different from that of typhus, and the delirium of acute inflammation is different from that of scarlatina. The poison of malaria is apt to induce distinct forms of mental disorder. Many poisons, such as opium, aconite, and Indian hemp, produce forms of mental conditions peculiar to each. It is one of the first points we investigate in any case of mental disturbance whether the internal organs and functions are in good working order or not, and whether there are any poisons circulating in the blood, and so affecting the brain. This "Toxæmic Theory" of mental disease is gaining ground every year.

Closely connected with the Mental Hygiene of disease are the facts which go to show that many diseases may be improved or cured through mental influences. John Hunter, a great surgeon and one of the most scientific and practical-minded men, said : "As the state of the mind is capable of producing a disease, another state of the mind effects a cure." The illustrations of this in the history of medicine are abundant. The doctor who neglects the mental condition of his patient in his treatment of him, no matter what the disease may be, is not a philosophical man and commonly is not a successful physician. The history of mesmerism and hypnotism is crowded with " cures " of disease, all of which may be traced to the influence of the higher brain on the whole nutrition of the rest of the body. Powerful mental attention is directed towards the disordered function and a powerful expectation of cure is thus roused. Especially in certain disordered nervous conditions, the accentuated suggestion and the rousing of action in other parts of the brain will dissipate disease. Unfortunately, mesmeric and hypnotic cures are notoriously haphazard and scientifically unreliable. They depend too much on the individuality of the particular physician and the patient, so that they cannot be subjected to definite rules. Especially the disorders of sensation have come under the curative influence of favourable mental conditions. An Italian doctor, Gerbi, stated that by using an insect squeezed between his fingers and then applied to aching teeth, he had been able to cure 401 cases out of 629. Long ago Sir Benjamin Brodie recorded a case of severe neuralgia which had prevented his patient from walking for years and which he had failed to cure by ordinary medical means. The patient happened to have a spiritual instructor of strong character and great faith, who in the name of the Saviour solemnly and earnestly told her that she should get up and walk, which she did at once. Many cases of defective action of the muscles and what are called " motor neuroses " have been apparently cured by strong mental influences. Epilepsy and palsies of many kinds have been thus removed. Sir Humphry Davy tells that he was taking the temperature of a man apparently suffering from paralysis by putting a thermometer under his tongue, and the patient, believing that this was an occult and effective mode of treatment, got up and walked and said he was cured when the thermometer was removed. All such cases, however, have been functional nervous disorders and not cases of

H

real organic disease. By the effect of mental attention, certain diseases of impaired nutrition, from warts up to internal tumours, from scurvy to dropsy, have unquestionably been cured by mental influences. This is perfectly explicable from what we know of the relation of the brain to the blood supply of the body. Through this "vaso-motor" brain function it can shut off or give an extra supply of blood to almost any part of the body if the proper stimulus is applied, and thus cure diseases which are due to an excess or too scanty a supply of blood to any particular part. Imagination, expectation, faith, hope, joy, fear, suggestion may all cure certain diseases. But for instances of this and a full treatment of the subject I refer my readers to my late friend Dr. Hack Tuke's charming book on *The Influence of Mind on the Body*. The most successful physicians have been men with great personal influence on their patients, this influence tending towards a firm faith in the remedies prescribed. Many such doctors have had that mental "magnetism" which tells so strongly, not only in medicine but in every relation of life. Such beliefs act as nerve tonics, and set the mental part of the brain into active exercise. This brings extra blood to it. The brain then acts on the rest of the body with every part of which it has relations, and thus we have the physiological apparatus for the mind cures of bodily disease. Quite lately there has been published a book by a Swiss physician, Paul Dubois, on the *Psychic Treatment of Nervous Disorders*. He seems to be a man of a strong, simple mind, vigorous insistent will, and a great belief in himself and his measures. He takes into account both the physiology and the psychology of the brain in those measures, and he frames his hygiene and his treatment accordingly. He thinks that in every nervous disorder there is a mental element; and in this he is not far wrong. He does not for a moment pretend that he cures all his cases. He begins by impressing the patient with the conviction of cure, and then he tries to make the general conditions of cure favourable. He does not despise rest, isolation, and very strict dietary rules. He recognises the influence of mind on the bowels as well as on the heart. He banishes hypnotic medicines to procure sleep. He cures constipation by mental and dietetic measures alone. He devotes much attention to what he calls the education and strengthening of the will. In short, Dubois pushes almost to an extreme Mental Hygiene and mental means of cure—I say to an extreme—because there are many people who are intensely desirous of being cured in such ways, who have unbounded faith in certain men and in measures that have an element of mystery and wonder in them, but such people are usually very disappointed and depressed when they fail to recover after such methods have been fairly tried.

Apart from any wonder-working measures and apart from men of special gifts there is a Mental Hygiene of bodily disease that can be applied on strictly scientific lines and by the application of which mental suffering may be diminished and disease averted.

The effects of many diseases are damaging to the brain and mind without producing technical mental disturbance. The memory is often greatly impaired after severe attacks of fever. The self-control is often much diminished after severe or prolonged illness. Notoriously, illness makes many people self-centred, exacting, unreasonable and forgetful of the comforts of others. The ego is disagreeably apparent while the altruism which had previously been learned and practised is forgotten. When the heart or kidneys, the lungs or the stomach, not to speak of the brain, have suffered from disease, it is often a long time before the effects are completely got rid of. This means often a poisoning of the blood and of the mind centres by deleterious products or a starvation of them by insufficient or badly made blood. In regard to all these things a Mental Hygiene and a re-education has to be done after the patient is convalescent, and it is marvellous the recuperative power of Nature in this respect even up to old age. The patient can do very much himself to hasten this process of restoration by adopting rational rules of Mental Hygiene.

There are many infections and poisons that impair the mental working, and should be specially taken account of. A medical friend lately consulted me about his feeling nervous, depressed, fanciful, self-centred, and unable to do his work and enjoy his life. I saw him a year after, and he said he had found out what was wrong. The drainage of his house had been bad, and he had thus been breathing sewer gas. When that was put right, all the worst of his symptoms disappeared, and he became cheerful and quite fit for work again. It is a well-known fact that the disease of the glands in the throats of children, called adenoids, renders them stupid, lethargic, and partially unfit for school work. The surgical removal of the adenoids commonly produces at once a mental brightening as well as a general improvement in health. The poison of malaria has often a markedly disturbing mental effect. Some people are active and happy in one climate and depressed and languid in others. An intelligent lady once told me that sleeping with open windows had quite dissipated a mental state of nervousness and discomfort which she had suffered from for a long time. Change of occupation will sometimes change the mental feelings greatly. A change of diet also has often a marked mental effect.

CHAPTER IX

THE HYGIENE OF MANNERS, PLAY, WORK, AND FATIGUE

Manners.—The psychology of manners is a difficult subject, yet the importance of good manners has been recognised from the earliest times. Good manners are of the East rather than of the West, but Greece soon picked them up, as she did everything else that was good. No one can read Plato's *Republic* without being impressed by the politeness of the disputants to each other. The educated classes in Greece at that time were evidently persons of good manners. Every one must have remarked on the good manners of the ancient Patriarchs as depicted in the Old Testament. The axiom of William of Wykeham that "Manners maketh Man" has been accepted as wise and truthful by the whole English race everywhere. The "softening of manners" has always been put down as one of the most desirable results of civilisation. Among modern nations, the Japanese seem to have attained the highest success in the cultivation of good manners, so that among them politeness has become hereditary and is practised by them all, from the youngest child to the oldest man. If manners maketh man, it must be remembered, however, that manners have themselves to be made. In most barbarous nations politeness, courtesy, and manners are little known. Among children of our own nation it cannot be said that manners are necessarily a part of their hereditary equipment. They need to be taught. Their importance in Mental Hygiene is twofold—first, the influence of the good or bad manners of one child on another, and second, the influence of the constant practice and habit of good manners on the mind of the child who practises them. Without denying that among the educated classes, children come naturally and by heredity by a certain tendency towards good manners and polite behaviour, yet it is certain that there are such children whose manners do need forming and who, if they habitually see rudeness of manner, will imitate it. Like morality in children, manners are chiefly the result of example, but being a more concrete and outward thing, they are more capable of being established by dogmatic teaching as well. This cannot be begun too young. There is no risk of any kind in teaching good manners. If rightly taught, and the reasons assigned to even very young children, it can have no effect but a good one on their Mental Hygiene. Good manners should imply altruism and a consideration for the feelings of others. To begin with, they are always a repression of the disagreeable in self. They also imply the exercise of the imagination, which is a faculty strong in young children. They lead to good habits of mind as well as good habits of body. They are a part of the discipline which is legitimate in childhood—a discipline which the child who is fine in the grain instinctively realises to be reasonable at even an early age. Good manners are also connected with the feeling of reverence for the old, the good, and the respected. The practice of them leads to so much evident commendation and approval from others that the child's self-respect and pleasure in life are increased. The practice of them also leads to the satisfaction of the child's love of approbation in a legitimate way. No one who goes into an Infants' school and watches the children playing but must see that the rude, boisterous children are also apt to be cruel and inconsiderate. Looked at by the physiologist, he sees that such children are forming a bad brain and muscular habit which will not be easy to be got rid of after it has been instituted in the brain cells.

Good manners have a muscular side, being connected with the pleasant use of the voice and body with the harmonious action of the muscles of the face. When children are ill, they are apt to forget their good manners. It is a great pity that it is not part of our educational process, from the Infants' school to the University to teach good manners. This is especially necessary in free and democratic communities. The sweetening of life that would thereby result is certainly one aim of a true Hygiene of Mind.

Play.—Play is a natural instinct in the young of all vertebrate animals. It assumes an endless variety of forms, but in some shape or other it is always there. It needs no teaching to appear, and therefore I call it an instinct and not an acquired character. It is most vigorously carried out by the strongest and the most robust. It has no immediate object in providing food or in protecting from danger, and yet it is evidently of the very highest importance in the development of strength and energy. Play is the real work of children. Froebel, a German schoolmaster, was the first to bring out its significance and its necessity in education. It is always associated with pleasure in a very high degree. It is commonly done in the air and sunshine. It is by far the surest index of organic health. It begins soon after free voluntary motion. It is so craved for, and its effects are so manifestly beneficial, that there can be no question at all that it is an organic necessity. We do not know how the young of the mole play, but if we knew sufficient of the life-history of that dweller in darkness it is certain that we should find play in some form just as in every other animal. No surer index of ill-health or ill-condition exists in a young animal than an indisposition to play. "No play no health" is a true axiom for the child.

Looking to man, play begins in babyhood, is a prime factor of well-being all through childhood and the school age, does not cease at adolescence, and among the healthy, who have their wants fully supplied without too hard work, it extends almost to the end of life. It becomes very closely related early in life to the saving graces of fun and humour. It is intimately connected with the great educative faculty of imitation. A child "plays at" every action and every piece of work that it sees others do. Physiologically, play means to a child exercise of the muscles, improved circulation of blood, inhalation of oxygen, better digestion and appetite, stimulation of all the glandular system, pleasant impressions on the senses and brain, a happy emotional condition and the acquisition of much knowledge that will be very useful in after-life. It becomes organised into games which do so much for the growing body and brain, as well as for the developing mind. It is a very social gift, because children always tend to play with each other rather than alone. A child who has the chance of playing with other children, and does not take advantage of this opportunity, is in a more or less abnormal condition. Play is literally the prologue and the preparation for the serious work of life. It is the most apt illustration of that " necessity to energise " which I have referred to as one of the organic necessities of the brain. Though thus natural and irrepressible, play can be greatly encouraged by wise parents and teachers so as to become a part of education, physical, mental, and moral. It is capable of direction and organisation greatly to the advantage of the child. Play that implies destruction of useful articles and beautiful objects, or that involves hardships or cruelty to younger or weaker children or animals, can be and should be discouraged, and so great moral lessons of tenderness and unselfishness can be taught. It can be used to improve the faculty of observation very early in life. To play at gardening, to play at baking, to play at dressing dolls may all be made educative in a high degree. Play is the great stimulant to the imagination in childhood. It is indeed doubtful if a healthy faculty of imagination could be created in its first stages except through play. The play world is, as every one knows, perfectly real to the child. This gives it a dignity and importance in the child's estimation. The talk of children is largely of play. The schoolboy and girl long for the time when lessons are over, in order to rehearse their play experiences. Adolescents talk of little nowadays except football, cricket, and hockey. Many grown men, similarly, golf all the week in many cases, and talk about their exploits on Sunday. It is quite certain, however, that play and the love of it can be overdone at all ages except early childhood. When so overdone it dissipates mental energy that should go to the serious work of life, and it gives a tone of frivolity to the later ages of life of which work should be the keynote. It consumes time which could be better spent in more serious pursuits. It lowers the intellectual tone and the seriousness of life. It leaves less time for reading and thought. Morally, it often tends towards selfishness and self-indulgence. During adolescence, especially among the wealthier classes in Great Britain and America, it is now distinctly limiting the output of useful human energy in those countries by being overdone. Play is, no doubt, a preparation for life, but it is far from being the only preparation. Excessive play and amusement bring their own punishment, for the young man and woman who thus fill up their time become sated and stale. The period of life in which high ideals of duty, increase of knowledge, a keen interest in literature, and habits of self-denial should be cultivated, may become, through excessive addiction to play and games, a barren and even mischievous epoch. The proper regulation of this play instinct is therefore a mental hygienic of immense importance. Fully to enjoy its pleasures and advantages it must, after the period of childhood, be intermittent and alternated with work. Though "all work and no play makes Jack a dull boy," all play and no work makes him an empty one. No play is so enjoyed as the month of it by the student or the professional or business man who has worked hard for the previous eleven months. Nature allocates her enjoyments largely as rewards for work done. No play-pleasure is so intense as the satisfaction felt at the end of a piece of good work done well.

For many years I have advocated playgrounds for our city children at all costs as being a necessity of life for them. Most cities have now parks and open spaces, but these cannot be used by many young children. There are few things more pathetic than a walk through the artisan quarters of a city on a fine Saturday afternoon or Sunday. All the small children are out and all are at play, but with only the streets and a chance contractor's bit of building ground to play in. An Act of Parliament making a playground compulsory for every block of houses containing five hundred children, at the cost of the landowner, would not seem an inequitable statute. Mrs. Humphry Ward's "Play Centres" are a hygienic measure of the most admirable kind, and full of promise.

The Hygiene of Work.—Those essential brain qualities or instincts which I have described as "the necessity to energise," and the desire to live, are the physiological bases of work, as well as play. Good work is got through the stimulus and by the regulation of those faculties. The philosophy of work consists in its necessity. The brain cell cannot in health cease to be active, except to a partial extent during sleep. It must transform its contents into energy of some sort. There must be some output of mind from the mind cell and of motor stimulus from the motor cell. The proper selection of work for the particular brain to do, and its regulation on physiological principles, is the basis of the hygiene of employment. For health, for happiness, and for efficiency, right work rightly done is the most important matter in any man's or woman's life. Nature abhors idleness as she does a vacuum. There is no more momentous question than the selection of the work to be undertaken in the early history of a life. In every civilised and properly organised community there is fortunately a great variety of employment for brain and muscle, and we know there is a great variety of talent in men. How can the congenial and suitable be brought together? How to choose at the proper time of life, how to educate for the special work to be done, how to regulate the amount for which the particular man or woman's brain and body is fitted, when to leave off when the capacity for work is failing, how to judge when disease or weakness demands a temporary cessation of work, and how to change employment so as to make it restful when such change is needed, are some of the most urgent problems of every reasonable existence. To solve them rightly there is needed not only ordinary wisdom and common sense, but in many cases very special knowledge of health, bodily and mental, fitness and temperament. I trust that in the future the medical profession will be able to aid the world in this matter more than it has done or been called on to do in the past. If to its present knowledge of physiology and health laws it would add somewhat more of practical psychology, of heredity, so strongly advocated by Dr. Archdall Reid, and of "human constitution" in the large sense of that term, a lack in our social life would be filled. The public and the State are entitled to look to it for some help in this matter which would be on the lines of the most recent development of medicine. To prevent being better than to cure, to get out of every man and woman what they can best give to the Commonwealth, to improve the race and to advance a step or two towards an ideal social fabric, are aims worthy of the most advancing of the scientific professions. On the other hand, work can unquestionably be made curative in many cases. Work under wrong and unhealthy conditions is, on the other hand, to body and mind, one of the great mental dangers of our modern urban life.

No doubt it will be said by many people that I am preaching a Utopia, that natural leanings and social and money circumstances must chiefly guide young people in the choice of occupation, that natural selection in some form will come in here, as elsewhere in nature, that few are really quite free in their choice of occupation, that most really great men took naturally to their special work, that special fitness is mostly latent at the early ages of life, and finally that there is commonly an adaptability to take to and in some cases to excel in occupations which are not the very best fitted for the special capacity of each individual. Those considerations are all so far true and to the point, but they are counsels of pessimism, haphazard or *laisser faire*, which do not tend towards the best that may be done for humanity or society. To follow them would not be to take advantage of what modern science can offer towards the good of mankind. They are unscientific, not only from the health but from the sociological point of view. They do not make the best of things in this world. The standard on which they are founded is low and unprogressive. They do not tend towards a further evolution for man. They are opposed to a higher civilisation. As a matter of fact there are few parents who do not exercise a choice in regard to the selection of an occupation for their children. They often feel the need of guidance in this and ask for it. Among the more educated and richer classes the cry of " What shall we do with our sons and daughters ? " is an urgent one. The great considerations which will help the doctor and the parent of the future in choosing an occupation for the young are health, defects, aptitudes, special leanings, opportunities, powers of resistance, bodily and mental conformation, tendencies mental and bodily to special risks and temptations and special mental, moral or bodily strong or weak points. In regard to health the family doctor could certainly help if he could obtain a good history of hereditary tendencies. He would warn off and encourage many young men and women away from certain trades and professions and give indications towards others. A narrow-chested young man or woman with a family tendency to consumption would not be sent into sedentary or indoor occupations. A lad of nervous constitution and heredity would not be set to pass competitive examinations in youth and made into a speculator afterwards. There are manifest indications in many of our city-brought-up boys and girls that they need to go back to Nature and lead country lives as farmers, surveyors, colonists, ranchers, or as sailors. It is simply marvellous what men and women may be made out of such material by the right sort of food, environment, and work. How much disappointment would be saved if the nervous young woman with no staying power or backbone could be prevented from going into nursing and medicine! For the neurotic, more especially, the choice of an occupation counteractive to their diathesis is important. I am persuaded, from my own experience, that if this was more frequently done much neurasthenia, nervous "break-downs," misery and mental disease might be saved. There are so many young people with manifest defects of intellect, of adaptability, of sympathy, of character, of manners, of firmness of purpose, of organising power, and of observation that the teacher and the doctor would be fools indeed if they could not help in choice of work. The natural partiality of affection of parents would thus be corrected by the real facts of science. If the well off would only accept facts about their children they would not strive so unreasonably, as they often do, to keep them in the same conventional social class as they are themselves, but would often make them into artisans, farmers, colonists, and clerks. What regrets might not thus be saved! Because a boy has been good at cricket and football should suggest not eminence in a profession but hard muscular work as his life's career. Some boys and girls have so little inhibition against temptation that it is mere madness to place them in occupations where severe control is needed to keep them right. No doubt English parents of the better classes have in a way been fortunate in having "the Church" as a convenient opening for the unspecialised. But that fact largely explains many of the Church's spiritual failures. Bodily habits and conformation often give wonderfully correct indications. The boy with big, effective hands, who can use tools early, is destined by Nature for engineering. There was often little doubt even from bodily indications among my fellow-students as to who were to take to surgery and who to medicine. It may be said with much truth that the parents who have sent their children from home and committed their whole training and education to the teachers in a public school from the age of nine onwards can know so little of their special aptitudes and defects that they are often unable to select a suitable occupation to fit their abilities. And equally the teachers in the Board schools are now so specialised in their work and know so little of the pupil's individuality that they cannot help as much as they might do in this matter. The greatest difficulty in making choice of an occupation for a boy or girl early in life, as the majority of our population have to do, is that no reliable indications of special aptitude are always then to be seen. On this point the practical physiology and heredity of the future may be expected to come in. Science may give indications where common observation fails—indications which may be invisible except to the trained insight.

It would be an interesting sociological inquiry to ascertain in modern society the real proportion of square men and women who have got into round holes and *vice versâ.* I have been looking over the list of my friends and acquaintances, and I think one may safely say that at least 20 per cent. have failed to find the work for which they were most fitted.

Occupation has a marked effect in moulding the mental and moral character, be it suitable or unsuitable. The mind and manners of the clergyman, the lawyer, the business man, the domestic servant, the citizen, the policeman, the soldier and the sailor, are all more or less distinctive. Surely no occupation and training was ever so effectual in obliterating every suggestion of originality and self-reliance out of the barracks or off the battlefield as that of the British soldier of the time before the Boer war. His original thinking power was nil and his sphere of action most restricted. That was why the employer of labour so specially shunned him when, after his discharge, he came asking "for a job." Yet many such men came back from South Africa alert and resourceful after their experience there. They had to be resourceful there or die.

But in the choice of human occupations, as in the choice of husbands and wives, the sphere of science will for long be limited. Nature settles many cases by strong leanings that will sooner or later be obeyed. Opportunity will not be denied in other cases, no matter what Nature says. Necessity limits the choice of occupation in perhaps the greater number of our people. Ambition will always try to set Nature at defiance. Ignorance and conservatism will complacently go on their stupid way, not seeing or hearing the voice of science. Knowledge must steadily work towards the better way for humanity in this as in all other things.

Fatigue.—Professor Mosso, of Turin, has lately written a most instructive little book on *Fatigue*, mental and bodily.[1] He has endeavoured, according to the methods of modern science, to measure and to record, in many accurate and most ingenious ways, the amount and kinds of fatigue to which human mind and muscle may be subjected. In this treatise I cannot refer much to his researches on muscular fatigue, except in so far as they serve to indicate mental fatigue. He fully recognises and proves, in various unexpected ways, the physical law of conservation of energy in nervous action. He shows that in fatigue there are very subtle brain-poisons produced in the blood, and changes in the temperature and in the muscles in consequence. He points out that headaches and nervous exhaustion are often the result of such poisons produced by over-brain work or over-muscular work. He shows that there are some people who can

[1] This has been admirably translated into English, and is published by Messrs. Swan Sonnenschein & Co. [EDITOR'S NOTE].

work their muscles or their brains and minds separately, but who cannot do both at the same time. He gives vivid examples of the physical effects of University examinations among the students. He shows that by the reflex action of disease elsewhere, the functions of the brain and mind may be retarded or interfered with. This may happen from such a simple disease as adenoid tumours in the throat. He shows that many unhealthy occupations, implying excessive labour or stress, will upset the mental working. The power of attention, he points out, may be specially affected by conditions of fatigue, and that modern "nervousness" probably results in some measure from the too great activity of the brain in modern life. He directs attention to the fact that consciousness, sensitiveness, memory, and reasoning power may all suffer from the results of fatigue. He gives most interesting examples as the result of the examination of his friends among the professors as to how their lectures and work affect their minds. His instances in regard to the effects of darkness and light, as to the relationship of over-strain and bad artistic work are full of suggestiveness. Wherever it was possible, he showed those results of fatigue by a graphic method. His diagrams are in themselves vivid pictures of what fatigue can do.

CHAPTER X

CHILDHOOD, FROM BIRTH TO 7 YEARS

The Order of Development of Brain and Faculty. The Hygiene and the Special Mental Risks of this Period.

I HAVE spoken of the ideals for mind and brain. How can those ideals be helped on in childhood? What sort of environment will best aid in their attainment? Those are questions of enormous importance to society, to the State, and more especially to the parent. Every increase of our knowledge in regard to them will, in the end, help to build up better practice. The first piece of important knowledge to be inquired into and to be used practically on many occasions is as to the heredity of the child. Were its parents healthy? If it has not a clean bill of health in regard to its ascertainable ancestry—and what child has the good fortune to possess that in our modern civilised society?—then the particular weak points must be ascertained. The boy is apt to take his chief features of brain and mind from the mother's side, the girl from the father's. Inquiries must not be limited to the parents, the brothers and sisters, and the uncles and aunts, but must be made in regard to the grandparents and their brothers and sisters. The first and second cousins too must be taken into account. The chief weak points to be inquired into are whether there was any mental disease, nervousness, epilepsy, idiocy, uncontrollable drunkenness, consumption, gout, rheumatism, marked eccentricity, hysteria, silliness, paralysis, want of force of character or vice.   The strong points in hereditary history should be inquired into as well as the weak ones. Longevity, size, muscular power, mental energy, originality, sound morals, self-control, are all most desirable character-istics in ancestry.   Strong artistic and literary instincts— the artistic temperament, in short—may be both a great danger and an enormous gain.   In any case its existence should be considered and taken into account.   As yet our power of counteracting a very bad heredity is limited, but it can do no harm, but good, to know that it exists and to face it up.   Thereby some of the dangers can be avoided and some of the temptations escaped.   It may be said generally that the child with a strongly nervous heredity or mental taint in ancestry should be fed on milk, farinaceous diet and fruits, certainly up to 7, and largely up to 25.   It should be kept fat.   Its faculty development should be repressed rather than stimulated. Undue excitement of all kinds should be avoided.   It should live much in the fresh air.   The winds of heaven not only cure consumption, they strengthen the nerves and promote nutrition at all ages.   The evil conditions to be looked for are—convulsions when teething, night terrors, stammering, backwardness of speech, eye defects, and special liability to a high temperature from very slight catarrhal or other causes of fever.   I have found that one child will become delirious during an ordinary attack of catarrh with a temperature of 99°, and that another will not become so at 104°.   The first was a nervous child ; and this indication of nervousness should be kept in mind by the mother and the family doctor.   A strongly nervous heredity, too, may result in idiocy and imbecility.   If an observable idiotic condition of head and intellect is seen soon after birth then there is no help for it but patience, submission to God's will, and infinite, but almost fruitless care, with the school for idiots to be looked forward to. Much may often be seen by a skilled observer in the formation and shape of the head, the facial and eye expression, the symmetry of the features, the shape and setting of the ears, as well as the normal formation of the body and the easy, graceful use of the muscles. Marked abnormalities in these respects are nowadays called "stigmata of degeneration." They are Nature's bad marks. Each one of them indicates some little defect in the brain-structure and working, but this may not affect the mental centres. Nature, within limits, is not always uniform, nor consistent, nor harmonious. Many a poor face and eye have a really good mental vehicle behind them, many an unlovely countenance has a fine mind at the back of it. Nature often appears to play tricks on us because we are as yet not fully acquainted with her laws.

The brain of a child at birth weighs 13·8 ounces, and at maturity 49·5. It increases between two and three-fold in weight during the first year of life, and rapidly attains almost its full weight at 8 years of age, though the body has only grown during that time a third of its adult weight. As we shall presently see, its mental functions are nil at birth, and most incomplete at 8. Therefore the brain may be said to have in childhood large substance but incomplete structure and immature function. It is in somewhat the same condition as a cotton mill in the course of construction, when its thousands of wheels and spindles and delicate machinery are made in the rough but have not yet a working connection with each other. The process of development in childhood is like that of the engineer who is gradually putting them in their places and fitting them to work in relation to each other. As we shall see, it is not till the age of 25 that the whole complicated and inter-dependent brain machinery is completed in its functions and can do its work in a perfect manner.

Order of Development.—It is most important to know and notice the order of development of the faculties of brain and mind.   It is one of the most astonishing facts to my mind, that until Darwin's time, with his marvellous power of seeing everything, his scientific instincts and power of coming to conclusions from his facts, the order of development of the faculties of childhood had never really been described in any systematic way, and this notwithstanding the very closest observation of children by loving and anxious mothers.   Was there ever any fact in a child's development and conduct too small for a mother's notice or too unimportant to excite her interest?   Her observation of what takes place in her child is not a thing of toil but of intense pleasure.   If all the observations of all the men of science since the beginning of the world were put together, the sum of them would not amount to a millionth part of the attention that the mothers of the world have given to their children. The rapture of a man of science when he makes a new discovery is a tame thing compared to the mother's joy when she sees her baby's first smile.   It might have been thought that we should have had nothing to learn about the development of children.   As a matter of fact, we had everything to learn, from the scientific point of view, until Darwin took it up.   The fathers and mothers had no doubt observed, the educationalists had dogmatised, the philosophers had speculated, and the religionists had theorised about the infant, but nobody had "set it down in order." The child's deformities had been put down to the mother seeing something disagreeable when she was pregnant. Its faults had been put down to original sin.   Its nervousness had been attributed to bad milk.   Publicists and statesmen did not concern themselves with the early

making of their people. Nature was supposed to take
the entire charge of the development of children up to the
ages when the schoolmaster and the policeman took them
up. She made them big and small, wise and foolish speci-
mens, irrespective of human intervention, natural law, or
the conditions under which they grew. Even yet, when
science is pervading the community, ask any ten intelligent
mothers who have each had six children, how many pounds
they gained in weight each year up to seven, or how many
inches in height they had grown, the chances are that only
one or two will be able to give anything like correct
answers. Ask them, further, the ages at which their children showed observation, power of attention, memory,
imitativeness, anger, or fear, and the certainty is that one
will get few scientifically correct replies. I should back
any enthusiastic dog fancier to give a far more exact
account of the development of his bull-pup and the
coming out of the qualities of courage and fidelity during
the first year of its existence.

Since Darwin's time there have been hosts of child
students and many good books on the subject have been
written, but his observations stand true at the present day
and marvellously cover the ground. He assumes, and we
must always assume it as the great fact in development,
that it is the brain which is the dominant organ ruling the
course of progress of mind and body and transmitting
hereditary qualities far more than any other organ. It
may be looked on as practically the child, all the other
organs and members being subservient to it. The appearance of its cells at babyhood as compared with maturity
I have represented in Fig. 6 a and b (p. 22). We believe
that the child has a mind apart from its body, yet it
is quite certain that without the body it could not think or
see or hear or feel or speak, and we should have no real
knowledge of its mind at all. Where the brain grows

rightly the mind develops naturally. Where the brain ceases to grow, or is arrested in its growth by some disease *in utero*, or some ancestral condition, the mind also ceases to develop, and we have idiocy resulting. If any of the organs of the senses, such as the eye or ear, or their centres in the brain, are absent or damaged at birth, we have a slow and mostly imperfect development. If the two dominant senses, sight and hearing, and the faculty of speech are absent, then we have the conditions of Laura Bridgman and Helen Keller. These girls were in such a condition that it needed an infinite amount of patience, skill, and science to educate them through the one sense of touch. If that had not been done they would have been in a mental state so backward as to be equivalent to idiocy. If there were many such children in the world they could not, as a matter of fact, be educated at all, and would remain "idiots by deprivation of the senses." At birth the child cries and moves and sucks and appears to feel pain as a mere automaton. Certain things, however, it does as well as it will ever do. It breathes, its heart beats, and the nourishment of its organs goes faster than at 25. The two first mental states that are developed in the child are a feeling of discomfort or ill-being when bodily or external conditions are out of harmony with its existence, and a feeling of well-being when those are favourable to it. Those two feelings it shares with the lowest of the animal creation.

Definite sensations of special pleasures through the senses are next seen. Food gives pleasure, and the person who gives the food is associated with this so that the emotions of attachment and love are observed. A child begins in a faint way to smile when it is about 45 days old. Its mind muscles then assume purposive action. (See Fig. 9, p. 85). This is the first muscular expression of pleasure. Its earliest exhibition of humour and amusement appears in about 3 months.   The vowel sounds of speech begin to be made at about the same period.   Imitation and curiosity, the great educative faculties of young children, appear about the fifth or sixth month.   From that time they may be said to spend their whole time in making physical experiments.   Anger can be exhibited at about 10 weeks, while violent passion may come on at 4 months.   There is no evidence that a child can distinguish one person from another until it is 4 months old, in spite of the strong and delightful belief of all mothers that their babies know them whenever they open their eyes.   Sympathy is shown at 6 months old.   Jealousy, the green-eyed monster, first appears at 15 months of age.   Anything that can be called reason is only seen after 100 days have elapsed.   Darwin's child smiled at his own image in a mirror at 4½ months old, and found out, by observation and reason, at 6½ months, that it was merely an image and not a real person. Next he saw his father through a plate-glass window. Through a reasoning process he naturally enough concluded that this was also a mere image, and treated it accordingly with contempt and neglect.

A child at about 4 months old or so will not do over again many times an act through which it has suffered pain.   Showing the contrast between man and one of the lower fishes, a grown-up pike dashed his head and stunned himself repeatedly for three whole months against a glass partition which separated him from some minnows, and then, after thus painfully learning that he could not attack them with impunity, when they were placed in the aquarium with him he starved himself in a persistent and senseless manner and made no attempt to eat them up. The first signs of moral qualities, sense of right and wrong, inhibition, took place in Darwin's boy at the age of 13 months.

Darwin says that he educated his child in morals solely

by working on his good feelings, and that the boy soon became as truthful, open, and tender as any one could desire, although at 2½ years he had shown "carefully planned deceit." No doubt the great naturalist was right in eliminating mere intellectual teaching and dogmatic education from the moral teaching of the child, but I think he omitted a very serious element in the up-building of his moral nature. That was the power of imitation, without which, I would say, that no constraining power of the feelings would entirely succeed. In moral education the knowing of right from wrong should always be associated in the child's mind with the doing of it by everybody with whom he comes in contact. No doubt up to 7 morals are more of an automatic, imitative habit, than of a real conscience. I have seen many examples of quick, nervous children being so permeated with notions of right and wrong through a constant insistence on them by anxious parents, that a sort of precocious and hyper-æsthetic conscience was created and moral ideas were constantly attached to non-moral acts. Such children I have known to be made acutely miserable by the idea that they had committed a serious wrong in taking too much jam for tea, with the superadded religious idea that there was great possibility of going to hell in consequence, if they died soon.

Any attempt to forestall Nature in developing that or any other of the higher mental or moral qualities is apt to be afterwards followed by paralysis of the qualities, thus fostered by a forcing-house treatment. There is no doubt that the moral sense has a hereditary basis. While all children have a certain tendency to deceitfulness and to do furtively what they have been told not to do, this is developed in some of them to an enormously greater extent than others. The children of the habitually criminal classes, of drunken parents, and of some of the insane, I have known to be hereditarily devoid of any sense of right and wrong. They seemed to take to deceit as a young wild duck takes to water. The children of gipsies, tinkers, and tramps are notoriously ill to train in habits of truthfulness and honesty. This defect has become in them virtually a diseased condition. There are in the history of Reformatory efforts, however, many examples of a re-creation of a sense of duty in such children, if put under right influences early enough, and if their environment has been of the right sort. This success has been most evident where the individual at the head of the school had placed himself or herself in immediate personal daily contact with such children and had that moral enthusiasm and magnetism of character which is given to some people. Moral action is intimately associated with the inhibitory or controlling centres in the brain of which I have spoken, and with their action. There is a real analogy between the two acts of voluntarily stopping a troublesome cough for a time and that of not appropriating a forbidden piece of food by a child. There is in both cases an act of inhibition—the lower being controlled by the higher. It is of great importance, then, not only for the muscles but for the morals, that inhibition should be cultivated as soon as its centres are developed in the brain. It is observed that after the first year most children exhibit signs of mental inhibition or control over their actions from some motive or other. Darwin found that some of the passions which have a strong moral relationship, such as jealousy, are very early developed.

The last point in a child to be developed is the general force of volition or will-power, to act as an independent being, the *ego*, as it were, asserting its power as a mental faculty. After the first year in a normal brain this develops very rapidly and goes on maturing till full manhood or womanhood is reached. It is no doubt the faculty above all others which makes one man great as compared with another. All men have it in some degree. The wills of some men are so masterful that, like those of Alexander and Napoleon, they subdue the world. It is one of the most difficult of all the parts of its education to treat this will-power in a child. We all want it to be made strong, but if it is cultivated for its mere strength, without reference to moral or altruistic considerations, we may be rearing a curse to humanity, the incarnation of Milton's word picture of the devil. On the other hand, if we try to repress it too strongly and successfully, the man or the woman may become a mere plastic cypher in the world, and so of little use. There is an old Scotch expression constantly used by the fathers and mothers of past generations in that country, of "breaking a child's will," though it was not really meant that the will to do good should be broken but the will to do evil. In trying to do this, however, the roughest methods of parental authority were used, often in a ruthless and essentially cowardly manner. The strong pressed the weak too hard, and many a man and woman have been thus rendered incurably facile or incurably deceitful. Really to "break the will" would be a device of the devil and would deprive the individual of his very highest faculty. Individual force of character and power for good are, of course, dependent on the strength of will.

There are certain faculties, curiously enough, that even in the child of 6 are stronger than in the grown-up man. Those are notably imitativeness, curiosity, a desire to make those about them laugh, and efforts to please those about them at all costs. The nutritive power in a child is stronger than in a man. It grows the first year of its existence far more in proportion to its weight than in any subsequent year of life. The brain grows far more in the first seven years of life than afterwards—in fact, as we have seen, it nearly completes its full weight then. It does not, of course, develop in its working power at this rate.

The attempts to stimulate the religious instinct in a child before 7 are, in my judgment, of a largely artificial character. Children are then psychologically unable to take in the abstract ideas of God and religious doctrine, but it is a very different matter, I would say, if we substitute the simple feeling of reverence for the good and for a religious life. The one is much less complex than the other, and will eventually proceed by slow but sure stages of development into the other. The one is the basal instinct on which the other has gradually reared itself in the course of the evolution of mankind. I would urge on all parents to try to create in their children a feeling of reverence for the old, for the good people whom they meet with, and for the great powers of Nature. I believe it would be easy to implant in children's minds a feeling of reverence for the sun, for beautiful scenery, for the sea and its majesty, for animals, for flowers and for grass. Such Nature-worship follows in the history of mankind on the mere superstitious fears of the primitive man, and if the child of to-day has to pass in body and mind through the same stages as its remote ancestry did in its gradual evolution, as is largely the case, it seems a natural thing for it to travel the same road in the growth of the religious instinct.

Speech Development.—The faculty of speech is, as I have already said, the most interesting and astonishing combination of a mental and bodily problem in existence. Its progress is surrounded by many pitfalls. It is highly under the influence of training, though it also owes much to hereditary aptitudes. Many physiologists and psychologists, not to speak of philologists, have studied this faculty of recent years. This is not the place to refer to the evolutionary aspect of speech and to the fact that all modern speech, all modern languages, can be traced up to about a hundred roots.   Speech begins by simple tones and gestures, expressive of feelings.   Those exist among animals.   Among low savages there are no abstract ideas at all and no words to express them, the whole number of actual words used by some tribes low in the scale of humanity only amounting to a few hundreds.   Among African bushmen and Hottentots there is evidence of the survival of an inarticulate system of sign-making.   Taine first studied carefully and on scientific principles the rising up of the faculty of speech in one of his children.   A child can cry and make a noise from the moment of its birth, but this is merely a mindless bit of automatism.   It first makes vowel sounds only.   At 3 months many such sounds are made, but they have no meaning.   It is simply practising its vocal organs as it practises its muscles by constant movements of its hands and legs. Consonants of the simpler kind are gradually added to the vowel sounds, and the child produces a series of simple cries almost as though it were talking a foreign language. The use of this gives great pleasure to the infant and the pleasure causes a constant repetition of this incoherent speech.   At 12 months, only the materials of language have been learned.   Children attach meanings to words uttered by others before they attach any meaning to words uttered by themselves.   From 12 to 18 months is the period when the first rudiments of real speech can be expressed by the average child.   Its articulation is poor at first.   The number of words are very few, and many single words do duty for a great many meanings. Thus the "Bow" means to most children not only the dog but all animals whatever at first.   There is a striking diversity in different children as to the time when speech appears.   One child may really "talk" at 15 months.

The speech faculty of girls is usually more quickly developed than that of boys. Another child equally intelligent, muscular, and in other respects as far forward, may not be able to speak till after it is two years old. I have seen remarkable examples of what I call postponed faculty —and few faculties are postponed longer than that of speech in a few cases. I know a girl who only began to speak at 8 years of age. By the age of 10 she could talk fluently. The postponement of speech is, however, in some cases a very serious indication of the arrestment of general brain faculty and of mental imbecility. I think far more could be done than is done by mothers and school teachers to make speech more articulate and more expressive than it often is. It is not only that we would thus acquire a more perfect vehicle for our ideas, but speech, like all muscular actions, reacts back on the higher centres of the brain and we should have keener feelings and more intelligence, resulting from the mere fact of better speech.

When we pass from the region of the normal to that of the abnormal we have, through brain defect and the explosive irregular outbursts of motor energy sent down by the brain to the vocal organs, the sources of much defective speech, from the lisp, so common at first with many children, up to the stammer which may make life almost unendurable to him who is afflicted by it, and to them who hear it. The effort required to speak is enormously different in different people, according to the perfection and size of their speech centres in the brain. It does not follow that a highly developed speech faculty always goes with a highly developed mental faculty, though undoubtedly the two should go together. Every evident speech defect or difficulty should be at once noticed, and the doctor called in at its earliest stages. There are now many methods of greatly improving the speech vice of stammering, even when it has assumed very bad forms, but it is much more easily treated at the beginning than when the brain centres have settled into this bad habit. Speech defects and difficulties are commonly accompaniments of idiocy and imbecility, and the chief means of coming to a conclusion whether one of those conditions of mental defect exist in a child.

Risks and Warnings.—Let us now consider some of the abnormal conditions which should be recognised, and many of which require attention or treatment. The brain of a child, receiving, as it does, millions of impressions and stimuli may be too reactive or it may not be reactive enough. When too reactive the faculties tend to be developed too soon, and in that case, not having sufficient power of resistiveness, the brain cells from being unduly stimulated are apt to become explosive. Such children start unduly at noises or sounds; they are too unduly excitable and emotional, they have fits of crying, screaming, and restlessness. The brain, in short, wants stability of action. If in a grown-up man or woman the "mind" cannot be dissociated from the brain, in a child they are still less dissociable. In a child the whole organism may be looked on as having a more distinct solidarity, the one organ to the other, than even in the grown-up man. In the child before 7 the body must be thought of first, the mind comes last, and, speaking generally, if the body is then properly treated the mind will largely take care of itself, in anything like a good environment. Education, in any technical sense, is then of really little importance, and the attempt to apply it often does harm. I believe that if children did not go to school before 7 it would make no difference in their future lives, as far as mere education is concerned. In short, the hygiene of the mind is then mostly the hygiene of the body. There are certain mental symptoms which, in a child, are undoubted danger-signals. If a child ever shows depression or mental pain, then there is certainly something wrong, some organ is disordered, the child is being poisoned by bad food or bad air, or some irritation is going on in its bodily processes. Studying the patients in the Edinburgh Hospital for Sick Children and making inquiries of the nurses, I found that in the delirium of fever most children exhibit a happy delirium, except in a few cases where there were injuries to sensitive parts of the body, such as take place in severe burns. The night delirium of such children was full of fears, terrible imaginary sights, and screaming as if in pain.

Looking still to the danger-signals, does the child grow and gain in weight at the normal rate? If it does not, then you will find that the brain and mind are puny as well as the body. More fresh air, more suitable food, and a careful examination to see if there is any disease, such as tuberculosis, are then urgently needed. There is a series of muscular symptoms of disease very common in childhood. The chief of those are convulsions, general all over the body, or local muscular spasms occurring in the arms or legs or about the face or head. Very closely allied to such conditions are undue restlessness, jerkiness, fidgetiness, slight St. Vitus' Dance, and hysterical conditions of emotional explosion. Muscular tricks and bad muscular habits, such as making faces, sucking thumbs, &c., are common enough in children, but are usually easily remediable if attended to. There are other conditions of a contrary nature but still marking disease, where you have stupidity, lethargy, slowness of movement, a diminution of sociableness, a lessening of the normal desire to please and a general lassitude of mind. Among the poorer classes the terrible condition called rickets, that arises from bad nourishment and deficient fresh air, is very common, and it affects the mind as well as the body. Undue nervousness and irritability in children always indicate that the doctor is needed, and that the conditions of life should be changed. Coldness of the hands and feet, with a bad circulation, are symptoms that should always be attended to.

Many children are subject to vague fears in the dark, which are often in words expressed by dread of the devil or hell. Such children are of the unduly nervous and unhealthily imaginative sort.

A child is so much all self that it seems ridiculous to talk of creating and educating it up to an unselfish state of mind. For most children there are no "others" in the world in the early stages of its life who have to be thought of or pleased or considered. Altruism and unselfishness are best taught by the association of a number of children together in the life of a family. The question of the use of rewards and punishments for developing good conduct in a child is one that needs much delicacy and discrimination. For a child to behave properly and stop screaming because it is going to get a sweetmeat can only be defended on the principle that you are thereby strengthening a good habit. Punishment in some form is absolutely necessary in the upbringing and hygiene of most children. It is getting out of fashion, nowadays, to apply this by making the child suffer bodily pain. It is rather used by depriving the child of something that it desires. Both forms of punishment are, I believe, applicable in a reasonable way and in a modified degree to different children with different constitutions and tempers. It should never be forgotten that in the early stages of a child's life, action follows sense impressions or feelings in an instant, "reflexly," without hesitancy, without reflection. It

K

is hair-trigger in its suddenness just as in animals. This must be kept in mind always before deciding whether any form of punishment is required. Children's actions are largely thus automatic. It would be as ridiculous and wrong to punish a child for such actions as to condemn your gun for going off when the trigger is pulled.

In regard to one thing I can speak with absolute certainty, and with no reservations, in regard to the bringing-up of children. It is that system, order, and punctuality should always be the rule of their lives. It should apply to play, meals, sleep, exercise, and such employment as children can do. For all children this orderliness is best. For many children of a nervous type and of an artistic temperament it may be their salvation in after-life to have acquired such habits of order. In reality, such habits should be regarded as in essence a part of the moral training of the child. For the children of our professional and educated classes who have had the advantages of education for many generations, and who are apt, therefore, to have become "fine in the grain" and rather nervous, orderly lives from youth to age may be the sheet-anchor of their health and happiness. It should never be forgotten that the nature of a child, as of a man or woman, is complex, not simple. No mere simple prescriptions and rules, however wise they look, will be applicable to all children.

The temperaments of children should be carefully studied. They appear early. There are two great forms of temperament which appear soon in some children. There is the nervous child, where the brain is somewhat over-developed, but especially where it is unstable in its action, where sensitiveness is too great, where reactiveness is also exaggerated, and in whom passion and emotion are too exaggeratedly or too easily expressed. Such children are often difficult to manage, are wayward, disobedient, and subject to gusts of apparently causeless passion and sulkiness; they are subject also to whims and groundless fears; they are fidgety, restless, and deficient in the elements of control; they are usually thin, often capricious about food, and they are subject to nervous ailments, such as chorea and convulsions.

The other temperament is seen in the phlegmatic, stupid child, unreactive, insensitive, slow in imitativeness, wanting in keen emotion. Such children are apt to be fat and awkward, and they tend to sleep overmuch; loud noises do not disturb them, they suffer pain with much equanimity, and the muscular expressions of their affections and passions are deficient.

Sleep.—Childhood sleep is the great healer of most defects that are remediable in a child, the divine restorer, the sovereign calmer. In the early stages of its life, up to its third year, one may safely lay down the rule—let it sleep as long as it will and encourage sleep in every way. I need scarcely say that the sleep habit should be made regular and punctual as to time. A sleepless child is always a nervous child, and is mostly an unhealthy one. As we have seen, during sleep the process of building up the cells of the brain goes on. Now in a child there is not only the wear and tear of brain action to be provided for, but also the steady growth of every cell, the formation of connection between different groups of cells by means of fibres. The electric batteries have to be daily made bigger and the copper wires to be increased and brought to many more stations. A child's brain, too, is apt to receive far more stimuli from the senses than can be written on its miniature brain. We require to provide that the evil effects of such stimuli shall be repaired and lessened through prolonged sleep. Each page should only take on the impressions of a few types at a time. If we applied more the printing would be blurred. The kind of sleep of every child needs to be studied. Some children sleep much more soundly than others, and are more difficult to awake. Temporary sleeplessness in a child means undue nervousness or disease. Nothing can be more troublesome or exhausting to the mother or nurse than a continually sleepless child. I have known idiotic children who, instead of going to sleep in the darkness, began to scream and became restless every night. The tricks of putting their children to sleep by the mothers of different nations have been very different, and in some cases very extraordinary. The cradle, the swing, perfect rest, rocking in the mother's arms, and many more have been in vogue. I believe it is best not to accustom the child to anything except a crib in a dark room. The doctor has often to be called in for sleeplessness, and he can sometimes help to restore the habit when it has been broken, by medicines and other measures.

CHAPTER XI

THE psychology of boyhood and girlhood has had many students. Not only have we had the classical pictures of *Tom Brown's School Days* and *Stalky and Co.*, but many Societies for the special object of child-study, those applying to early adolescence as well, and we have books innumerable "suitable" for boys and girls to read. They all naturally endeavour to suit themselves to the mind of the period and to put things in such a way that boys and girls shall be interested in them. If schoolboys and schoolgirls of the educated classes are not what they should be, it is certainly not for want of ideals placed before them. Every sort of adventure, every kind of "lesson," and every sort of predicament, good and bad, can be found in these books for boys and girls. Codes of public school life, the ethics of the boarding-house and the traditions of games so far regulate the lives of the scholars of this class. For the other and vaster classes who are taught in Board schools, there has been a singular deficiency of fiction or literature of an ideal nature. The man who could write another *Tom Brown's School Days*, where the scene is laid in an average Board school, would make the parent, the teacher, the scholar, and the State greatly his debtor. To touch with the light of fancy and romance, and so to inform with a high sense of duty, the five millions of our school children by means of a suitable literature—would indeed be a work that no genius need be ashamed to attempt. The practical effect of such a book would be worth thousands of sermons and tens of thousands of school lessons. Humanity even at that age will form its ideals, and the true ideal of a Board school boy or Board school girl has yet to be created. I trust that we shall soon see this enormous desideratum in our literature supplied. Authors innumerable have gone to the common life of the people for incident, for sentiment and for heroism, and they have found them there abundantly. It cannot be that in the lives of the children of those peasant heroes of literature there can be no ideals worth study and depiction.

Looked at from the combined points of view of brain and mind, the school age is first of all that of the higher co-ordination of mind and muscle. It is represented in the brain, not by actual growth in bulk and weight, but by the establishment of an infinite working connection of millions of fibres of mind cells already formed but requiring full development with motor cells also lying ready to be used. (See fig. 5, p. 20.) No doubt in the child before 7 this process has been already well begun, but it has not reached the stage where the mind wills and the brain at once at its bidding carries out accurate and complicated bodily movements of every sort. The muscles are rapidly developing, but they would be of little service if they were not connected indissolubly and for the whole of the rest of life with the mental apparatus, through which thinking, feeling, and willing are performed. A child of 8 cannot use effectively any instrument. But I have seen a boy of 15 in Cairo using, in obedience to his will, every finger of his two hands, every muscle of his arms and the toes of one foot, with such accurate co-ordination that he was producing, with the aid of a turning lathe, the most delicate balls and spindles to form beautiful meshrebiya work. He was turning it out with extraordinary speed and making as much money as the best hand in the manufactory. Each element of the complicated scheme in wood that he was constructing was like every other. The balls were of the same shape and size, holes were made of the same bore and depth, and the pins were made so accurately that they fitted, each into its socket, without any further dressing. Now this complicated process, needing skill and absolute accuracy, he had taught his muscles to perform in obedience to mental effort between the ages of 10 and 15. It is only at this period that the foundation of such co-ordination can be so perfectly acquired. This illustration shows what I mean by the co-ordination of mind and muscle at this period. It illustrates also how heredity comes in at this age. The Cairo boy was of a family and guild which for generations had done nothing but make meshrebiya work. A special aptitude had been created in their mental and motor nerve cells which had become hereditary, so that the training of this boy had been far easier for this work than that of ordinary children.

The ordinary co-ordinations between different groups of muscles, all being trained to do their work by the brain, do not often in this country assume the form I have referred to, but they are here equally real and equally important for the effective future life of our boys and girls. They take the form of being able to run and walk well, to sew and knit, to use tools, of being taught to write well, to speak clearly, with proper accent and emphasis laid on each word and sentence. Anyone hearing a deaf and dumb boy or girl who has been taught to read or speak will better realise how much the ordinary schoolboy and girl have learned in the way of using the fine muscles of the larynx, of the tongue, and of the mouth, all to act together and in harmony, to produce the intonation of pleasant speech and reading. So with writing. We all know how long a time it commonly takes to produce a beautiful handwriting. The achievement of the Cairo boy seemed to me more wonderful than that the English boy should be taught to speak and read and write, but in reality it was not so remarkable and delicate a process. Each little knob and pin of the meshrebiya work was scarcely as fine an example of nerve and muscle co-ordination as the recitation, with fluency and feeling, of a piece of English poetry, such as our well-taught boys and girls can easily do at 15, or than a well-written letter. The brain basis for these accomplishments exists in the shape of groups of cells, gathered in "centres" for the hands, the feet, and the voice muscles. There is, in fact, for writing, a special portion of the brain convolutions, which, if injured or deficient, no writing is possible. Then the whole carriage of the body, the power to play games, to leap and walk and run, and to express the feelings through the face and eye muscles, are all perfected at this period. A man or woman would be a poor, awkward, "feckless," and ineffective machine, but for the muscular co-ordinations learned during this period of life. Slowly acquired but delicately and constantly practised, they become a brain habit, and easy of performance afterwards. The right learning of these co-ordinations is the surest foundation of a hygiene of mind, and the strongest aid to mental health in the future lives of the schoolboy and girl.

The second great characteristic of the school age is allied to co-ordination. It consists of ceaseless muscular activity. This is why children at that age must have games, will shout and cry and scream, and are never at rest. To grow, muscles must be exercised, and to develop, the brain must be kept at work. To watch the dispersal of the scholars from a Board school is a great lesson to the mental hygienist. During the school-hours a somewhat unnatural inhibition has been enforced. The moment the outer door is opened it seems as if the safety valves were suddenly blown out, and noise and romping are indulged in without control of any kind. The cause of this is that the necessity to energise existing in the brain and the muscles, of which I have spoken, having been repressed for a time, must burst forth, while the inhibitory centres cease for the time to act. This is not only a physiological necessity, but it is the greatest factor of progress in the development of those children. I have already spoken of the hygiene of play.

The third great characteristic of the school age is its unreasoning fearlessness of consequences. Hughes, in *Tom Brown's School Days*, says that between 11 and 12 is "the most reckless age of British youth." In this I agree with him. The natural effects of certain conduct are not realised, and are therefore not acted on. Fear is one of Nature's great protective agencies. To rouse this faculty is, no doubt, the psychological explanation of the system of corporal punishments which prevailed so extensively in former times in all educational systems. Among many ancient peoples, such as the Spartans and the Romans, this was carried to such an excess that it became cruelty and tyranny. There is no doubt that if we turned out the scholars of an average school into an uninhabited island, and they tried to live the life of an ordinary community without the control of their elders, they would be most cruel to each other, serious accidents of all kinds would occur, they would set fire to their houses, they would eat up all their available food at once without the fear of starvation on the morrow, and their conduct would be reckless in the extreme.

The fourth characteristic of the period is its want of

power of origination. The schoolboy imitates but does not originate. Few new ideas occur to him. His plans are all founded on what he has seen or read about. In this respect he is in the condition of a low barbaric tribe. No real progress would be possible in a society with this deficiency.

The next characteristic of the period, which is allied to the last we have spoken of, is that of a cast-iron conservatism, strong, deep, unreasoning, stupid, often cruel, and unalterable till the period of life is past. Whatever a boy or girl sees others do, whatever school tradition is handed down, is imitated, stuck to, and regarded as a sacred rule of their lives. If a game is played one way, the idea that it may be improved is scouted, and its originator held to be an idiot. Where children live at home this is modified to some extent by their intercourse with parents and elder brothers and sisters, but in communities of boys and girls, as at the great public schools and large boarding-houses, this conservatism is absolute. It is, no doubt, one of the disadvantages of those institutions that this trait of character is apt to be passed on from the typical schoolboy age of which I am treating into the adolescent period of the higher classes and college life, when origination and "thinking for oneself" is possible. It thus becomes a repressive and retarding condition with them. It is one of the characteristics of the American and Colonial youngsters that the freer life enables them to shake off this habit of mind very soon after puberty. They learn to discard the schoolboy and schoolgirl cast-iron fixedness of ideas and customs, and to act for themselves more spontaneously. Individuality and resource are much earlier developed in those more free and more natural communities than among us. Hughes says, " Boys follow one another in herds like sheep. They hate thinking, and have rarely any settled principles." I agree with the first part of the sentence but not with the last, for they have the most settled principle of conservatism in the highest degree, and it leads to a universal and everyday practice. This conservatism of the schoolboy and schoolgirl is so strong and so marked that it must have a really beneficent end for the period of life in which it occurs. It punishes severely every departure from tradition, it sets its face against "blabbing" and tale-bearing, it tolerates and says nothing about bullying and cruelty. All this I look on as being the inchoate stage and the precursor of settled principles of action, and the resolute following of what is right, with the equally resolute avoidance of the wrong, which form the strongest element in the mental constitution of the late adolescent and the man of the right sort. It is an outcome of heredity which tends towards certain fixed beliefs and modes of action. Those codes are acted on till the reasoning power and the imagination have fully developed, before their rightness or wrongness, or expediency or their applicability is questioned and reasoned out. Every human being passes through this stage of physiological conservatism twice, the first during boyhood and the second in old age. Both, no doubt, are dependent on certain fixed laws of the development and the retrogression of the human brain. Both serve good purposes in a settled and civilised society.

The next distinctive characteristic of boys and girls, especially boys, is the extraordinary part which a spirit of adventure and romance plays in their lives, affecting their imagination chiefly, but also their conduct. There is no end to the castles in the air which boys and girls build. They play at life—another life than their daily routine of humdrum domesticity and school work —and for the time being this play is as real to them and far more pleasurable than if the events had been real. The fancy is very lively at this period. It cannot quite be called imagination, because imagination is creative. The boy's play-life is always founded on reading or hearing tales of adventure. We know that there is absolutely no limit to a boy's capacity for devouring *Robinson Crusoe*, Ballantyne, and Marryat. Unfortunately, no such classics for our girls exist. Lessons to many boys are simply disagreeable interludes between the times spent in vivid fancies which run riot and give unbounded pleasure. The imaginary adventures are mostly quixotic, foolhardy, and largely ridiculous. No doubt this state of mind is a highly educative one, if it is kept by work and discipline under reasonable control. It lays the foundation of the life, real and ideal, of the future in many cases. Even when the boy proceeds to build real castles in a solitary wood, when he launches his boat and imagines he is sailing to distant and delightful lands, even when he actually runs off to sea, such acts are often the preludes to overcoming practical difficulties in his future life, and to doing real deeds of daring. The schoolgirl's fancies are apt to have a different setting. She thinks herself a queen clad in most gorgeous robes. She imagines herself a lady of title with a splendid castle for a home, and servants innumerable to obey her commands. Lurking through the whole there is nascent wifehood, motherhood, and hero-worship. Her dolls are, in the early part of school-life at least, endowed with life and faculty. They help to materialise many of her fancies. They are her children, they are her companions, and she is seldom without an ideal knight-errant to get her out of difficulties, and to pay her an admiring worship. On this ideal characteristic should be built up at school a practical education for future real motherhood, by teaching the care of children, their needs, their dressing and feeding, their exercise, and play.

The next characteristic of boyhood and girlhood at the school age is a curious combination of frankness and reserve. A thoughtless person might imagine that a boy and girl—especially the girl—kept nothing to themselves; they are so outspoken, so talkative, and often so unconventional in speech. No doubt it is this which gives the impression of freshness in the lives of school children to older people, and makes them really useful and delightful to their elders. Among themselves this frankness is, of course, more marked than when with their seniors, but such frankness has a limit, especially among boys. Touch certain things and they shut up like an oyster. I quite agree with Kipling when he says that the "reserve of a boy is tenfold deeper than the reserve of a maid." This is entirely a natural brain characteristic, not the result of reason, not of the fear of consequences, and not even of being laughed at, although this last has something to do with the reserve of boys and girls. At the back of their minds there are things which are vague and awful, which they do not talk about. Deep religious ideas, certain matters between the sexes, and certain things of high romance and sentiment they will not talk of. When "Stalky and Co." formed a cadet corps, there was mixed up with the drill and the rifles the high ideas of serving their country in heroic ways, and when the fat, oily M.P. came and addressed them in the most commonplace words which instinctively vulgarised their sentiment, and when he at last reached the anti-climax by unfolding the Union Jack, they all felt most uncomfortable, somewhat outraged, and entirely unresponsive. The only charitable explanation that occurred to them was, "Perhaps he was drunk!"

The humour of boyhood and girlhood is peculiar to the period. It takes the form of fun rather than what can be called either wit or humour. It is constantly practised, usually at the expense of their fellows, in the shape of practical jokes or rough, inconsiderate speeches, which would be very cruel in the case of grown-up people. Pleasure and joy in life is longed for in boyhood and girlhood as an absolute necessity. It may, no doubt, be overdone, but to take it away from that period of life would be both a cruelty and a wrong. Joy and pleasure are the best tonics of the period.

The faculty of inhibition, in all its departments, over muscle and over conduct, is at this period of life imperfect and fluid. The moral character is only in the process of making. Conduct is regulated by rules, traditions, and the fear of punishment. How such punishments should be carried out is a difficult matter to say. No general rule, I believe, can be laid down. It depends on the social class, and on the nervous or non-nervous temperament of the boy or girl. If actual punishments causing pain cannot be used—and in nervous children they should not be used to any extent—then there remain the resources of deprivation of indulgences or setting tasks; but surely no more cunning device for making lessons abhorrent was ever devised than connecting them with punishments for ill-doing. For many boys and some girls there can be no doubt that short, sharp application of means which cause temporary but harmless bodily pain, is the best form of punishment. Children are in the evolutionary stage of savage man, and among all savages, and even among Eastern peoples, the stick, the whip, or some form of bodily punishment is universal, and it seems fairly effective for securing order and preventing the smaller

crimes. The quality of the motive must be suited to
the mental capacity of the individual to be acted on.
The end must be attained somehow.

There is one faculty of very different development in
different boys and girls which is of very great importance—
the simple one of learning to use their senses efficiently,
and of registering what those senses tell them. The
faculty of observation, in short, is one in which many
school-children are singularly deficient—most of them,
in fact. It is a faculty which is easily strengthened
in most cases if suitable means are systematically
employed. The development of it usually gives much
pleasure. It comes naturally enough to most of them to
observe what they see or what they hear, and to come
and relate it in definite descriptive words. This is
probably one of the best foundations of all education. The
girl or the boy who has been taught to observe accurately,
and to describe what has been seen or heard or tasted or
smelt, has a great advantage over others who have not
had the faculty of attention and observation thus educated.
It is simply marvellous how many grown people will
contrive not to see a thing, even though it is "before
their eyes," if the faculty of attention has not been
educated in them. This power of observation is the first
thing needed for most successful work. It is not only
good in itself, but by suggestion and association of ideas
it stimulates the intellect and power of reasoning. Its
presence may make all the difference between success and
failure in life, between effectiveness and non-effectiveness
in work.

This is naturally a very social age of life. The boy or
girl who is not social is not healthy. If they have not the
opportunity of mixing with other boys and girls they
readily take to older people, and in that way satisfy the
cravings of their social instincts. How those instincts are

ministered to at this period of life may make all the difference in the life of the future. The moral aphorisms current among all people in all civilised ages about the effects of bad company, " that evil communications corrupt good manners," and that the boy or girl is known by his or her associates, are all perfectly true. The social life of boyhood or girlhood can be so managed in many cases that the affection in that way created, and the good example shown, may almost antagonise " original sin." Wise parents know this well and do all they can in all sorts of skilful ways to carry it out. I used often to say to my friends that our garden was worth £500 a year to our children. In it they received their boy and girl friends— those whom we thought were good companions—and they played to their hearts' content under the very eyes of their mother. We made few inquiries as to how the flowers were trodden down or why the branches of the trees were sometimes broken off. It remains one of my most pleasant memories of life to people the garden with those noisy and happy social child parties. Regulation, not repression, should be the motto with parents and teachers for the social education of boys and girls.

There are certain characteristics of boyhood which are largely evil. Cruelty is one of those. I fear that most boys are more or less cruel and heartless in many ways. The way in which the fags were bullied in the English public schools in old times, the way in which a bad-tempered dog or a frightened cat will be pelted with stones, the real joy of cat and rat-hunting to a boy, the way in which most boys will abuse and strike and call evil names another boy who is soft or rather weak-minded or peculiar in appearance or dress, are all unmistakably of the evil one. The acuteness and the ingenuity that boys and girls exhibit in finding out the weak points of their schoolfellows, and the ruthless way in which those weak points are exposed and irritated is certainly of evil both to the persecutor and the persecuted. Boys' pets are commonly enough treated with much good-humoured kindness, but also with much unconscious cruelty. The hardness of boys' hearts in certain circumstances points to there being at this stage of life an element of unevolved barbarism in them. This tendency to cruelty, to unthinking hurt of the feelings of other boys and girls can undoubtedly be considerably modified by careful teaching, especially by taking as illustrations the hardships and sufferings thus inflicted on fellow-scholars or on animals.

The schoolboy and the schoolgirl should be well fed on a not too stimulating diet, should live very largely indeed in the sunshine and fresh air, should have plenty of open windows in their schools and in their bedrooms, and should have a very large amount of sleep—more than is often given in many homes and schools : ten hours for the age of 8, nine and a half to ten at 14, and I should put down nine and a half hours thereafter as not being too much sleep for the average schoolboy or schoolgirl. Unquestionably the ideal mode of education for both sexes, were all parents wise and firm and intelligent, and had they plenty of time and opportunity to devote to their children's up-bringing, would be home-life with day-school teaching. This at all events for the multitude, but with many exceptions where boarding-school or public school life would be for the best. The "knocking about" which all boys and girls at boarding-schools and public schools have to undergo has two sides to it. If one wants to realise the utter misery which a sensitive and highly intelligent boy may suffer through life at a public school, read the life of the poet Cowper. No one will convince me that the accumulated wisdom which the parents have acquired, and the family ties and amenities of home-life are not one of the best educative influences. I have no

L

doubt whatever that the general intelligence of the educated classes in England has suffered greatly through so
many of its boys and girls having lived a monastic life away
from home for most of their time.   It is always to me
pathetic to consider the way in which the boys at Rugby
were influenced so much for good by Dr. Arnold, when
I think that hundreds of those boys must have had parents
at home almost as wise as Dr. Arnold, quite as good in the
example of their lives and far more interested in them.
Education plus affection exhibited in daily life must surely
be a better thing than education minus affection and minus
intense personal interest.   The widely held assumption of
English parents that their duty has ceased and that of
the schoolmaster begins when their children reach 8 or
9 years of age, seems to me an essentially selfish notion.
It implies an incomplete conception of fatherhood and
motherhood.

The boy or girl during the school life should always be
plump, hard in the muscles, free from headache, cheerful,
and should sleep well.   The average growth from 8 to 15
for a boy should be from 2 to 4 lbs. a year.   A girl should
gain a little less weight during those ages.

Girls are undoubtedly more tender in constitution than
boys at this period.   They tend more to become thin.
They do not eat their food so regularly.   If of a nervous
constitution, they are apt to show some of the tendencies
to nervous diseases which I have mentioned, and they have
not the same strong organic craving for ceaseless exercise
and unlimited appetite which the healthy boy exhibits.   I
refer chiefly to town-bred girls and to daughters of
educated people.   To go into a country village and into a
country school the girls are, as a general rule, at that age
as rosy and robust as the boys, and in their play they are
often as vigorously rough and noisy.   This seems to
show that where the physical conditions and environment

are absolutely good the girls grow and thrive as well as boys during this period of life.

One will very naturally be asked by many parents and by all teachers—What about discipline, restriction, and steady habits of work, punctuality, rule, order, and obedience at this period of life? I am in favour of every one of them as hygienic agents, but not pushed to unnatural and unphysiological degrees. All those should be made into habits of life, and habits of life are not formed at once, but through repeated practice and steady but kindly and tactful pressure. The machinery for the practice of all these is being slowly formed and built up in the brain, and you do not expect such a piece of vital machinery to come out ready-made. It needs forming, fitting, polishing, and the effect of use to make it go properly and to do its work effectively.

I should certainly be asked by most parents and teachers in this country—What about religion? I cannot express too strong an opinion that religious tenet and religious sanction should be taught in the most careful way to the schoolboy. Better still, religious example should be exhibited in daily life by those in association with our scholars. But it should be taught in a way suitable to the apprehension of the brain that receives it. The facts about religion must be taught as other facts are. They will come in by and by in life to very great advantage, but it would be useless to expect that real religious feeling, in the highest sense of the word, can be experienced at the school age. The brain has not then acquired the religious instinct in anything like a full degree. It would really be an unnatural thing to see schoolboys and schoolgirls religious in the largest acceptation of the word. If religious facts and truths are taught, and if they strengthen and give sanction to moral habits, truthfulness, and the simpler virtues of school life, and arouse the feeling of reverence, that is all that can reasonably be expected at this age.

The making of manners, of which I have spoken in treating of child life, must be most assiduously followed during the school period of life. Good manners, as I have said, are not only agreeable to those near and beneficial for those round the scholars, but they react with powerful effect on the moral character and disposition of the boy or girl who practises them. I am strongly of opinion that the teaching of manners should be a part, and a very important part, of school life. Women teachers are naturally better for this part of school work than men. I have often been impressed with the difference of the children's manners in different schools, through care or the want of it in the different teachers. To see a number of schoolgirls in rude health but with good manners is indeed a pleasure. Boys are more difficult to teach in this respect. Naturally imitating the rude behaviour of their fathers, they need extra care and attention in this matter. They are very apt indeed to look on good manners as an index of softness of character and the want of manliness. Their ideals tend towards action and effort rather than to pleasant ways of saying and doing things. No doubt, the further north we go in the British Islands the less cultivation there is of good manners as a bit of life. One ought, perhaps, to except from this the Highlands and the islands of Scotland, where the pure Celtic and Scandinavian tradition is undoubtedly towards politeness.

One great risk of the school age is from over-pressure by hard and unsympathetic teachers striving to acquire personal credit or to earn as large Government grants as possible. If schools are ill-ventilated, stuffy, and either too hot or too cold, over-pressure tells much more against the health of the scholars than if they are sanitary. If the work of the day is ill-regulated with too long spells of attention in one direction and no interludes of play and fresh air with opportunities for the ebullition of high animal spirits and muscular work, the chances of the ill-effects of over-pressure are greater. In *Stalky and Co.* a boy who had been over-pressed was described as having "been hammered till he was nearly an idiot." Any want of orderliness and system in teaching and school work adds greatly to the risk of over-pressure, and forms a very bad training for the scholars.

Backwardness.—There is no practical risk of mental disease during the school age, but it is at that time that "backwardness" is first markedly observed. This means in most cases a badly constituted, unreactive, un-receptive brain, either from heredity or from very bad conditions of childhood, such as insufficient food, bad air, cruel usage, insufficient exercise, or irrational over-pressure. There are certain backward children who will necessarily be backward all their lives on account of the constitution of their brain cells. (See fig. 6, chap. ii. p. 22.) There are others in whom the backwardness is merely postponement in development of faculty. This latter backwardness is often of such a character that it looks like laziness and moral perversity. A few such boys and girls in a school or class are no doubt very trying to the teacher, and often the condition is misunderstood, with the result that great cruelty results from corporal punishments, de-privations, and insulting recrimination. The backward boy or girl suffers greatly also from the unthinking and cruel conduct of fellow-scholars. They are always the butt of the school, and much ingenuity of torture is exercised towards them. The condition does not amount to idiocy or congenital imbecility, but it is often of the same nature. Most really backward children should not be taught in classes with the average scholars, but should be taught apart, and their individual peculiarities studied. In London and some of the larger English cities special schools and special systems of education for backward children have been most properly instituted. Many such children have certain strong points capable of cultivation, with weak receptiveness along most of the line. They often show peculiarities in the form of the head and facial expression, their features not being symmetrical, and their movements awkward and generally lacking beauty and bodily presence. Those defects are now often called by medical writers " stigmata of degeneration." The presence of a degenerative process during development, leading to a large amount of bad stock in any people, is of enormous importance. It is attracting much attention nowadays, and has been the subject of two Royal Commissions.

Games.—The great risk of a want of proper system of games, gymnastics, and physical training during school life is that the scholars suffer in speech, in writing, and in the muscular exercise of the legs, arms, and body, and that the great process of co-ordination between mind and muscle of which I have spoken is not properly carried out. The consequences are a permanent lack of such co-ordination, with its results of awkwardness in gesture and manners, inharmonious, unpleasant speech, bad handwriting, and coarse needlework. " Handiness " if not developed at this period is very difficult to attain afterwards. The effect on the face and eye is that of a want of muscular sympathy and often positive ugliness. To attain anything like the physiological ideal of beauty and muscular harmony there must be constant and co-ordinate practice of the " mental muscles " of the face and eye during this period of life. There is great difference of opinion between the two schools of heredity as to whether such defects and marks of degeneration are transmissible hereditarily to future generations or whether they are simply confined to the generation that exhibits them. The school of heredity which asserts that acquired peculiarities are transmissible to posterity naturally fears that the race will suffer from the effects of such defective training during the school age. The school which asserts that no acquired peculiarities can or will be transmitted as naturally says that the next generation will be all right if proper training is applied to its individual members at the proper time. No doubt both doctrines are applicable to the awkwardnesses of the school age. In some cases they are undoubtedly hereditary, while in other cases they are as certainly " acquired " through want of proper training at the proper time.

Beer.—There exists a practice in many of the great English public schools and also in many homes even of our better-off classes to give beer as a part of the diet of schoolboys. This arose when beer was more universal as an article of ordinary diet than it is now, and before the effects of alcohol on the brain had been scientifically studied. I unhesitatingly condemn this practice out and out as being bad for the growing brain at this period and attended by many future dangers. Beer is not really a food in any proper sense, and it is certainly an unsuitable stimulant for this stage of life. It creates a taste for stronger liquors too. Tobacco, in the shape of cigarette smoking, is bad enough, but it is usually done surreptitiously, and not among the respectable classes encouraged. In many American States there is a law against smoking before 16 or 17. I would say there is more need for a law against alcohol in any form before that age. It shows how little the universal opinion of the medical profession, who know most about it, is able to overcome the old and bad traditions, that any school could give beer as a part of a dietary for boys at the beginning of the twentieth century. I do not believe in too much stimulating animal food for this period of life. I would give every boy and girl at least one glass of new milk every day, in addition to the ordinary meals. To many of them I would give two or three glasses. Milk is the article I should be inclined to give *ad libitum*. If fruit were attainable I should say the same about it. While my own children were growing up there was a dish of oranges and apples always on the sideboard, and no questions asked as to their consumption.

I have spoken of sleep in childhood and its importance (p. 131). During the school age it is almost, but not perhaps quite, of the same consequence. There are, of course, individual peculiarities and idiosyncrasies, where the time—$9\frac{1}{2}$ hours—I have recommended is too much or too little ; but that should be the average. We should have less weediness of growth, less nervousness, less tendency to hysteria and insanity in future life if this rule were followed.[1]

Diseases and Deficiencies of this Period.—The nervous diseases and deficiencies of this period of life almost all affect the co-ordinating power of mind and muscle. St. Vitus' Dance, epilepsy, asthma, sleep-walking, and several forms of squint and eye disease are apt to appear then. In idiocy the speech centres are incapable of development, and so speech is absent and cannot be cultivated. In the congenitally weak-minded and among backward and feeble-minded children speech defects and general co-ordination defects are very marked. In such persons the mind cells and the motor cells are defective, while the strands of

---

[1] In regard to the general health of our great public schools, I cannot do better than to recommend a perusal of Dr. Dukes' exhaustive treatise on *Health at School*, where the details of that momentous subject are entered minutely into. No parent can read it without profit and instruction.

fibres connecting the two are too few in number, so that a clear, pleasant speech and proper intonation cannot be acquired, while the writing is unformed, the movements of the body are awkward, the gestures are grotesque, and the face and eye muscles do not express properly mind and feeling.   There is often found a postponement of development of the co-ordinating faculties.   We see some schoolboys and girls who are poor in speech and awkward in movement and expressionless in face up to 10 or 11 or 12, and then there comes a sudden rush of development of those capacities, so that by 15 or 16 they have acquired them to almost a normal extent.

CHAPTER XII

ADOLESCENCE, BETWEEN 15 AND 25

THE period of life of which I am now to treat is the most important in life in its relation to the hygiene of mind. When one considers the enormous differences in the brain and mental life of the same human being in the different periods of life, it does not seem wonderful that each should need somewhat different principles and practice of Mental Hygiene. It would be very wonderful indeed, and somewhat incredible, if the brain and mind of a child of which we have spoken, whose chief characteristics are active growth, intense imitativeness in all directions, great inquisitiveness, quick, uncontrolled, unthinking response to stimuli, and marked immatureness in all its functions—if this period of life were subject to the same hygienic rules as that of the adolescent, after sex has asserted itself and manhood or womanhood is nearly reached. The prevailing activities of the two periods are entirely different; the one is chiefly trophic or nutritive, and the other is dynamical and developmental. Up to puberty there had been vast tracts of brain tissue which had never been put into active use at all. They had merely been undergoing the process of preparation for use. The enormous new development of the affective faculties, the new ideas dependent on those, the new interests in life, the new desires and organic cravings rising into a different and far higher region of imaginative and æsthetic life, all show that a fresh chapter in brain and mind life has been opened. With this new normal development of a higher life comes a special liability to previous kinds of abnormality in brain and mind, abnormality that may extend in character from a slight eccentricity up to an acute attack of mental derangement. There is, of course, no absolutely fixed line or short period marking the two eras of school life and adolescence. No exact age can be fixed, but for practical purposes we may say that the school age mind ends at 15 and that the adolescent period extends from 15 to 25. There is, naturally, much in common between the end of the school age and the first years of adolescence. The similarity of general mental lines between individuals of the same and of opposite sexes which characterises childhood and the early school ages now diminishes. Real sex differences of form and mind rapidly develop themselves. Those are accompanied by differences in every set of muscles, in every bone, in every internal organ and especially in the brain and its higher functions. In the man, after that time, the development is more in the direction of energising, thinking, discovering, ruling and ambition, while in the woman the direction is towards feeling, altruism, the protective instincts, sympathising, nursing, mothering, gaining approbation, and accentuation of the religious instincts. Looking to the brain itself, it scarcely gains at all in weight and bulk during the adolescent period, but in function it transforms itself from a lower to a higher plane in an extraordinary degree. It is during this period that the brain first exhibits some of its strongest hereditary tendencies. While such mental factors in human life as conduct and character are being consolidated, as they now are, it is no wonder that hereditary qualities for good or evil in different persons make all the difference between success and failure in life, even when the conditions and the environment are the same. It is then more especially that a man or a woman has to yield to the " tyranny of organisation," and but for Nature's two tendencies of which I have spoken, that of reproducing the normal and the favourable—in short, of natural selection—being then in most men and women stronger than that of killing off the unfit, humanity would have a poor time of it in after-life and in future times. Several authors, applying the ideas and facts of human adolescence to the history of the race, have described the Greek period as being the adolescence of mankind. The subject is now attracting enormous attention by psychologists and students of human nature. Stanley Hall has recently written two exhaustive volumes on the study of adolescence in all its relations. During adolescence in the woman the developmental process is still more important than in the man, for she then has to acquire the strength and other qualifications to reproduce the race. Hygiene is therefore of even greater importance to her than to the man. In the educated classes the higher sort of education only begins at adolescence, and goes on during the greater part of its duration. The principles and practice of such education are all-important to the woman's life. The doctors and the physiologists generally have not been satisfied with the principles on which the modern, higher education of young women has been conducted. They complain that hygiene, physical and mental, has not been the dominant note that it should have been. They feel that in their position as the priests of the body and the special guardians of the physical and mental qualities of the race, they are bound to oppose strenuously every kind and mode of education that in any way lessens the capability of women for healthy maternity and for the production of future generations of men and women, strong, mentally and physically. To think for a moment of Nature carrying out her process of the slow evolution of life from the lower ever to the higher, and that up to this point she has advanced, through a stringent natural selection and the elimination of the unfit in all ages, until she has reached modern woman, the goddess, the ideal of beauty, the highest source and embodiment of happiness—to think of this is firmly to resolve that neither the schoolmaster nor any one else must be allowed to upset Nature's ends and counteract her designs. I have already referred to the fact that Nature only produces her energies in strictly limited quantities, and that through the solidarity of the brain and of the whole organism, you cannot overpress or develop one organ or function without the risk of stealing energy from other organs and functions. If we set out at the beginning of adolescence to make every woman a Senior Wrangler and every man a Hercules, we stand a very good chance of turning out poor mothers and fools. I am not setting health and motherhood as being opposed to the higher intellectual pursuits if they are rightly gone about, and I am not arguing that such pursuits are necessarily incompatible with the higher principles of mental and physical hygiene. My thesis is not " Health and Ignorance " unconditionally. I am merely endeavouring to follow Nature in distinguishing between what is primary and essential to the race from what is, on the whole, not primary and non-essential. I would not say a word against the " higher education " of women if it is consistent with health of body, brain, and mind. I would merely emphasise the fact that this higher education has often been carried on at the peril of losing something higher still. It must be made compatible with the motherhood of the race. Woman's eager nature and greater conscientiousness during adolescence lead her on to take too much out of herself when she is being educated at many of our higher schools and at our universities. At that age she is not apt to realise her highest mission in life. The game seems so fascinating that the losses are not counted. Physiological hygiene and common sense have stepped in lately with much effect in diminishing cramming, over-pressure, competitive examinations, and overtime work in our higher schools for girls, and it was not too soon. If the American educational ideals of 40 years ago had been carried out, there would have been needed, for the continuance of the race in that country, an incursion into lands where educational theories were unknown and where another rape of the Sabines was possible. American physicians used to say that there were some schools in Boston that turned out young ladies so highly educated that every spare atom of their fat was consumed by the brain cells that subserve the functions of Mind. They told us that when those young women did marry they seldom had more than one or two children, that the primary curse of child-bearing was apt to be very hard on them and that they could not nurse their offspring from their own breasts. The energy that was needed for the race had been used up for the individual.

Looked at from a mental point of view, it can scarcely be denied by any one that the later years of adolescence from 18 to 25 are far more important than the first from 15 to 18. For years after puberty there is still much of the boy and girl mind. For this reason I find it difficult to give a description that will fit both periods. The girl at this time grows faster than the boy, both in body and in mind ; and while I have taken 25 as being a reasonable average for the end of the period in both sexes, there is no doubt that many women attain full maturity in mind and body a year or two before that age. The mental change that takes place from 18 to 25 refers to higher functions and, I think, is more interesting psychologically than that which occurs between 15 and 18. It is at this later period of adolescence that, for the man, life first begins to look serious, both from the emotional side and in action. It is only then that childish things are really put away. For the first time literature, in its higher sense, is fully appreciated. Poetry now becomes a passion—at least certain kinds of poetry. The very highest kind of all literature, however, is reserved for the manhood period after the completion of adolescence. The kind of novel that is enjoyed is always a good test of the mental and emotional development. The boy, as we have seen, enjoys Ballantyne, *Robinson Crusoe*, and Marryat ; the early adolescent takes to Scott and Dickens ; and later adolescents appreciate Tennyson and George Eliot ; while for the fully grown man Shakespeare, Thackeray, and the Bible are the most fitting mental nourishment. Go into a university and watch the demeanour of the first and fifth year's men. There seems to be a great gulf fixed between them. The fifth year's man treats his junior not as a mere boy, but as a different and inferior species. Watch the two in the presence of the opposite sex. In the one case you see mere shyness that soon breaks out into rollicking fun. In the other there is real sexual egoism, that most painful pleasure which consists of the half-conscious feeling that every person of the one sex is an object of the most intense interest to every person of the opposite sex of the same age. The events and possibilities of the future are reflected in vague and dreamlike emotions and longings. They have much pleasure in them, but not a little, too, of seriousness and difficulty as adolescence advances. The man feels instinctively that he has now entered a new country, the face of which he does not know, but yet that is full of the possibility of happiness to him. He has a craving for action. Ambition stirs him down to the innermost recesses of his nature, bringing out all his powers of body and mind. Longfellow's youth who vaguely cried "Excelsior!" was evidently at this stage of life. The reasoning faculty first gets full backbone at this period. The emotional nature instinctively shows a leaning towards the other sex that may quite swallow up all other emotions. Love between the sexes towards the end of adolescence is the intensest and the most unreasoning of human passions. The sense of right and wrong and of duty becomes an active principle, dominating the conduct. "Character" in the full sense is then crystallised. There are yearnings after an ideal and an intense scorn and hatred of evil. The purposes of life are then shaped. The impressions and the resolutions then formed affect the tenor of a man's or a woman's life, as a general rule, more than at any other age.

As Meredith puts it, "At the period when the young savage grows into higher influences the faculty of worship is foremost in him. At this period Jesuits will stamp the future of their changeling flocks : and all who bring up youth by a system and watch it know that it is the malleable moment." A little further on the same acute student of human nature describes another phase in his hero, Richard Feveril : "Richard gave up his companions, servile or antagonistic ; he relinquished the material world to young Ralph and retired into himself, where he was going to be lord of kingdoms : where Beauty was his handmaid, and History his minister, and Time his ancient harper, and sweet Romance his bride, where he walked in a realm vaster and more gorgeous than the great Orient peopled with the heroes that have been."

Thackeray, in *Pendennis*, draws with a master hand the different psychological eras of the adolescent and the phases of emotion and intellect that follow each other in due order as do the leaf and flower and fruit.

It is in the female sex that the period of adolescence has attracted most attention, especially among those most acute psychological students and delineators of character, the better novelists of the day. Art in its higher form has devoted itself to the depiction of the beauty of complete adolescence. No artist ever painted and no sculptor ever modelled a Venus before that time of life. Before that the love-making, the engagements to marry, and the broken hearts of women are not apt to be very serious affairs. At, and soon after that time, they become the cataclysms of a woman's life. Two pictures of adolescence have appeared in our recent literature, one of normal adolescence and the other of a pathological variety. The one is to be found in the " Gwendolen Harleth " of George Eliot's novel of *Daniel Deronda,* the other is " Lady Kitty " of Mrs. Humphry Ward's *Marriage of William Ashe.* Both rank among the acute and subtle studies of human nature. Looking first at Gwendolen Harleth, we see "she was powerfully swayed in feeling and action by the presence of a person of the opposite sex whom she had never seen before. She played, not because she liked it or wished to win, but because he was looking on." The subjective egoism tending towards objective dualism, the resolute action from pure instinct, the setting at defiance of calculation and reason, the want of any definite desire to marry, while all her conduct tended towards proposals, the selfishness as regards her relations, even her mother, and the intense craving to be admired, form a vivid picture of the mentality of adolescence. Witness her state of mind when Grandcourt first appears. "When he did arrive no consciousness was more acute to the fact than hers, although she steadily avoided looking towards any point where he was likely to be. There should be not the slightest shifting of angles to betray that it was of any consequence to her whether 'the much-talked-of Mr. Mallinger Grandcourt' presented himself or not, and all the while the certainty that he was there made a distinct

M

thread in her consciousness." The knowledge that comes "by instinct" to a young woman is thus described : "Gwendolen knew certain differences in the characters with which she was concerned, as birds know climate and weather." The sentimentality of this period of life is well illustrated when Gwendolen says, "I never saw a married woman who had her own way." "What should you like to do ?" said Rex, quite guilelessly and in real anxiety—he was an adolescent, early in the period. "Oh, I don't know—go to the North Pole or ride steeplechases or go to be a Queen in the East like Lady Hester Stanhope," said Gwendolen lightly. "You don't mean you would never be married ?" "No, I didn't say that. Only when I marry I should not do as other women do." The strong religious instinct contending with the egoism is thus brought out : "What she knowingly recognised and would have been glad for others to have been unaware of was that liability of hers to spiritual dread. Solitude in any wide sense impressed her with an undefined feeling of immeasurable existence aloof from her, in the midst of which she was helplessly incapable of asserting herself." The selfishness and craving for notice of the period is thus hit off : "I like to differ from everybody ; I think it is stupid to agree." She meant to do what was pleasant to herself in a striking manner, or rather whatever she could do so as to strike others with admiration, and get in that way a more ardent sense of living, more pleasant to her fancy.

Mrs. Humphry Ward's "Lady Kitty" forms a far less pleasant but to a doctor a still more interesting picture. She had a bad heredity, a bad example in her mother, and a bad boarding-school life in France. She was intense, brilliant, artistic, and dramatic in the highest degree, and her social talents were overmastering to every one on whom she exercised them. She fascinated and completely dominated one of the coolest-headed and typical of Englishmen, and when he married her she treated him in the most cruel and abominable way. As she truly described herself, "Of course I'm a vixen!" But as thought of by her friend the charitable and impressionable old Dean, "What a radiant and ethereal beauty!" "When the evil spirit was out of her she was all ethereal tenderness, sadness, and remorse. In this state she was one of the most exquisite of human beings, with words, tone, and gestures of a heavenly softness and languor." She allowed herself to be fascinated by another man than her husband, because he was adventurous, unprincipled, and poetic. Even her maternal affection for her partially idiotic, paralysed boy—a true hereditary example of a son of such a mother and an example of Nature's law of bringing a bad stock to an end—was spasmodic and unreliable. To be noticed, to be admired, to be talked about, to excite scandal, to punish her rivals and enemies was the breath of her life. No good principle really influenced her for long ; no religious feeling restrained her, and no fear of consequences prevented her from doing the most dastardly act that any wife could do to a most devoted husband. Yet after her fall "she is consumed with remorse night and day." The whole picture is perfectly true, but is that of a pathological mind. "Lady Kitty's" brain was constituted differently from that of the healthy adolescent girl. She was the victim of her heredity, her training, and her organisation. Few people have the wisdom to say in excuse for such a woman, as her mother-in-law did to her husband, "We will remember her bringing-up and her inheritance." Brought up under a better system of mental and moral hygiene, she would, no doubt, have been less interesting, but she need not have made such a wreck of her life.

In history and fiction few women have taken to the

higher learning with avidity during their adolescence. Shakespeare's women are certainly not of the learned kind, though learned women abounded in his time. Their youthful years were not taken up in getting book-learning exclusively. Their emotional nature was not dried up by the strain of intellectual work in youth. Their constitutions were not then spoiled by study. They had fair faces and womanly forms and warm affections and mother wit and keen discernment and vigorous reasoning, but nothing that we would call learning in one of them. Portia, who acted the most learned part of all Shakespeare's women, vehemently described herself as

"An unlessoned girl, unschooled, unpractised."

One of the strangest things in recent literature is this— that our most learned and most philosophical novelist of the nineteenth century, George Eliot, in all her host of female characters, never created a really learned woman like herself. Dorothea in *Middlemarch* had all the makings of the successful omnivorous young women students of the present day, intellectual, hyper-conscientious—as such young women so often are to their cost. " Her mind was theoretic and yearned after some lofty conception of the world. She was enamoured of intensity and greatness." She was self-sacrificing to a fault, she was open, ardent and not in the least self-admiring ; yet Dorothea was not highly educated in the modern sense. Perhaps a modern educationalist would say that this was the reason why poor Dorothea made such a mess of it and threw herself away, first, on a selfish, shallow old pedant whom she took for a great scholar, and then on the least interesting fellow in the book. Romola was in a sense a learned woman, brought up in the midst of books and in the atmosphere of culture, yet she took to love-making, marriage, self-denial, charity and religion, and discarded her books the moment her duty in them was done. She had no innate love of book-learning. She found no guide in it in her difficulties. It was no solace to her in disappointment. It was no resource when everything else had failed. It had not taken hold of her nature because it was not on the great lines on which her nature was built up. She and her father were as much alike as a man and a woman could be, yet to him his books were a perpetual joy all his life, to her their study had been a self-denial all through. We all know what Thackeray's women were—shallow, affectionate, and domestic, and little more, except when he created Becky Sharp, the worst woman in nineteenth century fiction. But whatever young woman is or is not, she has the power to fascinate young men. Hamlet and Ophelia, Adam Bede and Hetty, Lydgate and Rosamund, Deronda and Gwendolen, Romeo and Juliet—it is all the same story. But it may be said all this was wrong, the result of yielding to unlearned Nature's lowest affinities, and that many of those matches turned out badly both for the men and the women. If they had mated suitably, the world would have been better and they themselves happier. The physiologist and the modern psychologist will not rashly preach that Nature's affinities are wrong any more than they believe that the appetite is not on the whole the best guide as to the kind and amount of food that is good for us. When they find in Nature a marked masculine and feminine type of body and of mind, those types diverging strongly during the era of adolescence, each type with a different ideal, they conclude that the same type of education should not prevail for both sexes in this momentous era. This deduction seems to be backed up by natural fact, by the opinion of men of genius and by the evidence of history.

Many bodily changes take place during adolescence.

In the man the type is towards the Apollo, in the woman towards the Venus. The tastes for food and drink often change. Bread and butter and sweets no longer satisfy. Stronger and more stimulating foods are craved for. The carriage and walk change. For a man, football, tennis, cricket, and active exercise become a necessity. For a woman such exercises are less insistent. In both sexes sleep should be sound and long, fresh air should be craved for, and the craving should be abundantly satisfied.

We physicians find that the whole period is one of momentous importance for the health and happiness of the future life. The risks to body and mind are then, in many cases, very great indeed. We count it a fearful risk to run, not merely that actual disease should be brought on, but that a girl, capable of being developed into a healthy, useful, good and happy woman, if Nature's laws are obeyed, should, by unhygienic conditions or mis-directed education, grow into a maimed, distorted, bad, and therefore unhappy, woman, who cannot get out of the life she has only to live once all that it is capable of yielding to her. If the process of development is seriously interfered with or not completed rightly it is missed for life. Whatever is done then is final. Whatever is left undone is for good and all. If a woman is not well formed at 25, the chances are she will never be so. If she is not healthy then, there is a risk she will not attain perfect health afterwards. No acquirements, no knowledge, no intellectual pleasure can possibly make up for health in her after-life. There is an organic happiness that goes only with the harmoniously constituted body and mind ; without that organic happiness life is scarcely worth living. Cheerfulness is one of the best outward signs of this health, and what man, especially what woman, has not missed her vocation in the world who is not cheerful? There is no time or place of organic repent-

ance provided by Nature for some of the sins of the
parent and the schoolmaster. What is the use of
culture if it is to end with the present generation? The
actual list of bodily and mental distortions, defects, and
diseases that may arise during adolescence is manifold.
There may be mere arrest of growth and deficient nourishment of the body. The man or the woman, in this case,
is stunted and thin for life. Nature may develop on lines
away from her ideals. Instead of beauty there may be
ugliness. instead of harmony and grace of movement there
may be awkwardness, instead of staying power, brain and
muscle may be too easily pumped out. The digestion may
not work well, and who that has read Carlyle's description
of his own tortures will think lightly of indigestion? It
almost always affects the mental condition and the cheerfulness. There may be a sort of physiological laziness and
lassitude, in which exertion, bodily or mental, is not merely
not a pleasure, but a distress. There may arise actual
disease, such as epilepsy, asthma, anæmia, hysteria, neuralgia, nervous exhaustion, sick headaches, neurasthenia,
and other ills to which this time of life may become heir,
if the heredity to evil has been strong or Nature's laws
have been broken and hygienic rules of life set aside.
Mental and moral conditions, also, of the adolescent with
a bad heredity and unfavourably conditioned, may depart
from the normal, the higher brain function of mind only
being then affected, leaving the body apparently " healthy."
Bad temper and foolish, impulsive action, craving for
drink and stimulating drugs, perversion of the moral sense
and volition, perverted instincts, unfounded aversion to
relatives, deficient or changed social instincts, are all seen
during this period. Dissipation in every form may be
yielded to, coming in bursts like a disease. Family unhappiness of all sorts naturally follows such adolescent
mental changes.

The most grievous of all diseases—that of mental disorder—may, and often does, occur towards the end of the adolescent period. The transitory periods of depression to which I have alluded seem to have been very common indeed at this period of the life of many men of genius. Such appear in the biographies of Goethe, Carlyle, Cowper, Thackeray, Tennyson, and very many others ; even such men of philosophic type of mind as Hume and J. Stuart Mill being so affected. Suicide was often contemplated at the very time when those men should have been fullest of life. Carlyle's most vivid description of his own feelings, when he suffered from " Stygian darkness, spectre haunted," can never be forgotten by any one who has read it and knows its meaning. I would impress on physicians and the public that this is indeed a "critical" period of life. In other cases the mental disturbance takes the form of periodically recurring attacks of elevation of mind, unsettledness, and excitement, rather than of depression. I have called those types of mental disorder "Adolescent Insanity." Frequently the more serious of those bodily and mental disturbances are preceded by lesser ailments, which may be the danger-signals of more severe disturbances coming on, if they are not attended to. Such danger-signals often appear as headaches, sleeplessness, falling off in flesh, " queer " and uncomfortable sensations in the head, irritability or general feeling of " not being up to the mark."

There is a fact of importance that should be taken notice of in any book on Mental Hygiene. It is this—that you may use up by an undue pressure at one time of life the energy that ought to have been spread out over long periods. This is especially the case in adolescence. Through such over-exertion in study or games, too heavy a drain is made on futurity, and such persons wear out early or grow old too soon. There is another consideration which I believe to be important. One generation may, by living at high pressure, and thereby disregarding hygienic laws, exhaust and use up more than its share of the ancestral energy transmitted to it. It may draw a bill on posterity and not hand on to the next generation enough to pay it. I believe many of us are now having the benefit of the calm, lazy lives of our forefathers of past generations who stored up energy for us. We, in this too strenuous generation, are using it up. It has often happened in the history of the world, that families who for generations have exhibited no special qualities, blaze out into bursts of greatness for a time and then die out—like the two Pitts and Gladstone. This is seen among peoples as well as in families. The Mongols under Genghis Khan, the Turks when they overpowered the south-east of Europe, the Arabs when they conquered Spain, and the Spaniards when they overran America, all seem to be examples of this law. How often do we see a quiet country family, the members of which for generations have led quiet, humdrum lives, suddenly produce one or two great men and then relapse into obscurity again.

Lesser Mental and Moral Changes and Perversities of Adolescence.—The lesser mental and moral changes and perversities to which adolescents of both sexes are subject are specially worthy of attention, because they are so often neglected, so often misconstrued, and therefore no proper efforts are made to counteract them. The subjects of such changes have usually more or less hereditary tendency towards nervousness. They come of nervous families or of stocks in which drunkenness, eccentricity, genius, or insanity have appeared. The most common and, in my judgment, the most important mental change is that of a tendency towards depression of mind. It may consist simply of low spirits at times, especially in the mornings, and pessimistic views of life, which are quite unnatural for

that period of life.   Often the subjects of this depression
are troubled with headaches and have neuralgic tendencies.
The sleep is often neither so long nor so sound as it should
be.   The mental depression of which I am speaking is
really more or less marked mental pain.   It is strictly
equivalent to neuralgic bodily pain, so far as the functions
of the brain are concerned.   It is apt to be periodic in its
occurrence.   The sufferers from it are usually too thin.
They often have peculiarities in regard to food, not being
able to take certain things that would be very good for
them, such as milk and fatty foods.   Study or work of any
kind cannot be properly engaged in while the depression
lasts.   Work is no longer a pleasure, as it should be.
The social instincts are diminished.   Friends are not so
welcome.   Games are not gone at with zest.   The eye, the
countenance, and the walking often show a lack of nerve
and muscular energy.   The appetite and the digestion are
not so good while the condition lasts.   What should be
realised about this is, that although it may be slight,
although the sufferers may be able to pull themselves together with an effort, yet it is unnatural—it is first cousin
to actual disease.   In many cases it may be helped greatly
by proper tonics, medical measures, rest, changes of scene
and air and other means.   In other cases there is a
lethargy or stupidity, so that the young woman or lad
ceases to care for, or to show intelligent curiosity in anything.   There is no actual mental pain or depression.   In
other cases it takes the form of an a-social condition at
this, which should be one of the most social of all ages.
The social instincts seem, for the time being, to be almost
paralysed.   In other cases there are causeless changes
in the emotional nature.   There is a felt aversion to, or
suspicion of, father, mother, sister, brother or friends, for
which no reasonable cause can be assigned.   There may
be an entire disregard of the feelings of relations.   In other

cases, again, there is a general "incompatibility" of temper developed, irritability in social intercourse, so that the sufferer "gets on" with no one, is cantankerous and suspicious, even quarrelling with friends, and making enemies everywhere. Or, again, the adolescent period may be invaded by impracticable and foolish scheming, projects wanting in common sense being continually hatched. Stupid plans are formed and odd purposes carried out, which astonish friends, who remark, "I did not think So-and-so was such a fool." Occasionally, again, a frothy, sentimental sort of religionism develops. It is usually emotional, often of the aggressive, uncharitable —"I'm a good man ; you're of the devil" type, and is unassociated with doing the plain, homely duties of life in a routine, satisfactory way. Occasionally the moral sense is invaded and the self-control lost, so that we have sudden immoralities contrary to the tenor of the former life. Perverted trains of thought seem to seize hold of the mind and affect the conduct. Such changes often cause great misery in families. Their real nature is commonly misunderstood and their kinship to actual disease is not often suspected. The subjects of them are blamed and scolded instead of being medically treated. As illustrations of those conditions, I once saw a young man, about the end of the adolescent period, whose mother had been nervous and his father healthy. He was of average ability, he led a fairly good life, but he began to leave his work for days without any reason except that he said he could not possibly go on with it. Then he began to stay in bed half the day and did little or nothing the other half. Such "laziness" had not been his habit previously. Spells of it came on periodically. He could talk quite rationally, and he sometimes bewailed his condition. Outward pressure on him to do work when in this state simply caused pain and irritation. He would take two hours to his bath and dressing. He could not sit down to a meal regularly. His bodily health and condition were not satisfactory. He always felt better in the fresh air, and through sending him to the country, where he lived an outdoor life, and had a good deal of exercise, plenty of milk with nerve tonics, he came round in about a year or so and resumed his ordinary healthy condition. I knew a young lady who, up to 14, had been as ordinary children, but who since that age had been the despair of her teachers and the distress of her mother. Quite clever, intelligent, and not given to gross vice of any sort, she had exhausted all the arts by which disobedience, lying, perversity of every kind and outrageous unconventionality of dress and conduct could break her parents' hearts. She seemed to be without affection, except towards tramps, animals, and oddities. She always professed sympathy with the bad, the low, and the unfortunate. Respectability was an unpardonable offence to her. She was most ingenious in her ways of shocking her parents and her friends by her words and actions. Yet she was well read, she could pass muster amongst strangers as a clever, interesting, and original girl. She at last married a robust but respectable clodhopper, entirely out of her social sphere. She had children, and became a happy and careful mother and a frugal farmer's wife, but she never regained her affection for her parents or her relations. She was an example of "reversion" to a lower type.

Occasionally such changes as I have described take the form of a craving for drink or drugs. Their effects are intensely pleasant to such persons whose inhibition is weak. It is a curious fact, not well known, that almost all the most hopeless drunkards, those called "dipsomaniacs," begin their excesses in the adolescent period of life. This uncontrollable craving for drink is often seen in members of nervous families. No higher motive will arrest it. Honour, truthfulness, and self-respect are lost. Taken altogether, such cases are very incurable. At present the law gives us no means of dealing with them by early restriction and treatment, as we can with disease. As showing that this period of life has to do with the condition, and that it is of the nature of disease, the cases that recover usually do so between 25 and 30. There are other persons who at this time of life take to lying, and do all kinds of criminal acts, some going even the length of murder. Criminal statistics show that most first convictions of crime are between the ages of 16 and 21. I long ago described this "adolescent criminality" as one phase of the nervous liabilities of this period of life.

CHAPTER XIII

ADOLESCENCE (*continued*)

Hygienic and Preventive Facts and Measures.—I would begin my remarks about prevention and direct hygienic measures in adolescence by saying that there are many individual men, such as I have described, in whom the evil states of body and mind are inevitable and from the beginning quite incurable. Nature has thus set her seal on them as being of the "unfit." Such are all the idiots and congenitally feeble-minded, most of the epileptics, many of the adolescent insane, and a certain proportion of the lesser mental distortions. In many of those classes their brains pass rapidly into a condition which renders them a burden to society and a care and responsibility to their relations. Such have always a strong nervous or insane heredity. A fate is thus laid on a man or a family against which there is no striving. But taking a large view of the subject, we see that while there are degrees of taint in all such cases, our first duty is to try and estimate its strength. It may be an irresistible force, or it may be a very minor tendency which can be counteracted and its effects overcome. The greatest problem of life is being solved during adolescence. The mind and brain are striving after perfection, and heredity is undoubtedly the most important factor that affects those subtle developmental processes. The first thing a rational parent, a wise doctor, and a reasonable advanced adolescent himself should do, is to look the question of heredity fair in the face and try to find out all the facts about it. It should never be forgotten that there is a good heredity as well as a bad, and that even when a bad heredity exists in some department of brain or mind, there may be good heredity in other respects which may largely counteract the bad. In spite of Galton's brave and scientific effort to make every family of education keep accurate family histories as to its bodily and mental qualities, his far-seeing advice has not been taken to any extent. A scientific sociology would dictate that hereditary defects, mental diseases, and nervous defects should be intimated and registered as infectious diseases now are. That may come some day, but meantime some reliable and useful information can usually be got in regard to the history of most families, if trouble is taken. Truthfulness is seldom practised in admitting facts about bad heredity, or mental diseases, or defects. We have to inquire as to the history during life and the causes of death of the grandparents, the parents, the uncles and aunts and cousins. If we could go further back still, it might be useful in some cases, for there is a curious law of "atavism," through which peculiarities, mental and bodily, good and bad, prevailing in progenitors, may pass over a generation or two and appear in grandchildren and great-grandchildren. For instance, I lately ascertained in regard to one of my patients that there were several other cousins and second cousins insane. The family came from a secluded district, and I had the help of a very intelligent and interested relative in ascertaining the facts as to the family history. I found that for three previous generations there was an absolutely clean bill of health, as regards the graver nervous diseases, in all but one slightly eccentric weak-minded grand-uncle, who did not marry. But in the

great-great-grandfather's family there had been several
cases of suicidal melancholia, which was the disease the
insane great-great-grandchildren suffered from.   Here was
a stream which had been replenished by four new streams
through marriage.   The patients affected had received a
special tendency to mental disease, which had lain
dormant, as a mere potentiality, but yet had been exis-
tent as a something, and had been transmitted by three
generations of nervously sound people.   Even the scientific
imagination fails to grasp in any definite way what such a
series of facts really means.   The only explanation that at
first occurred to me was that the environment and circumstances of my patient had changed from that of her
country Highland ancestry.   She had had no trials or
special difficulties, but she had become a city woman.
The weak point, however, of this explanation of mine
is, that her cousins who had also become insane had been
subjected to no such change of environment.   We must
probably assume that there are but few, if any, absolutely
healthy families, each member with the *corpus sanum in
corpore sano*, and no one of them with any tendency
whatsoever towards any hereditary disease.   I would
impress on every one who consults a doctor on such a
matter, first honestly and thoroughly to inquire into the
heredity of the patient and thus to bring the facts
candidly under the doctor's notice.   There is a strong
human nature tendency to do otherwise and to minimise
the facts, or to shut one's eyes, or to deny them.   The
same rule should apply to the preliminary inquiries when
marriages are thought about.   It is a crime then to conceal
bad heredity, which I have often seen lead to much unhappiness and recrimination, and to the avoidable pro-
pagation of a bad human stock.   As yet there is little
" health-conscience " among mankind in this matter.
   A very striking fact it is, that we all, as living organisms,

may thus carry within us tendencies, instead of actual observable features, mere potentialities, instead of facts. There is much need to find out about those ancestors and connections of ours, whether by temperament they were nervous or phlegmatic, what sort of dispositions they had, whether they were moral or immoral, drunken or sober, whether they were unstable or wanting in balance, or solid and reliable, whether clever or stupid, whether they were explosive in mental or nervous action, whether they were steady-going and unexcitable, and whether they had or had not an average control in speech and action. We have to ask what diseases they suffered from? whether any of them had had asthma, sick headaches, convulsions, epilepsy or neuralgia? how far mental disorder had prevailed among them? We must ask about their tendencies to consumption and rheumatism and gout, whether many of the children had been liable to die early in life, or whether longevity had been generally prevalent? There is a fact in disease which must be kept in mind in making such inquiries, that there exists an interchangeability between different diseases in different generations. A gouty father may have a melancholic son; an insane father may have children subject to neurasthenia, to epilepsy, or to become tubercular.

We must next look, with the help of such skilled advice as we can get, at the conformation of the body and of the head of the adolescent, at his upper palate to see if it is round arched, or Gothic in shape, at his nutrition and at the way the bodily functions are performed. We must ask how the instincts, the appetites, and the mental faculties are unfolding themselves during the period. Is the great function of inhibition keeping well to the front of every other faculty during development? If not, there is undoubtedly a danger. Control is the regulator of the higher faculties, and should precede them in time of first

N

appearance.   Does higher motive come in the regulation of life and overcome lower motive?   Is there educability in method, punctuality and order in life?   Is the higher kind of veracity developing itself?   Do the natural desires towards social intercourse, towards the other sex, dominate the conduct, or can they be controlled at will?   Are there any idiosyncrasies of mind or body? How are the religious instincts progressing?   Are they invariably associated with duty and with right states of emotion?   Are all the social instincts healthy?   Are ideals of purity, honour, and righteousness being slowly built up as pillars in the fabric of life?   Are the poetic and artistic feelings keen or absent?   Are the imaginations of the earth earthy, or are they inspired by high ideals of beauty and love?   Many of those questions suggest their own answers in the way of prevention, or, as we doctors say, prophylaxis.   We must first see that the body in all its parts and functions has a healthy environment and lays a good foundation thereby for the higher brain action.   There must be supplied a great abundance of fresh air, by night and by day.   Of that there cannot be too much during growth and development. The more oxygen that is breathed by the lungs the redder will be the blood corpuscles, and the more of them will be produced in the bone marrow and the blood glands. Thus the brain will be rightly stimulated to do its work. Adolescents cannot do without fresh air, even if at later periods of life it may be safely scrimped.   The muscles and the heart and the blood-vessels must all be strengthened by exercise.   There is no antidote to many forms of nervousness equal to an abundance of air and exercise.   As to food, it should, of course, be in amount what is needed to repair waste ; but I am convinced, and most of the medical profession are coming to this belief, that most of the comfortable classes and many of the higher-paid artisan classes in Great Britain eat too much at all periods of life except childhood. I believe that they also do not always select the best food to eat. I am satisfied that, speaking generally, Americans, English people, and Colonials eat too much butcher meat. To see the quantity of beef that a public-school boy of 16 or 17 will daily consume is, in my judgment, to condemn the amount. It must never be forgotten that every particle of food that has to be dealt with by the stomach and the digestive apparatus, more than is really required to supply growth and repair, has to undergo a series of complicated chemical changes, all requiring an output of energy from the organs and vital forces. This means waste of precious force which should have been reserved for really useful work and growth. The chemical changes, the metabolism, may be imperfect and its products may be poisonous, thus causing an auto-poisoning of the system. It is to be admitted that Nature does generally provide an excess of energy, more than is needed for the daily service of healthy organs; but she can be overpressed, and is, in this matter, constantly overpressed in the classes of which I have spoken. This over-pressure, if it is practised at all, should not be a constant daily thing. Nature only provides for intermittent excesses. Such over-feeding tends towards periodic sluggishness of the higher brain working. One cannot think when the force that ought to have gone towards thinking is being used up by the over-pressed digestive organs, or when the brain is being poisoned by toxins from imperfectly digested or unassimilated food. It tends also towards the development of a certain kind of nervousness in those of a neurotic constitution. It leads to a premature development of the reproductive and sexual instincts before their higher control is established. It lays the foundation of rheumatism, gout, and kidney disease. The stomach and the appetite, through getting into a bad habit, come to demand more than the body and the brain need. I believe that a healthier diet for adolescents would be more milk, more cereals, more fruit, more sugar, and more vegetables, with less animal food. The Japanese showed us how work and fighting can be done on what we call "low diet." I expect their system will soon become the fashion, and be followed by us. The scientific gymnastics of the present day—such as the Swedish system—which are in many ways scientific, supplement ordinary games, exercise, and sports. No doubt, during the boy period, between 7 and 15, the co-ordination of mind and muscle, ordinarily called the training of the muscles, has mostly taken place, but it must be kept up by constant practice ; and there are higher and finer developments of this co-ordination, such as performing on musical instruments, fine handiwork, the graces of deportment and gesture, using the voice in singing, and the muscular expression of the emotions generally, which have to be perfected during adolescence. This perfection can only be attained by the steady practice of those co-ordinations. In regard to the use of such things as tea, coffee, tobacco, and alcohol in any form, which are not strictly foods, the greatest care should be taken not to use any of them in any degree that can be called excess during the period. In fact, young men should not begin to smoke nor to use alcohol until their beards are grown if they strictly obey the law of Nature and follow her lead, while no young woman should then or afterwards drink, or smoke, or swear, or take to strong tea. The brain cells, during this precious period of development should not be constantly stimulated by anything that cannot properly be considered as food. It may be that the majority of adolescents of a race that was perfectly healthy and lived in the country could take an excess of beef and a certain amount of tea, tobacco, and beer with impunity ; but it is certain that the descendants of the city-born, those of nervous constitution, those with a tendency towards insanity, consumption, and actual nervous diseases, should avoid those things if their lives are to be as healthy and useful and happy as is possible, and if their children are to be free from nervousness.

Competitions.—One of the practices now much in vogue in the higher schools and in colleges is that of the competition of one scholar with another through the "examination system." Sometimes this competition is terrific. It becomes so keen as to put every girl who is in the foremost rank in a fever heat of emulation before the examination. It suits the schoolmaster very well, because it is a great stimulus to work. He is not always as interested as he might be in the health or the special nervous constitution of his girls. He does not regard them from the physiological or hereditary point of view. He does not know that the mother of one of his scholars died of consumption, that the father of another was insane, that neuralgia was hereditary in the family of a third, while another had convulsions as a baby. His training has not taught him to know or to notice the meaning of narrow chests, the absence of fat, quick, jerky movements, headaches, want of appetite and disinclination to bodily exercise. It is the most nervous, excitable, and highly strung girls who throw themselves into the school and college competition most keenly, and they, of course, are just those most liable to be injured by it. Girls take a personal animus more than lads, and do not take a beating so quietly. The whole thing takes greater hold on them, and is more real. When I used to lecture to a class of girl medical students it was almost pathetic and a little amusing to me to see the desperate anxiety that all exhibited to take down everything I said. Their looks were earnest, their attitude expectant, and their minds appreciative. I should have been better pleased had they paid somewhat less attention when the subject treated of was not very important nor specially interesting. Young women at adolescence are apt to have in large degree the feminine power of taking it out of themselves more than they are able to bear for long. Now when this power is called up for months for such a purpose as a college education, with many competitions throughout its course, the body not having attained its full size and shape and still growing, the brain and faculties only maturing, it should not be surprising if the result is disastrous towards the end of adolescence. Womanhood is apt after such an education to be entered with a handicap. There is too little joyous feeling bubbling over in life. The sources of vital energy in the brain have not been replenished sufficiently by outdoor recreations, fresh air, and the right kind of food. Blood has not been formed in sufficient amount. Nature has not got the material nor the force to build up the form towards the fair woman's ideal, and therefore personal beauty and grace of movement have not been attained to the extent that might have been. A store of latent energy, sufficient for future use, should have been laid up all this time, for woman's special work, for motherhood, and for the race of the future. Mind cannot grow except by growth and development of brain. Brain will not grow except through proper environment and conditions. The muscles will not harden but by having plenty of blood and exercise. The fat, that most essential concomitant of female beauty during adolescence, will not form in the proper way unless the blood is rich. Fat is to the body what fun is to the mind, an indicator of spare power.

The average height for the lad in the well-fed classes at 15 is 60½ inches. By 25 he should be 67 inches. The average height of the girl should be at 15 about 61 inches.

At 25 she should be about 63 inches.   During that period
of 10 years, the boy should have gained at least 14 lbs. in
weight and the girl 12 lbs.   That growth in height and
weight does not take place all at once.   For the girl there
is a spurt shortly after 15.   For the boy there is apt to be
a spurt later on.   Now height and weight are most important expressions of energy, of growth, and the best
index of health.   They show that nutrition is going on
normally or is being interfered with.   If it is so interfered
with then every rule of hygiene demands that the reason
for this should be ascertained.   Those seem gross bodily
facts.   Some one may ask, What have they to do with
Mental Hygiene?   Normal body growth usually means
normal brain development, and normal brain development
means healthy-mindedness.   If we could, as a matter of
fact, keep our lads and girls healthy in body, to a large
extent the brain and mind would take care of themselves.
Once fully formed as a woman, she can then stand much.
She is capable of taking up any *rôle* that falls to her,
whether it be teacher, daughter, or mother.   Whether she
is an actual mother or not, she is infinitely the better for
having the full capacity of motherhood.

To me it seems inexcusable that simple lessons in
hygiene are not given in all schools, and more advanced
lessons in this science given in every higher school and
university.   What great public school for boys and girls
has a special teacher of health, whose instruction all must
attend?   The money and the time given to teaching music
to scholars with no ear, and classics to unclassical minds,
would be infinitely better spent in physiological and health
instruction suitable and interesting to all if rightly taught
and illustrated.

Sleep during Adolescence.—Dr. Dukes, of Rugby, in his
Health at School, has in regard to the amount of sleep
needed by early adolescents spoken most weighty words

as the result of his great experience and keen observation. Dr. Acland has written strongly in a similar sense. Recently the heads of the medical profession have considered it their duty to make a serious pronouncement as to the amount of sleep needed by the schoolboy and schoolgirl during early adolescence, and as to the insufficiency of the hours of sleep allowed at most of our public schools. The whole profession of medicine is at one on this point. I have already spoken of what sleep means to the brain cells and as to the necessity of sufficient sleep at the earlier ages of life. I can only say now that during early adolescence, and even up to the age of 20 or so, the time for sleep should not be less than from $9\frac{1}{2}$ to 10 hours. This especially applies to all youths doing brain work.

Sex Difficulties during Adolescence.—I shall devote a special chapter to sex hygiene, more especially in its mental aspects throughout life, but I cannot omit here to emphasise the fact that the hygiene of the sex question is one of the most important that has to be faced during adolescence, especially during its earlier stages. It is most difficult, it is often urgently pressing, and in many individuals it is paramount. If early adolescence can be got through without the breaking of the laws of Nature and morals in regard to sexual conduct and impulse a tremendous risk has been avoided. The management and the control of the sexual instinct at that age is, perhaps, the most urgent question during the whole life in the case of many persons of both sexes, but more especially in the case of lads. The risks are not only bodily but intensely mental and moral. An instinct of overpowering force is let loose by Nature in many youths before its natural controller, inhibition, physical and moral, has acquired the strength necessary to check its unnatural ebullitions. An unbroken horse has to be managed by a weak and an inexperienced rider. Nature's innate gift of modesty, her organic repugnances, the moral feelings of right and wrong, the strong instinct of manliness and womanliness and the power of religious teaching are all needed in a high degree to act as controllers, and they all fail often enough. When emotion, imagination, and strong animal impulse are all one side it needs a strong rein to curb them. What I have been urging as to proper diet, much exercise, games and steady occupation all point towards the right solution of the developing sex question as much as to keeping up of the general health. The magnetic force of a strong man's influence, such as that of Arnold at Rugby, no doubt is a powerful force for good, but that cannot be got every day. I am in favour of plain speaking by the family doctor as one means of safe enlightenment and as a deterrent influence. He alone has the physiological knowledge to speak with scientific authority. He has not the diffidence of the parent in talking of such matters, and the boy prejudices against the teacher do not exist in his case.

Regulated and natural social intercourse between the sexes, especially in the shape of family life, is one of the most powerful outlets and regulators of sex impulses. There lies one great danger of the monastic life of public schools. A lad who loves home and is much at home is far safer than one who sees little of real home life. Mother and sisters and young lady friends of the right sort fill up a gap and satisfy a natural social craving that tends to the expulsion of the gross and animal. Sex cravings are transformed into social feelings. The " expulsive power of a great affection " comes in as a powerful hygienic force. A subconscious shame and reasonableness as to baser impulses arise in a strong and natural way and act as powerful inhibitors. Control is much easier because the direction of thought and emotion is carried into other channels.

The Moral Sense during the Period.—The moral sense has, like every other mental faculty, a brain basis. In the lowest animals there is very little moral faculty to be observed. No doubt, when animals become gregarious, there are certain necessary relationships of one individual to another which gradually appear, as evolution proceeds, until we reach the moral faculty in the human being. Taking the dog, as having the closest association with man of any animal, and being intelligent and imitative in a remarkable degree, he has an unquestionable sense of right and wrong. There is an enormous difference in this development in different dogs. Some are always endeavouring to do the right thing after they have been taught, while others will be constantly disobeying the law of right and wrong and clearly realise when they break it. I have now a very intelligent well-bred Gordon setter who strives with all his might to carry out his own simple ethical code of steadiness on his birds and obeying the whistle, and when he breaks it his look of guilt and penitence is pathetic to a degree. When a puppy is present he will not eat his meal, however hungry he may be, till the youngster has had his fill and stops eating. In the child of two there is little manifestation of moral sense. There is no feeling of the " ought " in it and small sense of guilt on account of any breach of law or custom. From that time its rudiments begin to appear. During childhood and the school-boy time of life, nothing is so constantly reiterated as what ought to be done and what to be avoided, what is right and what is wrong. This constant teaching, with the examples of doing right and avoiding wrong in its parents and teachers, has a great effect, no doubt, in the creation of the moral sense. There arises a feeling of duty, but it is during later adolescence that this feeling assumes a large and dominating position and becomes associated with the emotions, with the intellect with the will and with the religious instincts. This, however, implies a moral heredity and a brain with the innate capacity to take up this great function. I have known many children and many boys and girls at the school age who never could be made to *feel* that there was a compulsion on them to do right things. They had, in fact, no brain basis for the moral sense. They were moral idiots, and very troublesome members of a family. I knew a little boy of ten who was always trying to put the cat in the fire and who dropped his mother's watch coolly down a well. He grew up at adolescence to be a very troublesome young man indeed, requiring never-ceasing watching, and by that time it was fully recognised by his parents that he was not "responsible." He was sharp enough intellectually and acquired school learning fairly well. I have known other cases where the on-coming of the moral sense was merely delayed. After puberty they acquired the faculty for the first time. It is a well-known fact that many of the children of the criminal classes and of drunkards and of the insane are practically without a sense of right and wrong. This lack had become hereditary in the class from which they sprung. Punishments do little good in such cases. Exhortations are lost on them and even good moral example is not instinctively imitated.

In regard to the development of the moral faculties by teaching, it may be summed up in this—"Obey the Ten Commandments." The moral sense, as we have seen, began its cultivation in early childhood, and receives a very strong impetus during boyhood, but it is during adolescence that the faculty of inhibition, which represents the moral sense, is fully developed and becomes a dominant part of life. Example is, no doubt, a powerful agent in its building up. Literature of the right sort becomes an extraordinary stimulus also. I do not mean treatises on ethics or homilies on conduct, such as were chiefly believed in during the eighteenth century. I rather mean good biography, poetry and fiction. Fiction, like alcohol, has, however, its dangers. It must be a real literature, and exhibit art in its composition. There are, of course, plenty of good examples, but I need go no further than Scott's novels as rising to the standard I have indicated. Those novels, combined with a reasonable number of the more modern psychological novels of character rather than of incident, and good biography, are the safe mental and moral literary diet of the adolescent. To establish a conscience, to cultivate self-control, to make the sense of duty dominant in life, to give the idea that law and rules must be obeyed, to create a sense of discipline, is the very highest and most important duty of the teacher and parent during adolescence. All this is closely allied to the religious sense of sin, but it is not the same. No doubt example, the following the lead of others, the inner feeling of pleasure when right is done and temptation overcome, all tend to build up the moral faculty. There is formed, in the developing condition of the adolescent, an ideal—even a passion—for beauty. The imagination comes in and protects from wrong courses by creating pictures of the real beauty of right conduct and of the unattractiveness of law-breaking. There is a moral enthusiasm roused at this time of life in favour of right and against wrong. The daily habit of doing the one and avoiding the other writes itself on the brain cells and their action, and becomes a permanent record. This moral sense attaches itself to actions of benevolence, justice, and self-denial, on the one hand, as things to be imitated, and to meanness, untruthfulness, jealousy, evil passions and anger as things to be avoided. No doubt the punishment and the disapproval of the evil, with the approval of the good, help in the process of conscience-making. It certainly does not do to begin too early in life a too stringent process of creating this sense until the brain basis is there and the power of inhibition exists. Especially is it desirable not to create a false moral standard. To try and make a child believe that taking too much jam is really a wrong act, that hitting its still younger brother when in a passion is a very dreadful thing—all this tends to establish a precocious ethical standard that often is very hurtful as life goes on. I have sometimes noticed a precocious sense of right and wrong to be followed during adolescence by a sort of paralysis of the faculty. A healthy young man or woman, well exercised, is always apt to have a healthier sense of right and wrong, and virtue is easier of practice than in the nervous, thin, or hyper-æsthetic person. A sane conscience is part of a sane mind, and on the whole goes with a sound body. In many persons acting by instinct is swift, easy, and pleasant. Such persons are usually of the artistic temperament. The knowledge of right and wrong in them may be quite well developed, but action from instinct is so strong that the moral brake cannot be put on in time. It is in such persons that the cultivation of the moral sense during adolescence should be very assiduously attended to, for it is often their weak point. They always try to do what is easy and pleasant, and for them to do right, if it is not pleasant, is specially irksome. It is most important that in them a definite moral ideal should be formed, that the imagination should be brought in, and that the altruistic faculty should be exercised. Some such persons are so intensely instinctive that motives, in a rational way, have little power over them. Wrong action soon becomes a brain habit, and the sense of right and wrong becomes callous and unreactive. In certain departures from mental health, such as occur in melancholia, the sense of right and wrong becomes hyper-æsthetic, so causing a torture to its owner. In other conditions of mental disease the moral sense is the first faculty to be lost. No doubt, in the course of human evolution, a high moral sense was the last to be evolved, and in the dissolution of the higher mental power, which is the essence of insanity, it is the first to be lost. We have cases of mental disorder with high intellectual power, but no moral control; this we call "moral insanity."

The Religious Instinct in Adolescence.—James has, for the first time, at least in ordinary English literature, given us a scientific study and analysis of the religious instincts, their expressions and their psychological meanings and relations. I believe that his study is on the whole a true one, and it is certainly very instructive. This is not the place to follow the evolution of religious instinct and religious practice, from its first dawning among primitive man, up to its elaborate manifestations in our modern civilised communities. That it is a universal and a most powerful determinant in human life is undeniable. That it really arises in the individual in a definite and almost complete form in adolescence is, I think, absolutely manifest, both from a study of physiological psychology and from a study of the history of religion itself. There is no instinct more radical in man, but, on the other hand, there is no instinct so cultivable and so capable of being moulded into different forms by dogma, by tradition, by example, and by strong emotional feelings. The religious instinct has a very obvious and close relationship to emotion, to imagination, to morals, to æsthetic feelings, to the social instincts, and to sex. The feelings of reverence and of awe and the consciousness of the infinite in man are vague but most powerful parts of his nature. They are subject to law, even if that law is difficult of formulation.

All normal religion is a highly emotional stimulus. It is a means of education in many ways; it is the only pure ideal that half the world has access to. It has proved an intellectual stimulus, and has roused a metaphysical frame of mind in some of the most vigorous nations, such as the Germans and Scotch. It leads to refinement of life more than any other agency. It stimulates benevolent and altruistic feelings and practical efforts above all other human instrumentalities. It fights gross vice and immorality. It reaches the poorer intellects as much, or even more, than the highly cultivated. The faith which is its essence has " removed mountains " and " turned the world upside down," will take no refusal and see no obstacle that it cannot surmount. It seizes on the higher part of man, and condemns, perhaps unduly, his lower part. It " giveth life " to multitudes who were mere animals before it came into their lives. It rouses hopes that never die. It affords examples to lure men on to better lives. It and art are the only great spiritual forces. It feeds imagination and may stiffen self-control. If all this be true, then to treat of the Hygiene of Mind without including a consideration of the religious instinct and its effects would be to omit one of its most powerful factors.

The chief hygienic idea in regard to the religious instinct is that it should be tied indissolubly to duty. Without this association its effect on life and character is apt to be small, and it may, in many cases, be even harmful. The religious instinct should take its due place and order in the natural developmental scheme of adolescence. Let it be cultivated, but always in association with control. Eliminate from it egotism, obtrusion, frothiness, hallucination, and sex ideas. To give its sanction to the moral sense, to do acts of altruistic benevolence, to accept the Judgment-Day text, " I was sick, and ye visited me ; I was naked, and ye clothed me," St. James's definition, " To visit the fatherless and widows in their affliction," and the prophet's definition " To do justly, to love mercy and to walk humbly with thy God," would seem to be the rational outcome of all the great religions in the world. No doubt the practice of humility and of self-denial are, and should be, specially connected with the religious instinct. All religions have been character-ised, especially during adolescence, by special crises, con-versions, excitements, ecstasies, fervours, revivals, vivid symbolism and mysticism. Such emotional intensities are not to be thought lightly of or scoffed at. It is according to psychological law that any instinct may burst forth suddenly after lying in a latent form. They may vivify and give an entirely new turn to life and conduct.

Some of these phenomena are, however, closely allied, or are very easily connected with mere selfish feelings of pleasure, and with the natural enthusiasms of the female sex in youth. They readily lend themselves to the ecstasies of ordinary love between the sexes, and they may develop selfishness in a high but very subtle way. From the point of view of the Hygiene of Mind, they all need most careful looking after, and in some cases require discouragement and repression. Such emotional inten-sities are dangerous to the highly nervous, the intensely imaginative, the unstable, the explosive in mind, and the essentially unreasonable in mind, because they tend towards the pathological in such persons, while it is in them that they are most apt to appear. In such persons they unquestionably may lead to mental disorder, to selfish religious sectarianism, and even to vice, natural and unnatural. It is natural that the expression of the religious instincts should call in the aid of music, beauty, and symbolism, but there is always the risk that those things should minister simply to the emotions and to selfishness, and should divorce the instinct from duty. The great aim of the religionist, if he takes Mental

Hygiene into account, it seems to me, should be to make the religious instinct a habit of life rather than an occasional pleasure, so to leaven society with it that it should not be the exclusive possession of a few, and that thus its great powers over the individual man and body politic shall be naturally handed down from generation to generation instead of being a personal affair of spurts and spasms.   A reasoning basis should surely run through all its dogmas and practices.   The apparent antagonism of some of its formulas to natural law should now, when science has assumed so great a position in human life, be minimised as far as that is consistent with its essential substance and its practical application to the needs of human nature.   The unessential accretions which surrounded all religions in the superstitious and unscientific times of the past should be gradually got rid of as human nature will bear it.   The spiritual comforts and consolations which it offers to the weak, the needy, and the dying are sufficiently real to stand on their own merits without being paraded as reasons why the strong and the healthy, who do the world's work, should be called irreligious and materialistic if they refuse to swallow the dogmas of old superstitions and exploded beliefs.   Let the religious instinct, in short, be treated like any other part of the psychology of man, as being subject to law and compatible with reason.   That will not weaken its sanctions or lower its ideals, and will not lessen its consolatory power. No scientist can admit that right faith can be inconsistent with or contrary to right reason.   Man cannot live without religion ; therefore it is the more important to avoid its counterfeits and to lay its foundations on health of body and soundness of mind.   It is far too precious a support to a good life to rest on any false or pathological basis— at least, if we look on religion as an important means of Mental Hygiene, these views are sound.

o

Balance of the Mental Faculties.—As I have so frequently had to say, the mental faculties, the appetites and instincts and bodily powers all have a normal and mutual relation which, as a hygienic measure during adolescence, should be assiduously cultivated. There exists an average mental balance between the different faculties without which a man or woman is morbid or unsafe. If from natural causes or by educational pushing a man has high intelligence without much will, or keen emotion without much inhibition, or overmastering will power without the moral sense, or vivid imagination without common sense, or intense social instincts without much conscience, or fervid religious instinct without much sense of duty or altruism, the results will be bad for society and for such unbalanced and one-sided persons themselves. At all events, if there were too many such one-sided people in any society or State, the steadiness and harmony of a progressive civilisation would be impaired and endangered. Many of the bad laws, of the evil customs of society, the religious persecutions, the fanaticisms, the oppressions, the cruelties, the sectarianism, the fruitless social efforts and the crimes of men and nations have resulted from unbalanced mental conditions. There can be no doubt that the greatest comfort in life is attained by the individual through this balance. It naturally leads to a calm and philosophical conduct of life ; it saves the waste of mental and emotional energy ; it guards against frothy religionism, hurtful spurts of emotionalism, and the fanatic temper. It helps its owner to see the true relationships of life, and to look to the end of a course of action from its beginning. No doubt natural brain qualities and temperament chiefly determine the capacity to attain brain balance, but very much can be done by teaching, by following good example, and by personal effort. The tendency nowadays is to run into mental specialism, to yield to enthusiasms, and to show originality by taking up fads. Life is like a juggler keeping up six balls at once in the air—none of them must be neglected. Balance of faculty is certainly one of the important aims of a true Hygiene of Mind, and it can best be attained during adolescence.

Every kind of nervousness and mental instability tends towards a want of balance of faculty. True sanity is largely tested by the presence of this quality. Nothing is more striking than the examples of such want of balance in states of partial mental disease. I have now a patient who is learned beyond most savants, even in many specialisms. He is well read beyond most men. He is liked by all his friends. He talks in a most interesting way on most subjects; his judgment is sound on almost all matters outside himself. No one in one interview could say he was even partially insane. Yet his conduct of life has been utterly disastrous. He has no true affection for his wife and children, and has neglected them in the most scandalous way. He cannot keep an engagement or pay a debt. He cannot help drinking to excess if he has the chance, though when kept out of temptation he has no craving for alcohol. His personal want of order and untidiness is indescribable. His intellectual power is, in fact, overdeveloped at the expense of his emotions and inhibition. He has no sense of responsibility, no regrets for wrong-doing—indeed, is "never in the wrong." Such examples of what I describe as unbalanced faculty are common enough if looked for. They could, many of them at least, have been saved from this by right mental hygienic training during adolescence.

The process of adaptation to new environments in all living beings is always accompanied by many individual failures. It seems to me that many of the nervous diseases of adolescents are examples of this law. Brains of ancestral primitive constitution that would have stood well enough the simple life of a primitive age break down in the effort to adapt themselves to the conditions of our modern and complex civilisation.

CHAPTER XIV

MANHOOD AND WOMANHOOD. 25-55

THE Mental Hygiene of the fully developed man and woman is not so important as the hygiene of adolescence, not because there it has less work to do, but because the flux of growth and development is over and the brain and mind have nearly reached such stability as the individual is capable of. Physiologically and psychologically we have to do with mature faculties, with an organism whose mental resistiveness and reactiveness have almost reached their maximum, whose beauty, mental attractiveness, and physical perfection cannot be much improved by any measures that may be taken. We have to do with fully developed sex, the full capacity for the reproduction of the species, and the strength to do effectively the world's work. Mentally we have cognition, reasoning, emotion, will, memory, imagination, ambition, passion, all in as high a degree as the heredity and training of the individual make possible. Inhibition of all sorts in a normal individual should be strong. The full power to apply experience to help life's future work should exist. We should have the masculine and the feminine characteristics, each fully developed. The man excels in cold reason, in courage, in originality, and in physical activity. He can do the work of a profession, can make money, and those should be a pleasure to him from the power they give him. He can fight, can sail a ship into unknown seas without fear, and he can rule other men ; he can exercise a trade, can compel the grudging earth to yield her fruits, making Nature and her laws his slaves by mechanical inventions. The woman has developed more on the lines of sympathy, emotion, of wanting to please those she loves, yielding to man's wishes, delighting in being the mistress of a household, and loving children passionately. She is the centre of the home-life, and revels in the knowledge that she is so.

Heredity, good or bad, has set its mark on both the man and the woman, but it is no longer an advancing and uncertain process. Its effects may come out in many ways, both in strengthened and weakened defences against enemies from within and without, but we do not take so much account of it as an ever-present source of danger, arrestment of function and of degeneration as we have had to do during adolescence. If proper inquiry has been made, and proper antagonistic hygienic measures have been adopted, heredity is not so much of an unknown quantity as in the earlier stages of life. It is not so much a shadow coming out of the darkness, the aspect of which may be either fair or terrible. In fact it has done its worst or its best, and we can now reckon more surely on its future.

Manhood and womanhood, as things commonly go in the world, and for most people, imply hard work, stress, disappointments, and success or failure in the main efforts of life. In a healthy and well-developed man or woman this striving is, on the whole, bracing and healthy ; at all events it can be endured with reasonable equanimity. From a hygienic point of view, we need to ask, How can the powers of mind and body naturally inherited or developed be best conserved and made the best use of for life's work ? Enjoyment and happiness must by no means be excluded as a part of the life of the future. This perhaps is not quite so essential a means of development as in childhood and boyhood, but without it, in many cases, it would be vain to apply every other kind of hygienic agent. The seriousness and settledness of life of the period, with the bracing of every nerve and sinew to do work, to gain a reasonable position in society, and to enjoy a fair amount of happiness, is itself a tonic agent of no mean value. A superficial view of life, changing purposes, a want of strenuousness, neither tend to success nor to happiness. Other great questions are : Do weak points exist in brain or mind? Where do they lie? What part of conduct or work do they affect? How can they be best avoided or antagonised? Those weak points must be known by the man and woman themselves, and do not need to be known by others as in the case of the more helpless periods of life. " Know thyself" is an axiom of enormous hygienic service to be frequently applied by every reasonable man and woman. Frequently enough knowledge exists, but the wisdom that applies it may not be there. Regrets, vain enough and useless enough, may be the only result of the possession of such self-knowledge. It is quite certain that few men and women have the absolute choice of their place in life and work and climate and friends and companions and their general environment. To most it is a case of making the best of what is possible. Nothing is more certain than that fair health, an averagely working brain and fair mental power, may all be improved, retained and used to the advantage of the life of those so equipped in the case of most persons whose heredity is not very bad and their luck average. It is also certain that those things may in many cases be voluntarily weakened or lost, and that this makes all the difference between success and failure, usefulness in the world and being an incubus on society. Men and women have far greater responsibility than in the earlier ages, because on their health and on their action depends the future of the race. Selfishness in adolescents may not do so very much harm ; undue selfishness in men and women means an unorganised society and national decay. Fatherhood, motherhood, citizenship have necessarily a large strain of altruism running through them, and some cultivation of this setting aside of self is probably the first and the highest duty of all men and women as a mere measure of hygiene. The idea does not occur to many men and women that this is so, but that wrong conclusion results from want of thought or want of teaching. It is part of what the moralists call the discipline of life. That discipline may be hard or easy, according to the temperament of the individual.

It is a most fortunate thing if, during the latter period of adolescence, an occupation in life has been selected which really suits the capacity of the individual and goes with his innate tendencies. It is always hard to change a line of life, and it means worry, wasted time and labour. I believe that the " preventive " doctor of the future will be called in most cases where a young man or a young woman is about to select an occupation in life. A good deal of failure and a good deal of unhappiness would thus be avoided. To turn a man, strong in muscle, ardent in temperament, full of sanguine life, into a sedentary lawyer is so manifestly against Nature's indications that it should be avoided. To send a studious, nervous, thin-skinned man into the army would probably, in most cases, be putting the square pin into the round hole. To set the man with a bad nervous heredity to mental work, where the brain is exercised rather than the muscles, and where an outdoor life is scarcely possible, may be the unmaking of him by depriving him of his one chance of escaping his hereditary enemy. To put a hard-headed, calculating, un-sympathetic, business mind which takes chief delight in bargaining, in not being overreached, and to whom the chief joy of life is making money—to put this man into the medical or clerical profession is usually a mistake. He is apt not to love science for its own sake, not to hunger and thirst after knowledge, and not to have sympathy with human weaknesses. It is one of the greatest of hygienic studies to find out what a man is best suited for.

There are many dangers of mature life. Overtaxing strength of body and mind, over-exertion, especially to those of sanguine temperament, is always a risk. Ambition that overreaches itself comes into many lives. I have just met one man in life, a very strong and active man he was, full of energy in all directions and business-like in everything, who told me that he had never felt tired in his life. He did not know the sensation, and he therefore could not help having a dash of contempt for people who got knocked up by their work. He was a hard man, hard on his wife, hard on his children, and harder still on those with whom he had business. But he broke down in brain and died long before he ought to have done through sheer overwork, leaving a great fortune to children who had not the most grateful feelings towards their father who made the money for them. At the present day there can be no doubt whatever that a certain amount of nervous instability, best understood as "nervousness," is too common in our city populations. The great fault of the nervous man usually is that he is not punctual, systematic and orderly enough in his life and his business. The assiduous practice, until it became a habit, of this one minor virtue would enable him to get through his work with comfort and die in peace at a good old age. The nervous are apt to be irritable when a little tired, to take too much out of themselves when that is not really necessary, to be sleepless, to have indigestion and to be thin. Like the melancholy man, the ordinary nervous man should try in every way, through suitable food and through systematic periods of rest to carry a comfortable amount of fat.   Mrs. Carlyle wrote to a friend after she had had a month's rest from housekeeping and from the temper of the great philosopher, " Thank God for that blessed stone of fat !—it has made a new woman of me." Some men and women, so long as there is no special stress and trial in life, go on quite well, doing their work effectively, but they have no spare energy laid up in the shape of fat or nervous tone, and so they live always on the edge of a precipice.   The pessimist or the hypochondriac may be so by reason of his organisation, and nothing could have saved him from it, or he may be so through neglect of obvious health rules and of a reasonable Mental Hygiene.   Such people do not get the most out of life, and they often become a nuisance to their friends and relations and a dead weight to society.   Some nervous people are liable to sudden collapses, slackness in work, getting jaded long before holiday-time, and becoming stale and irritable.   Unquestionably in many cases such conditions might have been avoided.   Then to go to the other extreme.   The over-sanguine, boisterous and rash man might, if he studied his own constitution, largely curb himself from over-speculation and excitement if he knew himself well enough.   There is no doubt that there is a mental gymnastic that can be and should be practised by reasonable men who wish to keep their mental faculties correlated and under control, just as bodily gymnastics do for the muscles and the internal organs.   One such mental gymnastic recommended by my friend, Dr. George Wilson, is for every man for some period of each day, short or long as opportunity occurs, calmly to look at the sky or the hills or big trees or sheets of water, absolutely excluding every other mental impression, while the great things of nature are thus got into the life.   Most men will find this will add a little to their conscious equanimity and make them more able to resist the pin-pricks of life. Another mental gymnastic closely allied to this is to indulge frequently in a quiet bit of solitude and communing with oneself. Most of us nowadays read and speak far too much and think too little. The cultivation of conscientiousness or a strict sense of duty, of a tender conscience in regard to all things, big and little, that have any relation to duty, is beyond any doubt one of the highest moral hygienics that any man can aim at. The difference in the way in which the work of the world would be done, as compared with the way in which it is done, if every worker cultivated a reasonable dash of conscientiousness would be enormous. Paradise regained would not be too strong a description of society under those circumstances. A reasonable cultivation of the religious instincts in mature life is quite as important as the development of those instincts in adolescence. For a blend of religion and morals, few grown men could do much better than a regular perusal of St. Paul and Marcus Aurelius, while if the religious mood happens to be more intense, St. Thomas à Kempis's *Imitation* will serve well as its pabulum. For most people, regular exercise in the fresh air, some outdoor game or sport at times, change of scene and occupation occasionally are very necessary as hygienic measures for the brain and mind. There are, no doubt, a few exceptions, who do best to run in one groove and who are utterly upset if disturbed or taken out of it. Many men and women bring on mental irritation, depression, laziness, and unfitness for work by a disregard of the commonest rules of health in regard to diet, sleep, bathing, and the improper use of food or alcoholic stimulants. The brain has ramifications everywhere, and has feelers down to the finger-ends and in every organ, so that no part of the body is misused without a mental penalty. There is a solidarity all through life as there is in the working of every part of the brain. If "one member suffer, all the members suffer with it." A man who knows himself ought to know his strong and his weak points, and knowing them he can afford to take much out of the strong faculties and members and to spare the weaker ones. I once knew a man who did a great amount of work in life and was reasonably happy in the doing of it, who had an immense capacity for acquiring knowledge, an extraordinary memory, and a good literary capacity. But he was very irritable, very sleepless, very susceptible to noise and distractions of all sorts, and he was a man in certain respects with a very weak will. All those things he thoroughly realised, and, being a man of wisdom, he so arranged his work that he produced a large output of effective scholarship. He left the whole of his affairs—housekeeping, travelling, social intercourse—to a very sensible wife, to whom he submitted all the minor details of life, and so contrived to get round his weak points without either suffering or taking too much out of himself.

The minor virtues and the minor vices are often of as much importance in human life as the greater ethics. The cultivation of geniality, contentment, taking an interest in small things, trying to get on well with people, trying to practise the adage that "a soft answer turneth away wrath," doing his best to bear fools gladly, patience, tolerance, and practice of the humanities—all these things, physiologically calming to the brain and will, yield much happiness and an enormous avoidance of friction. If at the same time the man will try not to be in a hurry and will repress as well as he can the smaller jealousies, vanities, egotisms, unveracities, irritabilities, uncharitablenesses and criticisms, he has a much better chance of a satisfactory life than other men with much higher powers, ideals, and aspirations. No doubt "moderation in all things" applies to more than meat or drink. Most men and women of experience in life, and who have had trials and difficulties, learn much wisdom in the conduct of life in regard to such minor matters. The man who habitually makes a fuss about small things has an element of foolishness and lack of philosophy in him which often shorten his life. The bore, the egotist, and the universal critic come to be cursed and avoided by all sensible men. The saving grace of common sense is not one, unfortunately, that can be acquired by any amount of care or resolution. It is innate, and if it is not there nothing can supply its place. Common sense and real wisdom, fortunately, do increase towards the latter part of manhood and womanhood in most people. The fool who will not learn by being "brayed in the mortar of life" is evolutionally "unfit," and equivalent to the vermin and smaller pests of nature that are instinctively avoided or killed at sight. Every kind of virtue has its brain basis. Every time it is practised an impression of it is written on the brain cells. Every good practice in morals and life is necessarily in accordance with the laws of brain physiology. It represents something that is good for brain life and health. Looking to the mental action of the brain it cannot be dissociated from the good effects of food and muscular co-ordinations. Both render the brain more fit to do its work, to resist its enemies, and strengthen its defences. It thus becomes more fit to live in the struggle for existence..

As yet, mental and moral health and capacity do not admit of exact measurement or being stated in mathematical formulæ. They do not submit to the exactitude of physical science. We have no exact psychometer, and it is doubtful if we shall ever have one. This must always give a looseness to Mental Hygiene. A man feels a bit run down ; he is conscious there is something weak and wanting in him, but he cannot, from the subjective side—nor can we, from the objective state—precisely measure the amount of his brain fatigue, nor always tell the precise nature of what is lacking. Mosso's mechanical modes of showing the amounts of muscular energy and co-ordination that a man·can exercise, in full vigour or after fatigue, are about the nearest that we can as yet come to state the problem in a scientific way. I met the other day, on our way to dine with a common friend, a hard-worked professional man. He said to me, " I feel a bit slack somehow, my work takes it too much out of me. I can't exactly tell what is wrong, but I know I am suffering somehow from overwork and worry. I was going to take my strychnine tonic if it had not been for this dinner to-night. I know that will pick me up, and I shall be all right for the next few weeks." A state of nerve fatigue and mental exhaustion that may be treated with equal effect by a few doses of strychnine or a good dinner with a cheerful talk must necessarily be a very difficult thing to understand. The reactiveness of my friend's brain was in a healthy condition, but the two sorts of stimuli that were capable of acting on it seemed to be as wide as the poles asunder, yet were equally effective. Both could determine more blood to the brain cells, and both stimulated those cells towards healthy action.

The Mental Hygiene needed by the head-worker is essentially different from that required by the hand-worker or the mere routine worker at a desk. In the head-worker the principle should be to stop for the time being, and at regular intervals, the working of the higher brain cells. Often it is well to put the motor cells into action for a time and take muscular exercise almost in excess. To some such people a change of occupation is the best rest. As life goes on, however, with the head-worker I should certainly not advise him to overdo the output of muscular energy, and I should recommend much sleep and bodily rest. Some men have a pleasant way of taking rest and getting into sound and refreshing sleep by simply shutting their eyes, and by visualisation and imagination combined going over the pleasant parts of their past life. I can usually do that by repeating in imagination a trip up the Nile I once took with its novel and interesting details. I am usually asleep before I have got to Assuan. Others, again, have not this visualising faculty. They must actually see the fine scenery or the ocean in its beauty. They must go to theatres for their rest and to concerts for recreation. For the hand-worker or the man of routine the proper recreation is to go in for reading, discussion, and thinking more. I once knew a man whose work five days and a half in the week was an exciting rush of business, and he gave his brain rest and passed into a weekly Elysium by going to the British Museum every Saturday afternoon to study Natural History.

How enormous has been the wastage in the past through neglect of a reasonable Mental Hygiene! How great has been the loss of human effort thereby! Pitt served his country only twenty-five years, and died at 47. No physician now doubts that the port wine which he drank in such quantity brought on his hereditary gout, and that this, combined with his strong nervous heredity, killed him prematurely. No one who has read his life doubts that had Pitt fully known the consequences and taken account of the constitution he inherited, he would not, for his country's sake, have drunk that bottle of port a day. It may be said that Burns knew quite well that his excesses would shorten his life. It is very doubtful if he did. The drinking customs of the time were so universally accepted, and the scientific risks so unknown, that no young man could well have set himself against them. Robert Louis Stevenson undoubtedly brought on his lung disease through disregard of Nature's laws by exposing himself in his donkey rides to exposure that he was not

fit to stand.   If Keats had only had philosophy enough
to laugh at *The Quarterly* and to take better care of his
health, what additions to the highest English poetry might
we not have had!   Had wrath, intemperance, pride, and
superstition not shortened the life of Alexander the Great,
how different might have been the history of the ancient
world!   How wise Charles the Fifth showed himself in
laying aside his crown and retiring into the calm of a
religious life when he felt his powers declining!   A medical
reading of history and biography has yet to be done.   The
world will certainly some day look at men's lives and
actions largely from the point of view of their heredity and
brain constitutions.

Mental Hygiene of Womanhood.—The hygiene, and
the rules suitable for a man do not apply all along
the line in the case of a woman.   She has duties
thrown on her in life and special capacities to do them
entirely different from man.   Those duties are of such
supreme importance to the race that in certain respects
they are of more value than anything that falls to the lot
of man.   She has special weaknesses and special strength.
Her nervous and mental organisation is more delicate and
more complicated than that of a man, and it cannot be
said to be quite so strong.   Her periods of periodic "illness"
necessarily handicap her in many ways.   In certain respects
she has to be ever on the alert, to exercise more cunning
in a good sense, and to repress certain instincts in a way
which is often exhausting.   The necessary repressions of a
woman's life in civilised societies constitute, in fact, one
of her serious strains and dangers.   Her peculiar duties of
child-bearing and nursing are attended, at least in civilised
life, by dangers and risks of exhaustion and disease.   The
life and conditions of the wife of a working man who has
six or seven children in a few years, who has small means
and little help are, in my judgment, the very hardest of any

human being in our modern social system. She gets little out into the fresh air with its healthy influences. During her child-bearing she is creating human beings with all their capacities of body and mind—the highest and hardest call of organic life. She has to keep the house going whether she is fit for it or not. At childbirth she has too little help, too little rest, and runs many risks of infection from microbes and in other ways. During the nursing of her children she commonly has not a single night of continuous sleep. She has little social recreation. In the ordinary course of the upbringing of a family she will have illness among her children, and perhaps her husband may be sick or out of work. Nature, in such a case, has indeed to provide extra-ordinary compensations in the shape of maternal affection and a sense of duty to lighten up the dark, but not exaggerated picture I have drawn. The kindness and the charity of the benevolent scarcely touches the vast problem of how to make the lives of our working women hygienic and reasonably happy. It is probably the highest and most difficult social problem that exists in our urban life. The solution of it would act for good on the race to an incalculable degree.

The sensitiveness and the sympathy of a woman, her greater nervous reactiveness, in short, takes it out of her in a large degree. The unmarried woman has also special risks in her life. The absence and the repression of family life, of motherhood, and of physiological altruism must always be a strain on her. Except when she has the good fortune to be a maiden aunt, a well-employed, effective nurse, or housekeeper to a bachelor brother, she always has something wanting in her life. Woman is not so hungry as man. She craves such things as tea, which are not real food, more than he does. If she ever takes to alcohol or dangerous drugs to give her stimulus and comfort she comes under their power more than man

P

and suffers degradation sooner. She is much more subject to neurasthenia or prolonged nerve exhaustion, that modern disease of civilisation. The uncivilised woman is often as healthy and nearly as strong as the man. Woman has not attained through civilisation that adaptation to environment to the same extent as the man. Of recent years I believe we have been on the right lines in encouraging our girls of the better classes to live in the fresh air and play games like their brothers, and the grown woman is realising that thick boots, physiological clothing, and a fresh-air life are not unbecoming to her sex and are very good for her health and happiness. The curious feeling of rivalry which nowadays is felt in some cases, and written about between the two sexes is one of the most preposterous and unscientific feelings that was ever expressed. It should be strenuously resisted by every sensible man and woman. Each sex has a place and a work which the other cannot do. Each is necessary to the other, each completes the happiness of the other. One of the tasks of the practical sociology of the future will be to find out the true spheres and work of each sex, and to regulate our social system in accordance with that knowledge. No doubt this is now being done, but in Nature's rude but sure way of the survival of the fittest, which necessarily entails the suffering and the extinction of the unfit. Greater knowledge and a rational hygiene should in this matter certainly "improve on Nature."

The ideal woman has been often depicted in literature. In Proverbs we have one picture in which industry, governing power, and household management are the keynotes. From St. Paul we have another, and in the *Arabian Nights* we have one quite different. In modern fiction and biography we have many pictures and many ideals, good, bad, and indifferent. Woman is certainly undergoing evolution in modern times faster than man. It is not for want of advice or ideals held up to her if her evolution and her Mental Hygiene are not further advanced.

She now presents a much greater variety of mental features than of old. She has far more scope for her capacities, she is trying innumerable new spheres, she is in the stage of experiment, she is often dissatisfied with her position ; and discontent is said to be the mother of progress. She has many ambitions which her sex did not in former times cultivate. It is clearly not yet determined what aspects of her are the fittest to survive. All this means that the woman of to-day is in a more trying position mentally than ever before in the world's history. So much is expected of her, and she tries so much that beyond a doubt a Mental Hygiene is most necessary for her present happiness and her future evolution. Efforts to originate schemes, ideas for new modes of life cannot be done without a certain stress for which, in individual instances, at least, her organisation is not fitted. There are certain characteristics, however, which neither she herself nor man will ever be content that she should be without. Modesty, attractiveness, sympathy, practical helpfulness, unselfishness, devotion to the weak, and the religious instinct, no ideal woman can ever be without. All those imply a sound mind in a sound body. Her sympathy and her strenuousness, whether in work, social dissipation, or play, must not be overdone, otherwise she will become neurasthenic. Her nerves must not be too much irritated, otherwise she will become neuralgic and thin. Her appetite, her digestion, and her power of nutrition must not be allowed to run too low, otherwise she will become irritable, depressed, and get old before her time. Her natural instincts must not be too severely repressed, otherwise she will show discontent and hysteria. Her sphere of life must not be narrowed too much, otherwise she will become petty-minded and a gossip. She must not be too much indulged, petted and flattered, otherwise she will become capricious and selfish. Her religious instincts must not be too exclusively cultivated, otherwise she will run into clergy-worship, symbolism, and saintliness of a disagreeable and useless sort. If religion in a woman is too much divorced from the practical things of life it is apt to run into ecstacy and hallucination. But for the practical side of her nature being strong and having room for exercise, St. Theresa would certainly have passed over the line of sanity.

Husband and Wife.—The true and full psychology of the married state has yet to be written from the point of view of modern science. Its hygiene, bodily and mental, has yet to be formulated. We have pictures innumerable in literature of married life, from the brutal characterisation in the *Kreutzer Sonata* up to the ideal poems of life of our great authors. Any society which can seriously discuss a recent question, "Is Marriage a Success?" must be in great need of a scientific education. The conditions of the married state have undergone, since Christian times, marked evolution, and that process is going on rapidly at the present time. The instinct and the practice of all great civilisations mark it out as by far and away the greatest of all social institutions. It is that instinct which has produced the inclination of modern times to pass the old theories of marriage through the melting-pot, because it is not always an ideal condition. Theorists, pessimists, and revolutionists have therefore asserted that something was radically wrong in its theories and practice. Many thoughtful men and women are of opinion that really successful marriages, if universal, would do more for a country, for society, for morality, and for individual happiness than everything else put together. Different countries and civilisations have different theories of the married state. It was a slavery among bar-

barians, it was animalism in many countries of the East, it was mutual helpfulness among our Teutonic ancestors, it was a merging into one individual according to St. Paul, and to modern scientific sociology and psychology it is one of the chief problems of life. History shows that woman is easier satisfied and more adaptable in regard to marriage than man, for she seemed to be fairly happy whether as a slave wife, a paramour, or a joint worker. The "revolt of woman" is an idea of purely modern times. Nature, religion, and custom do so much in regard to marriage that it well may be asked whether science can help in this problem. There have been many quasi-scientific theories as to the conditions for successful marriage. It has been described as a question of similar, opposite, or complemental temperaments and dispositions. The theory that love was all in all and that reason has no place in the matter is the commonest, and perhaps the most dangerous theory of all. In some modern countries the wishes of parents, who arrange the whole matter between the young man and the young woman, seem to work wonderfully well. The *dot* is fixed, love is assumed to come afterwards as a matter of course. On the whole, the American woman seems to have evolved most and is freest in her choices. The scientific and the eclectic theories of modern times assume a very large assortment of qualities and conditions for a scientifically sound marriage state. Love previous to marriage is seen to be, if not essential, yet the natural basis of most unions. Bodily health, suitable ages, conformability in education and social experience are all assumed to be necessary for the average case, but exceptions are admitted in all these. Few differ in laying down as essential that respect, a touch of adoration in the man and a dash of idealisation in the woman, a special unselfishness as regards the interests and wishes of the other, a give-and-take quality, a mutual consideration and helpfulness, a partnership, a friendship, a comradeship—if these are combined, then a union for life will be a safe arrangement for both parties ; but it is admitted that there is an element of risk in the matter always. No human prevision can anticipate how two human beings will combine into one life. Love may be and often is a name for passion. Indeed if there is no passion in the love that is consummated in marriage there is an essential lack. Experience of this must lead to disillusion and to actual dislike. Marriages founded on mutual intellectual and literary tastes have often been sad failures. The power of mutual adaptation is a natural gift about which too little has been said as a condition of scientific marriage. The power to fuse love into a pleasant and helpful comradeship is too little regarded. The mere sense of duty, apart from emotion, and apart from religion, is too little looked to as an element of scientific marriage. The physiological aspects of marriage are often present to the physician but are not a suitable subject of discussion in a popular work. The hygiene of the married condition implies the consideration, not of one mind, but of two minds in a peculiar and most intimate relation to each other, always acting and interacting on each other, separate in a sense but not free.

Nature, if properly interpreted, provides in sex itself the best and the most effective hygiene of the married state. The conscious cultivation of the strong points of each by husband and wife and the conscious admiration of the strong points of the partner is always one of the best measures of hygiene. The safest marriage always consists of a mutual admiration society of two. I have always held with the late Professor Laycock, who was a very subtle student of human nature, that a married couple need not be always together to be happy, and that in fact reasonable absences and partings tend towards ultimate and closer union.

Biography shows marvellous exceptions to any general rules that can be laid down. Tom Moore got all the flattery and all the charms of a brilliant society in London, and his wife lived in the country and got none of it at all, yet she seemed to be perfectly satisfied and happy. Rousseau seemed to find happiness of a sort in married arrangements that defied all reasonable anticipations.

The number of " love marriages " where every circumstance was in favour of a happy union for life, but which have turned out failures, has been innumerable. The royal marriages of old were arranged on every principle but that of the mutual affection of the couple, and yet a very considerable proportion of them, probably more than half, turned out to be averagely happy, some of them ideally so. Woman is so constituted that it takes in most cases a great deal of neglect and even positive cruelty to make her entirely unhappy as a wife. If she has children they naturally become the centres of her affection, and she feels less the loss of it in her husband. Which sex suffers most from incompatibility, unfaithfulness, and lack of conjugal affection it is somewhat difficult to say, but I think the female sex suffers most and says least about it. Speculations have been entered into as to the proportion of successful and happy marriages in modern times, but there are really no definite data on which to found any certain conclusions. I would give it about three-fourths. The question naturally arises, What is the best thing to be done if there is an entire loss of affection and utter incompatibility of disposition or an actual repulsion ? The answer of the Church of old was that there was no remedy. The answer of Milton and modern society, especially in America, is that divorce and separation are justifiable and expedient. So far as science has any say in the matter —and it has a large say when all is done—the answer would be, that as a man and a woman have only their lives to live once over there can scarcely be any moral or religious consideration that should tie two human beings together indissolubly when the effect is continuous unhappiness and absolute interference with the ends of life. Law and sociology, however, would have a great deal to say as to the risks of applying such a principle. The obvious interest of children comes in as something that cannot possibly be got over. The great moral of this momentous question is this—that marriages should be most carefully considered and due time taken before they are entered into. One of the factors in solving the problem has been far too little inquired into hitherto. The heredity of each of the couple who are thinking of being married cannot be too closely scanned. An unhappy husband—a good man—once said to me, "Ah, if I had only thought of my wife's mother, whom I knew very well, before I took the final step!" To conceal bad heredity, as is so often done, should be regarded as anything but a venial sin. There are few things indeed in ante-nuptial lives that should be concealed before marriage is entered into. They are always found out afterwards, and are often the bane of married life. There is no doubt whatever that engagements should be of reasonable length, so that each should know the other and mere passing gusts of emotion should have time to die out. Science looks forward to the time when such an evolution of insight and knowledge together should have taken place in both sexes that they shall know definitely whether any one individual is really suited to become the husband or wife of any other. The theory of "marriages being made in heaven," no doubt, represented the vague conclusion that the most important social arrangement among mankind must, like all else, be subject to definite laws—at least that would be the scientific explanation of the adage.

The birth-rate in all civilised countries is found to be

going down, and in some cases at an alarming rate. This is especially the case among the educated, the well-off, and the intellectual classes. It means that the gains of the evolution of centuries are being lost or thrown away, and that they must be recovered slowly and painfully, and with much risk afterwards from the unevolved strata of society. It means that social and conventional arrangements are overpowering Nature's basal laws. The very latest investigations, published in 1905, clearly exclude natural causes to a large extent for this result. The restriction in the number of children among married people is in the main selfish in motive, and is of evil omen. It undoubtedly results, in many cases, in bad health, a hardened moral nature, and a very a-social state of mind. It is the acme of selfishness and of bad citizenship. Nature, in many cases, inflicts on it severe punishment. There is something wrong in any society where it exists to any extent. Ignorance and its effects are responsible for much, but not for its entire prevalence. It is the duty of science and hygiene to step in, in this matter, and before it is too late. France stands out as the worst example of the common practice of the voluntary restriction of families among modern nations, and she has suffered the greatest punishment in a stationary population, and a tremendous fall in power.

CHAPTER XV

THE DECADENT PERIOD, FROM 55 TO THE END OF LIFE

The Climacteric.—Mental Hygiene comes in at the period of slow decadence from 55 to the end of life more than in the middle period and less than in the earlier periods. There are unquestionably slow but great mental and brain changes during this period. Those changes affect all the faculties, more or less, but especially those of emotion, energising, and memory. The great instinct of the reproduction of the species weakens and dies. The affectiveness changes in its object, and shows greater intensity from the mate to the progeny. Losing their imaginative force, their fire and their fierceness, poetry and love tales then cease to have the power to set the brain on fire. Action of all kinds gradually ceases to be so pleasurable for its own sake as it has been in the earlier periods of life. The reasoning power does not necessarily lessen, indeed it often strengthens till age is fairly well advanced, when there occurs actual decay and atrophy of the brain cells in senility. The " wisdom of age " is a human quality so universally recognised from the earliest ages that it not only must exist as a fact, but must have greatly impressed mankind. Conduct becomes more directly and universally under the influence of reason and fact rather than emotion and impulse. The subtle interest of the society of the other sex is less electric and overmastering. Life becomes slower mentally and physically. A genial contentment takes the place of a striving ambition. Courage lessens, and a certain indefinable sadness sometimes comes in. Shakespeare well depicts the early stage of the period, when he makes Antonio, the former active merchant, say—

> "In sooth, I know not why I am so sad :
> It wearies me ; you say it wearies you ;
> But how I caught it, found it, or came by it,
> What stuff 't is made of, whereof it is born,
> I am to learn ;
> And such a want-wit sadness makes of me,
> That I have much ado to know myself."

No doubt, the course of human affairs has often been changed, battles have been lost, and great projects unaccomplished because this mental condition came on the makers of history. At a later period of life still, when old age has set in, the changes in mental faculty are still more marked. All this mental change is accompanied, and is accurately enough expressed, if we could read it, by the changes of mental expression in the face and eye, of gesture, of walk, and of appetite. The form alters, especially in women. Certain internal glands lessen in bulk, the red blood corpuscles diminish in number, the nutritive energy of every tissue is less, and in certain respects the defences against disease are lowered. The voice changes towards the end of the period, the heart and the arteries lose force, and the brain begins slowly to shrink. Where the heredity is good, the health average, and there has been no special exposure to stress, over-exertion, privation, or disease, the whole process of decadence should be slow, gradual, and normal, with no cataclysms and few dangers if the circumstances and environment are favourable. Those conditions, however, are seldom fulfilled all of them together. The difference between a normal and an abnormal or diseased decadence is often great and striking. As I pointed out, when treating of the earlier periods of life, the brain faculties appear in a certain regular order. So in decadence the decay of faculty should follow a definite order and law of dissolution. It is the unequal and abnormal kind of dissolution that gives trouble, and that should be known by those who practise Mental Hygiene among the elderly. The earlier periods of decadence, perhaps, admit of more affective hygiene than the later. Those earlier periods are called climacteric. The "grand climacteric" period was fixed at 63 by the classical authors in the man. They were not far wrong, except that there is no one year of life to which it can be strictly confined. It is an epoch rather than a sudden event. In reality, and looked at with the modern physiological eye, we must put it down as covering at least five years in both sexes, this occurring seven or eight years earlier in the woman than in the man, and even to those general rules there are many individual exceptions. Some men grow old at 30, and die of old age at 40; other men do not grow old till they are 80, and do not die of old age till they are 100. There are animals low in the animal scale that die at once after the reproductive act is carried out. The meaning of the climacteric biologically is therefore clear enough. It is the departure of one great function and a slow lessening of all the others. The rules of its hygiene, therefore, must be absolutely founded on those facts. The intense energising, the ceaseless thinking, the overdoing of all kinds of work and enjoyment, which might be allowable if not continued too long at a time, during full manhood and womanhood, can no longer be safely practised when this period has commenced. All output must be lowered to the capacity of the producing mechanism. The way in which some men and women suddenly collapse at this period either results from bad heredity or too much overpressure for the period, or both combined. The weak points are beginning to come out, and must be carefully considered and allowed for if the remainder of the life is to be as effective as it can be and as happy as the lowered energies permit of. To those for whom it is possible, a distinct rest-ing-time about this period, a change of scene, a long voyage, a deliberate slackening of business or professional engage-ments, and a considerable change of diet are all desirable, and may make all the difference in attaining that green old age which every one would like to enjoy. To adapt, in fact, hygiene to the physiology and psychology of the period seems not only common sense but a duty which all men and women owe to themselves. The tendency among the strong and the healthy is to resent Nature's sure law of decay and to disregard her danger-signals until it is too late.

There are certain obvious and well-known mental dangers of the climacteric which have attracted the atten-tion of all observers of human nature, though the subject has not been systematically treated from the combined mental, moral, and bodily points of view. Some of those dangers and risks are capable of mitigation, others are not so. Perhaps the most common of all the mental changes which take place at the climacteric is the *tedium vitæ* of the classical authors. This may exist in every degree from an almost imperceptible loss of interest in living and all that it implies, up to the complete cessation of the love of life. That love of life and the constant effort to preserve and prolong it is the radical instinct of all human beings and of all the animal creation that is in a normal con-dition. It is impossible to imagine the existence of life in any higher form if this instinct were not a strong and essential part of it. It is the basis of all the interests and pleasures of living. It is the foundation of all the exertions which men and animals undergo to secure food and drink and air and pleasure. It is the root incentive to improve the environment which has been the basis of civilisation and the main stimulus of human evolution so far as that has been brought about apart from fixed natural conditions. That love of life is keener in its earlier periods because the pains and penalties, the stresses and disappointments of life have not been felt. It is strong enough in matured manhood and womanhood, but in many circumstances and by many individuals doubts are sometimes theoretically felt as to the *cui bono* of living. Those transitory points of interrogation do not really affect society materially. When the climacteric comes, it is different. The conscious intensity of life is felt to diminish. Its interests are not so absolutely overmastering and death not so absolutely abhorrent. The philosophical tone of mind and the theories of the Stoics, which included the idea that death is as much a natural part of existence as birth, are then beginning to be realised and to affect the feelings and even the conduct. No doubt the Stoic philosophy never took its origin among men who were young. The *tedium vitæ* often implies an instinctive feeling that work, exertion, and effort are not always entirely worth the doing. Physiologically and psychologically, energising by itself is no longer felt to be so necessary. *Tedium vitæ* often leads to a lowering in the desires and ideals. Pleasures that cost little and imply small exertion are preferred to pleasures of the higher sort that need some strenuousness to attain them. The well-off man and woman at this period often take, in a larger degree than in the earlier periods of life, to the pleasures of the table, because they are easily attained and imply no exertion. For the same reason I have known many people take to alcohol then, because in them it seemed to be the simplest way of reviving some of the intensities of their former lives or of deadening the regrets which the conscious absence of those intensities created.

In some persons at the climacteric there are apt to arise what may be called obsessional feelings—that is, strange ideas come into the mind apart from the will and often contrary to volitional effort in a somewhat dominant and irresistible way. They come like strangers unbidden to a feast. Sometimes such ideas are merely theoretical, in other cases they tend towards some kind of action of an unreasonable kind. A man gets an idea that his account-books of last year contained an error or that he had not posted a certain letter, or that he might have done something which would harm a friend. He does nothing and nothing comes of it. Or a woman takes it into her mind that she had neglected some duty in regard to a dead child, or that her thoughts had wandered to improper subjects during her prayers, or that she had not educated her children in the right way. Sometimes such obsessions or " imperative ideas " cause much unhappiness. Sometimes when they are exceedingly imperative they may go the length of leading to suicide. Persons with brains that have been highly educated and that are of a metaphysical, reasoning, and questioning character are most apt to suffer from this obsessional or ultra-critical state of mind. In its early stages and in a minor degree it can often be reasoned down and so got rid of. It can often be laughed at even when half believed. Or it may be the prelude to actual insanity. I have known many women at the climacteric take most preposterous and obsessional notions as to gentlemen paying attention to them and proposing marriage. If such an idea remains a mere theory, kept to herself or merely communicated to her intimate friends, it is all very well, but I have known it result in very unpleasant persecution of the supposed lovers and in most ludicrous acts with serious consequences, such as giving the two names to have the banns proclaimed in church, taking a house in the name of the imaginary lover or ordering a large supply of groceries or furniture for their common use.

Turning to the emotional and affective life, there are always changes, to a greater or less extent, at the climacteric. The general intensity of the emotional life is, as I have already referred to, lowered. This takes many forms, the most common being undoubtedly a lessened conscious affection between husband and wife. It is well indeed if by that time a friendship, a comradeship, a mutual helpfulness and dependence have been so firmly established that the passion and the lessened emotional fervour is not so much missed. Conscientious, sensitive women often deeply deplore this lessening of conscious affection, and it causes them much unhappiness. It often takes the form, where there are no children, of an almost pathetic and constant effort to be helpful, to anticipate needs and to persist, in season and out of season, in being in the presence of the mate. The lessened emotion is thus sought to be made up for. I cannot say that I have ever seen maternal affection in any way diminished even at the climacteric or through its influence. There is no doubt that between persons of the same sex, close friendships of the previous life are often less cultivated at this period. Men and women who have seen each other every day or every week during the previous life are content with a monthly visit or a casual meeting at the club. In the male sex it is often felt to be necessary to spend more time and to get more dependent on such games as whist or bridge to pass the time and to make life tolerable, independently of its affective interest. In short, the tone of life is rather lower emotionally, after the climacteric has set in. It is notorious that new friendships, especially of the more intimate sort, are not nearly so apt to be formed after the climacteric as before. There is, in fact, a lowered intensity of social instinct as well as of emotion. Social functions often become a bore. The instinct of gregariousness is lessened.

The failure of memory which old age brings undoubtedly begins first to show itself at the climacteric. Names are forgotten. The things of yesterday do not grave themselves so deeply into consciousness and do not rise by representation so vividly. Persons with whom you have a somewhat slight acquaintance are not so readily recognised nor their names remembered.

The will power, the originating faculty, is certainly lessened at the climacteric. Great deeds, involving intense and persistent will power, are less frequently seen. It is not so great and conscious a pleasure to command others. Purposes are more easily departed from. There is a greater tendency to ask the opinion of younger men and to act on it. I do not say that the negative exhibition of will power which is called obstinacy is lessened ; it is, in fact, sometimes accentuated and more unreasonable than before.

The faculty of speech is diminished. Fewer words are used to express meanings and the general literary faculty is lessened. Up to manhood and during part of that period, speech and words are all the time increasing in perfection and number. After the climacteric they gradually undergo a shrinkage.

The imagination and the poetic faculty undergo a very great change and sometimes an entire obscuration at this period. Some have gone the length of saying that no poetry was ever written by a man over the age of 50. But this cannot be quite true when we have in our minds the poems of Wordsworth and Tennyson written long after that age. But the form of the poetry undoubtedly under-

Q

goes a change then, and it is doubtful if such men as Byron and Burns, had they lived, would have produced any characteristic poetry after that age.

There are present in many post-climacteric people vague feelings of organic bodily discomfort which are difficult to analyse and impossible to name. They do not amount to pain nor to unhappiness, but there is a something which interferes with the full enjoyment of life and which means that the processes of nutrition and the working of the great internal organs connected with digestion are not done as well as before and no longer give conscious satisfaction. This feeling is often connected with a newly developed constipation of the bowels and with the diminished keenness of the appetite for food. The modern school of pathology would be inclined, I think, to account for this by assigning as its cause an incomplete metabolism in the tissues of the body and a slight amount therefore of an "auto-intoxication." All recent physiological and medical study and experience go to show that the diet should be materially changed in amount and in kind at this period of life.

Sleep tends to change in character and to diminish in amount at this period. It is not so deep, it is more dreamy, and there is often wakefulness earlier in the morning.

There is a condition of chronic grumbling and dissatisfaction with everything which is frequently characteristic of the climacteric, especially among the better-off classes. It represents an incapacity to take pleasure in and to be satisfied with the things which formerly filled up life pleasantly and with the usual humdrum routine work of life. You see people with everything apparently that heart could wish get into a dissatisfied and often restless condition. Nothing pleases them. They are always criticising their neighbours. Nobody can do anything rightly for them. If there has been anything of the cynic in the man he then becomes more disagreeably so. Very often such persons have been of an active, managing disposition, who have had a good deal of their own way and were never satisfied without this, but who did their work well. Something seems to have gone wrong in them in a chronic way. Neither their pleasures nor their work in life seem to satisfy them and the new things they so constantly take to do not last long in the satisfaction they give.

Perhaps the most serious of all the changes that are apt to occur at the climacteric is a tendency to an actual depression of mind, with much increase of foreboding and fears for the future. There is a tendency to "vain regrets." There is a feeling of deadness of the emotional nature of which men are conscious rather too acutely and are alarmed at what is going to happen to them. There is often also a sort of "cloudiness" of mind and feeling which seems to prevent them thinking clearly, feeling pleasantly, and coming to decided conclusions in their business and the affairs of life. The brain seems befogged and depressed. Often there are curious perverted sensations in the internal organs with an organic "distress." With those mental feelings there is usually a great loss of appetite, a want of enjoyment in food and drink, sleep-lessness, a loss of flesh with a tendency to a bad colour and darkening of the skin in tint. The "freshness" of complexion is lost.

The true hygiene of the climacteric ought, no doubt, to have been begun in the previous stage of life. Over-work, over-worry, idleness and aimlessness, love of over-eating and drinking, and too little exercise during the period of manhood and womanhood all tend towards a disturbed climacteric. When any of those mental symptoms that I have been describing do actually appear there are three

measures that, above all, may be effectual for their mitigation or cure. Those are an extra abundance of fresh air,
change of scene, and an alteration of diet so as to make it
less stimulating. To many such people fresh air seems to
be a specific. While out in the air, especially bracing air
with sunshine, they feel like their former selves. All the
little mental peculiarities disappear for the time being.
No doubt this effect is got through the oxygen of the air
giving just the right kind of stimulus which the brain
needs for its proper mental action. It accentuates all
the nutritive processes of the body, and makes the great
internal organs and glands work more actively to complete the conversion of the food into living tissue. Along
with the fresh air a certain amount of exercise, but not too
much, is needed.

Exhausting walks or cycle rides should be avoided. For
a man there are probably no two such suitable exercises
as golfing and fishing. They seem to supply just the
amount of muscular exertion needed to exercise and rouse
the mental power into a steadily pleasurable feeling. The
change of scene of which I have spoken should certainly
not take the form of rapid and exciting travelling. That
becomes wearisome, to many people involves worry, and is
too much of a mental exertion. Probably the popularity
of the Scottish " Hydropathics " is owing to their extreme
suitability for persons in the gentle down-grade of life. It
always struck me when I have seen the visitors to those
establishments that such persons formed the majority of
them. There has been a right popular instinct in
placing most of those high up on a hillside or by the
seashore. I have noticed that the most popular and
most frequented " Hydros " are placed where the air is
bracing, and there was little temptation to life's more
exciting pleasures. No doubt sea voyages of the right
kind, and with reasonable luck in the company and the

weather, fulfil in a high degree the conditions for improving the mental tone of the climacteric and preventing further mischief in man or woman. The sitting and walking on the ship's deck all day with the superabundance of ozone which this implies, and the absolute purity of the air, all tending to hunger and sleep, are most admirable mental restoratives.

There are many natural waters and watering-places whose effects are hygienic and curative, by improving not only the physical but the mental tone of the climacteric. This is better understood in Germany than here. Those waters should be of the tonic and chalybeate kind, and in some cases those containing sulphur are good in their effects. But so much depends on the temperament of the patient, on the constitutional diseases to which he is subject, and on his former mode of life, that no general rule can be laid down applicable to any individual as to taking courses of natural waters. One can only say that they are often exceedingly effective in restoring a sluggish, unhappy climacteric dyspeptic to a better state of brain and mind.

The non-stimulating diet, and that in not too great abundance, takes less out of the waning vital forces, and stimulates the nervous system less than the too great amount of flesh diet to which our leisured, professional, and better-off industrial classes in this country are accustomed. So many people also have hereditary tendencies towards gout and rheumatism that it is desirable that the nitrogenous diet and proteids should be diminished. The climacteric is a time when certain hereditary diseases are apt to show themselves. The natural defences of vigorously acting nerves and energetic nutrition are then getting lowered, and so everything must be made as favourable to health as possible. Fruits, vegetables, cereals, and fish are the typical diet for the climacteric. Dr. Haig's theories in regard to diet and uric acid may not be universally applicable, but they are more so at the climacteric period of life than at any other. Excess of alcohol is especially bad at this period, but, on the other hand, I think for certain persons light natural wines and weak beers, used in a dietetic form and in strict moderation, are undoubtedly beneficial as tonics, and aids to digestion as well as mild nerve stimulants.

Nature provides that there is a period of mental peacefulness, calm, and health, with even a reasonable amount of energy of the right sort in many cases, between the crisis of the climacteric and the beginning of old age. Especially in the female sex there is better health enjoyed at this nondescript period of life than has existed for twenty or thirty years previously. Many of the dangers and excitements of life have passed ; its passions have abated, and the powers of judgment and control have asserted themselves over emotion and impulse. Much good work, especially of the judicial and benevolent sort, is done at this period of life. If strenuousness is not so great, caution is enormously increased. The experiences of the former life are applied in a really effective way. Much happiness may be enjoyed if a too keen enjoyment is not expected or strained after.

Old Age.—Normal senility is the purely physiological abatement and decay in the mental functions going along with the brain shrinkage and the lessening of energy in all the other functions of the organism which mark the last part of life. Its full psychology has yet to be written. No doubt if every one had a constitution with no special hereditary weaknesses, and that had been subjected to no special strains, all the functions of mind and body, except the reproductive, would decline gradually and simultaneously, and death would take place, not by any process of disease, but through physiological extinction. Physiological senility means typically no reproductive power, a greatly lessened affective faculty, diminished memory, lessened energising mental and bodily, lowered imagination, little adaptability to change, dulled emotion, slow mental action, less vigorous speech, impaired muscular co-ordination, changed expression of face and tone of voice, fewer blood corpuscles, a poorer nutrition, a tendency to disease of the arteries, lessened bulk of the whole body but notably of the brain, which alters structurally and chemically in its elements, the cells degenerating and the nerve currents becoming slower. In the young man there is an organic craving for action, which not being gratified there results organic discomfort; in the old man there is an organic craving for rest, and not to gratify that causes organic uneasiness. The three great dangers to normal mental senility are hereditary brain weakness, disease of the vascular system and toxic irritation of brain structure. Until the organ has begun physiologically to lose its structural perfection and its dynamic force the pathological phenomenon that we call senile mental disease is not developed. Heredity to insanity is less common in the case of senility than in any other form of mental disease except general paralysis, but there is this fallacy—that the facts about heredity are further back and more forgotten in this than at any other time. An old man's living relations are few and his ancestors' histories far off. It is a certain law of nervous heredity that the stronger the predisposition the sooner it manifests itself in life, and the weaker it is the later in life it shows itself. To have survived, therefore, the changes and chances, the crises and penalties of life with intact mental function till the age of 70, means only slight neurotic heredity or a great absence of exciting causes of disease. It is impossible to fix an age at which physiological senility begins. Some men are older at 50 than others at 70. I believe that in some cases neurotic heredity assumes the special form of early senility—that is, of early wear-out of purely organic staying power. Most congenital imbeciles and idiots grow old soon. Many of them die of old age at 30. Very many races of men grow old early, like the Kalmuks and Hottentots, but roughly speaking, among our race, one does not usually call a man old till he is over 65.

In King Lear we may find almost every mental symptom of old age. It is often felt to be coming on.

> " 'Tis our fast intent
> To shake all cares and business from our age;
> Conferring them on younger strengths, while we
> Unburden'd crawl toward death."

Well it would be for many old men if this intent were carried out. Those near them see the change both in character and temper—

> " The unruly waywardness that infirm and choleric years bring
>   with them."

And Goneril says—

> " You see how full of changes his age is."

Those sudden changes and loss of affection were vividly expressed in regard to his favourite daughter—

> " I lov'd her most, and thought to set my rest
> On her kind nursery. Hence, and avoid my sight!
> So be my grave my peace, as here I give
> Her father's heart from her ! "

The way in which old men must often be treated is put by Goneril in a vivid way when she says—

> "Old fools are babes again ; and must be us'd
> With checks as flatteries."

His forgetfulness, suspicion, irritability, impatience of contradiction, and his impulsive violence, are well exhibited when Lear says to Oswald, whom he had known very well—

> " My lady's father ! my lord's knave : you whoreson
>   dog ! you slave ! you cur.
> *Oswald.*   I am none of these my lord ; I beseech your pardon.
> *Lear.*   Do you bandy looks with me, you rascal ? (and strikes
>   him)."

The extreme mental confusion that sometimes occurs in senility is well expressed :—

> " Does any here know me ?—This is not Lear: does Lear walk thus ? speak thus ?   Where are his eyes ?   Either his notion weakens, or his discernings are lethargied.—Sleeping or waking ?—Ha ! sure 'tis not so.—Who is it that can tell me who I am ? "

The impulsive, unreasoning action appears thus—

> " Darkness and devils !
> Saddle my horses ; call my train together.
> Degenerate bastard !   I'll not trouble thee :
> Yet have I left a daughter."

The sudden emotionalism is often seen—

> " I'll tell thee !—Life and death ! I am ashamed
> That thou hast power to shake my manhood thus ;
> That these hot tears, which break from me perforce
> Should make thee worth them."

Often the old man realises that his mind is giving way, as when Lear pathetically says—

"O, let me not be mad, not mad, sweet heaven !
Keep me in temper : I would not be mad !"

" We are not ourselves,
When nature, being oppress'd, commands the mind
To suffer with the body."

" O fool, I shall go mad !"

His loss of memory appears everywhere throughout the play. Certainly when age and its infirmities go on to such mental dissolution as affected Lear, we may well say like Kent in the death scene—

" Vex not his ghost : O, let him pass ! he hates him,
That would upon the rack of this tough world
Stretch him out longer."

We must not take King Lear as representing ordinary old age. Fortunately, its common mental manifestations are far milder than the old monarch exhibited. His condition was of the aggravated and pathological sort of senility. The dramatist had to deepen the shadows in order to bring out the tragedy more forcibly. All the features are there, but we must tone them down to get the picture of the ordinary old man of everyday life.

As in childhood and youth the faculties first appear in a certain order, so in old age they commonly abate in regular sequence. The memory is unquestionably the first great faculty which shows signs of diminution, especially the memory for recent events is lessened, though there is much truth in Cicero's opinion that old men "recollect everything in which they take an interest."

The brain cells will not take on impressions so deeply or so readily as in the former life. As a matter of fact the power of keen attention is diminished, so that things are not seen by the inner eye of consciousness so vividly as before. The memories of the older things that occurred earlier in life are often vivid enough. The impressions that were then made were so deeply cut that they are not readily lost. So much of what we have to remember is pure memory and nothing else, with no connection of ideas, that it is no wonder things are forgotten when the brain cells have become less sensitive and shrink. Most names of things and persons are merely tickets, meaning nothing in themselves and not exciting any ideas or suggestions, and so making little impression. If every Mr. Brown was brown in colour, and every Miss Black was dark, there would be no difficulty in remembering their names. The next faculty which fails in natural order is the originating power, in a far deeper degree than during the climacteric. This always implies much effort and output of nervous energy, and it is therefore natural for it to abate at this time. There is a greater tendency to put off doing and thinking about things, and the effort to originate is often really painful. The strong exercise of will power is next impaired, not that its negative obstinacy always goes. Sometimes, as I have said, this is increased. But to impress one's will on others, to make it overcome difficulties, to put obstacles out of the way by its means, is certainly a greater effort in old age than at an earlier time, and is less forceful. With will, the power of control naturally becomes lessened. Self-control, inhibition, mental and bodily, being on the whole the greatest thing in man, cannot be expected to survive a shrinking brain. Emotion suffers abatement at the same time as inhibition. The actual keenness of feeling is not so great. Emotion does not carry a man away with a strong and irresistible wave as it used to do. The old rarely feel with the same intensity the loss of friends and children and wives and husbands as the younger do. The control over the exhibition of emotion is, however, much lessened, and therefore some people think that the old feel more. They do not do so. They merely show it more. They are more emotional through lack of power to conceal it. It is notorious that the very old will weep and laugh at little. This, in fact, is a sign of advanced age. It is also a sure sign of many of those gross brain changes which are classed under the name of "softenings of brain" and paralysis. An old man, who is also paralytic, weeps at the sight of his friend or the sound of his name. He also laughs, in an uncontrolled way, at the least suggestion of what is ludicrous. The intellect is the last faculty to disappear or weaken. It does weaken if a man lives long enough, but it commonly lasts out most of the other faculties. Possibly, the very highest and most difficult form of reasoning, especially in regard to abstract subjects may be diminished, but a man of 75 or 80 will often come to the soundest conclusions from the facts put before him, when his memory is far gone and his energising power is much impaired.

All those mental and bodily changes in old age can now, through our most recent modes of microscopic examination of the brain, be seen to be accompanied by and co-related to corresponding deteriorations in the mental vehicle, the cells of the brain. By the naked eye there can be seen a general shrinkage in the size of the brain, and usually a great change in the blood-vessels that supply it with nourishment. This general atrophy of from 4 to 6 ounces corresponds to the lessening of mental force and the loss of memory. The cells become blurred in outline at first. Then a number of them begin to waste and look like " ghost cells " (fig. 10 *a*, *b*), and then finally disappear. The numbers of fibres passing outwards from each cell lessen and, as it were, "fall off," so that the connections of each with its neighbour cells lessen. The "nucleus," or central body of the cell, its most im-

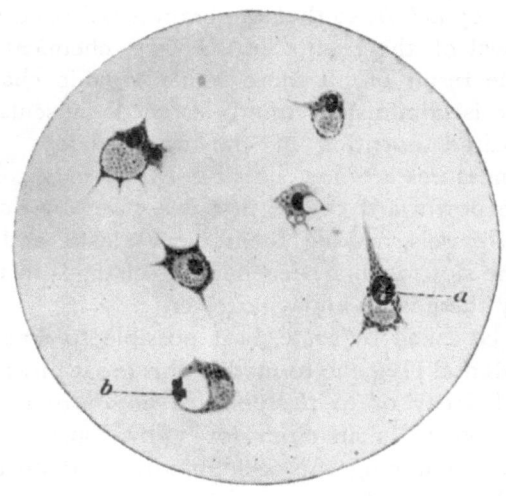

FIG. 10.—SIX EXAMPLES OF DETERIORATED CELLS FROM THE BRAIN OF AN OLD MAN OF 80 IN THE STATE OF EXCITED DOTAGE.

They show various stages of deterioration, degeneration, and shrinkage corresponding to the deteriorated and damaged mind of their owner. Not one of them was fit to be the vehicle of sound mental operations. *a*. Is least degenerated. *b*. Is most so. The others are in intermediate stages of damage. Those cells may be compared with figs. 2 and 3, pp. 16, 17.

portant part, is the last to disappear, but it often gets displaced and pushed to one side. Various degenerations take place in the contents of the cell, some of them getting masses of fat in their substance, some becoming "granular," and some acquiring little masses of a dark brown or black substance—the "pigmentary degeneration." The blood-vessels that supply the cells assume a clear look— the "hyaline degeneration"—and become inelastic, or they get partially blocked, so that the blood current that pours through them is lessened in volume and force. In some cases the drainage channels in the brain are partially obstructed by *débris*, so that the brain is poisoned through non-removal of the results of its own chemical action. The whole result of all those senile organic changes in the brain is diminished mind, lessened muscular force, and impaired nutrition of the whole body. Certain medical measures are now possible which may somewhat arrest the downward course in a few cases by acting on the blood-vessels, making them more elastic and patent. But for the slow, regular, degenerative changes in the cells in senility there is no known arrester.

It will be asked by some, Is it possible to do anything through Mental Hygiene to modify this great physiological process of decay or to postpone in any way its mental manifestations? Is an elixir for "slow-consuming age" possible? Something can undoubtedly be done to make old age happy and even useful. Every one with any experience and observation of life has seen old age that in all respects was delightful, as also old age that was unpleasant and almost intolerable. Whence the difference? In the one, through good heredity, a fortunate life, and favourable environments before and at the time, the process went on in a gradual and physiological way. In the other, through bad heredity, an unfortunate anterior life or unfavourable environment, the condition was one of explosiveness and irritability, with many troubles and responsibilities to all who had to do with it. If a man has had a reasonably good heredity, has been moderate in all things, has had some philosophy, morality, and religion in his life, if he has seriously fought the evil and cultivated the good, and if he has been reasonably fortunate in the general circumstances of his life, then we anticipate with confidence that he will exhibit the better and the happier side of old age and "live out his time," a comfort to himself and to others. Shakespeare does not help us with the hygiene of old age as he does with its symptoms. That was not his business, nor was the knowledge of the time sufficient to enable him to take the scientific view of the decadent brain and mind. He only mitigates it by "honour, love, obedience, troops of friends." Some of his old men are wise, but all are senile in mind, more or less. Some are "full of wise saws and modern instances," and some, like Polonius to Laertes, may give advice to serve a man in every difficulty of life. Yet still the conduct is that of old age. There are certain hygienic rules which, if practised, will help the attainment of the normal old age in a large degree. Probably the most important of these is to select and carry out occupations in life suitable to the period, to give up exciting and harassing work, to take to routine, easy occupations, to cultivate hobbies that do not imply too great exertion, to be wise enough to know when to give up the things that cause stress at the proper time. If old age receives honour and respect, and has not perhaps "troops of friends" but a few choice and intimate acquaintances, they exercise an extraordinarily soothing influence on the brain. Cicero says: "For what is more gratifying than old age surrounded by the studious attention of youth?" That comes, as a reward of wisdom, unselfishness, and benevolence towards the young in the former part of life. The typical environment of old age consists of a quiet home, sons, daughters, and grandchildren, not necessarily living in the home, but frequently accessible. Thus is attained Cicero's wish: "I like to see an old man with something of the youth." Thus opportunities are afforded of using for the good of others life's former experiences, and so making the world a wiser one through those experiences.   This undoubtedly has been one of the modes of human evolution.   Think how much is lost if a man of vigorous mind has no opportunity of handing his large experience on as he becomes old!   What an amount of practical wisdom such a man must have acquired!   In ancient times, this seemed to be more realised than now.   The Old Testament, and especially the Book of Proverbs—that summary of the everyday wisdom of the time—is full of reference to the value of the wisdom of age.   Cicero would not have written his treatise on old age except Roman society had appreciated the value of that time of life.   He says: "The old man does not do the same things as the young man ; no, but he performs much higher and better duties," though he admits old age "will never be anything but burdensome to a fool." His eulogium of farming, of going back to mother earth, and her soothing processes as an occupation, a resource and a solace for old age, may well be taken to heart in modern times.   His summing up applies more even to us than to the Romans, for we know more of Nature and her laws than they did.   " Here lies my wisdom, viz., that I follow the best guide, Nature, as a god, and am obedient to her laws."   " A youth of labour with an age of ease" is Nature's rule.   The life of the old, at least until near the last, should not be without some variety.   The frequently quoted adage, " Try and keep young," is a good one.   It is best carried out by seeing young people, by efforts to sympathise with them, and even by following at times and in a mild way some youthful pursuit or game.   A gentle contentment with life comes naturally enough to normal old age.   The very opposite state comes to the explosive and pathological variety of it.   It is marvellous how happily nowadays many men and women of 80 get through the twenty-four hours. I met such a man lately, who had led a busy, intellectual, and practical life, and I asked him, "Doesn't time hang heavy on your hands?" "Not at all," was his reply; "I never was so busy in my life, the days seem too short for me." He had, in fact, resumed hobbies and work of the right sort which he had not had time to do in his younger and busier days. Loneliness is certainly bad for the old. The brain and mind need the right sort of stimulus, and if they do not receive it they fall into a moody, selfish isolation. There is one trait which I have seen in some old people which is the cause of much misery—a jealousy of the young. The unreason of this is only equalled by its evil practical results, because it alienates and sends away just those social elements that might be helpful and hygienic. Much may be done by the old for their mental equanimity through right treatment of the body. Gentle exercise, fresh air, not too great exposure to cold, right diet, well cooked, non-stimulating, and easily digested, will do much for the old man's or the old woman's mind. I preach much milk, little flesh, and a very small amount of alcoholic liquor of any sort—though I am bound to say that there are some conditions of old age where the heart and the circulation are weak, or where the digestion and appetite are not good, in which some natural wines or ales or even a little good whisky, well diluted, certainly aid digestion and produce a feeling of strength and gentle stimulation that seem obviously good for the individual. No doubt, for the rich nowadays, when travel is made easy and the sunshine of Southern Europe or Northern Africa is accessible during the worst of our winter and spring, old age may thus be prolonged and helped. A saying of the first Lord Brougham used to be quoted, "that he would never die of old age if he got to Cannes in time every

R

year." Certainly his villa which he built there seems to come fairly close to a sunshiny Paradise for an old man. There are certain medicines of the gently sedative sort which, when rightly applied by the medical art, have the power to tide over irritability, and conditions of explosiveness and insomnia ; but, speaking generally, the less physic taken by the old the better. I am largely at one with my now venerable friend, Dr. George Keith, that "a simple life" is good for all ages and all conditions of men and women, but that it is especially good for the aged. He himself, not far from 90, hale, hearty, and cheerful, is an admirable example of the application of his own practice. His *Fads of an Old Physician* will well repay reading by every one who is approaching the older period of life, and his *Plea for a Simpler Life* has evidently made a deep impression on thoughtful people in this and other countries.

CHAPTER XVI

SPECIAL SEX QUESTIONS

A BOOK on Mental Hygiene that did not discuss certain questions relating to sex and sexual life—however delicate such questions may be—would not be complete. The reproductive instinct is the second strongest power in all the animal world. Therefore its study and right regulation is a consideration of great importance. Modern medicine and psychology are much concerned with such questions, and have come to decided conclusions about some of them from the scientific point of view which, to some extent at least, the public should know. Their honest treatment is not unattended with risks. "Where ignorance is bliss, 'tis folly to be wise." The mean between a dangerous ignorance and a prurient knowledge is difficult to steer. To some natures, and at certain periods of life, such knowledge seems to be overpoweringly suggestive of evil-thinking. Yet Science can scarcely accept ignorance on any important matters that deeply concern the health of men and women as being safe. Most men and many women have at some period received information about sex questions that was not knowledge, and have accepted, as facts, what was not true, having thus been misled and injured. Sex and all that it implies is so great a thing and so much knowledge about it is taught by Nature herself that Science is bound to step in to supplement. A sexless world would be a joyless world. Emotion, passion, beauty, art, imagination, poetry, valour, and chivalry are all mixed up with it. Even religion and morals have the closest relations to it. All religions have fought it or yielded to it. Many of the early Christians called it accursed, yet had in time to idealise womanhood in the cult of the Virgin and make her a chief feature in their devotion. Science treats sex in the cold light of passionless knowledge, yet feels that there is something behind which is not fully elucidated by its methods. History emphatically points to the decadence of mighty nations as being specially connected with departures from natural and moral laws and practices in regard to sexual relations. All degenerate nations are sexually corrupt. The coming in of riches and luxury has always had such dangers in every people of which history tells. St. Paul begins his greatest Epistle not by any exposition of the Christian faith or doctrine but by a scathing denunciation of those who gave themselves " up to uncleanness through the lusts of their own hearts to dishonour their bodies between themselves." There can be no reasonable doubt that a right solution and treatment of the reproductive problem is one of the keys to individual happiness, to social cleanness, and to national longevity. The sense of self-respect in the individual, his freedom from morbidness of feeling, his power of control, depend largely on his harmonious and natural reproductive development in youth and on his having conformed to natural law in his conditions of life and practices during that period. Premature or unnatural exercise is found to be most dangerous to the perfection of its proper development and to the end for which the function exists, viz., a strong, healthy race of the future. Such premature or unnatural exercise is equally fatal to the perfection of the emotional and moral qualities which are tied to the body functions. Proofs abound as to it being a physiological law that neither reproduction nor sexual function should be exercised till full bodily development is completed. Neither desire nor a certain capacity is the test of fitness here but the organic completeness of the whole organism. Developmental nutrition should have ended before reproductive output begins. There is only one natural mode of gratifying sexual *nisus* and reproductive instinct, and only one truly social arrangement—that of marriage— while there are many unnatural methods. Science, sociology, and Christianity are at one in their conclusions and prohibitions. If natural law is not obeyed we have emotional instability, impairment of manliness and of such social virtues as modesty, purity, control of imagination, and true chivalry. It will be observed that I am not now pressing any conventional or moral rules or any social or religious dicta, but the laws of body and mind and purely scientific facts. If those laws are broken we find arrested nervous energy, less capacity for work, tendencies to nervous excitement with frequently arrested growth of the body. We also find unnatural attention to reproductive trains of thought that seem to defy voluntary control and to paralyse more healthy mental occupation. There is less freshness of mind, less mental staying power, and less is made out of life. There is often also a tendency to actual nervous disease thus induced. The strong and natural tendency towards games and open-air exercises in youth that so powerfully help bodily and mental development is lessened. The power that has been wasted is the highest of all the bodily energies, and if energy is wasted in one direction it certainly diminishes the sum of force, mental and bodily, that remains. Nature will not be set at naught without exacting her penalty. Tainted hues are given to innocent subjects, social intercourse between the sexes—

that most delightful and hygienic of all social charms—is apt to be poisoned, the ideal of one sex in the mind of the other is lowered. Sin has been introduced into paradise. Nature has punished the law-breaker by leanness of soul and grossness of feeling. Even the pure ideals of motherhood, sisterhood, and brotherhood, on which the highest social life should be founded, are rendered less pure, for the youth whose ideal of womanhood has been formed on that of his mother and sister is almost safe against his lower passions so long, at least, as he "wears the white flower of a blameless life." He instinctively recoils against lust as a dishonour to them. To say that unlawful gratification is often mentally harmless, and that unnatural sexual practices are inevitable among the young, is to say that Nature in this matter has contradicted herself. To say that indulgence in youth is good for the health and that restraint is bad for it is contrary to fact and medical experience. Avoid the beginnings of evil is the essential thing in the matter. Well did St. Paul say "God" or Nature as many would now say, "gives up" the unnatural practiser of lust to his evil ways. Control over sex thoughts, imagination, and desire is best helped by diverting attention to other things, or by transforming the sex energy into the forces of work and thought. Like all forces it is capable of transmutation into other forms of energy. Constant and regular muscular exercise, games, and cold bathing convert it into muscular energy—hence their supreme importance in school life. Our foods are usually too great in amount and too stimulating in quality. The well-off and well-fed are far more apt to fall into evil practices than the ploughboy. Then the gross and animal may also be transformed into the ideal and poetic, as black coal is converted into luminous electricity. If a high social tone, a lofty ideal of woman's position in life, a strong sense of obeying law, and sound, strong muscles are all sedulously cultivated, there is far less fear of undue domination by lustful feelings and practices. Work of every honest kind is Nature's antidote to half the sex evils and dangers that weaken body and mind. Self-denial is a virtue that strengthens by exercise but is rapidly lost through indulgence. Looking over the biographies of some of the most gifted men and women, and reading between the lines, the Scientist sees the havoc made by uncontrolled sex feeling. An example of the highest form of idealisation of sex and love, linked with nature, is seen in Burns' song of "Flow gently, sweet Afton." He idealises Nature and his love ; but in the song Nature is only the setting, woman, the picture. He begins by saying he is to sing his song in praise of "sweet Afton," but he at once changes the note to love and his Mary. The poem is as psychologically true as it is beautiful—

" Flow gently, sweet Afton, amang thy green braes,
Flow gently, I'll sing thee a song in thy praise;
My Mary's asleep by thy murmuring stream,
Flow gently, sweet Afton, disturb not her dream.

Thou stock-dove, whose echo resounds through the glen,
Ye wild whistling blackbirds, in yon thorny den,
Thou green-crested lap-wing, thy screaming forbear,
I charge you disturb not my slumbering fair.

Thy crystal stream, Afton, how lovely it glides
And winds by the cot where my Mary resides!
How wanton thy waters her snowy feet lave,
As gath'ring sweet flow'rets she stems thy clear wave."

Nature and woman—but woman first ! How different would Burns' career have been had the purity of that song been the keynote of his life !

The poetic by temperament, the nervous and the unstable by constitution, are those who, especially in youth, have most difficulty in living rightly. If there is any taint of melancholy there is apt to arise in after-life a terrible retribution for sexual sins in the shape of exaggerated ideas as to permanent harm done and a remorse that is morbid.

While I have thought it my duty to speak plainly as to sex risks and evils, I am equally bound to point out that the harm done to the brain is often temporary and remediable. Sensible people can usually be made to see this, but on the minds of the nervous people of whom I have spoken there is apt to be cast a glamour of sex imaginings, a morbid fascination that is most difficult to cast aside. A straight fight against it is not always the best way, but through diversion, healthy bodily work, an outdoor life and a literature of a passionless hue, the mind can be turned to healthier channels. I have known natural science, mathematics, engineering, farming, all used to fill up the spare time and direct the attention from such morbid domination. Evil and unnatural sex excitement and practices unquestionably infest many of our schools for both sexes. Especially in the semi-monastic aggregations of boys in our public schools is the evil sometimes rampant. Bad teaching for example, and the somewhat unnatural life away from mothers and sisters and female friends, all tend towards this evil. I was inclined at one time to think it was especially prevalent in such schools in England. But recent accounts by reliable medical observers in Germany and America, where there are few schools on our model, make me doubt this. In the Latin countries, in spite of the energetic efforts of the Roman Catholic Church, it is equally bad or worse. It certainly can be prevented and controlled, but that cannot be done by any " system," but by the unceasing vigilance and supervision of individual masters, by creating a right "tone" in a school and by the introduction in some cases of strong, manly, and religious motives of the right sort. The appeal to manliness and the effects of suitable instruction by the right sort of person, with the close attention and supervision referred to, are on the whole the best counteractions. I strongly advocate, as I have said, that the family doctor, guided by the parent and the teacher, is by far the best instructor and monitor. The knowledge should be given early in adolescence or late in boyhood, but the development of the individual boy must be taken into consideration. The precise amount and kind of knowledge cannot be stated in any accurate way. Each doctor would take his own way of giving it. It should be direct and perfectly intelligible, and the evils and dangers of breaking the law of one's nature emphasised. Shame, fear, and a sense of right should all be appealed to. If boys were as well looked after as girls are at home by their mothers the evil habit would certainly be avoided in most cases. It is often acquired and taught at such early ages that there is no knowledge of its meaning and effects. A lad, healthily constituted in body, mind, and morals, does not tend to come under its influence to any very hurtful extent for long, and in late adolescence, when the faculty of inhibition has come fully in, its effects are fortunately forgotten in most cases. There is a natural organic repugnance which arises and conquers the evil. It is in the cases of lads—and girls too—of a nervous organisation and heredity, where a deeper hold is laid, where the control is quite lost, and when exhaustion of the vital powers takes place. In such it seems to take possession like an evil spirit that will not be exorcised. Quack advertisements of a suggestive kind are responsible for much harm. It is a strange sort of ethics which enjoins a newspaper proprietor to preach righteousness and denounce thieves, and yet pocket hundreds a year from such vile sources. Those are the youths who very specially need early care and watching. The quality of brain and constitution of the subject is the true explanation of the differences or of the harm done by those evil habits. Much may be done by medical management as well as by knowledge and by the strengthening of the faculty of inhibition. The dangerous stage is when the sex feeling has arisen—and that is often prematurely developed—and the inhibitory faculty and moral sense have not developed in strength enough to control and regulate it.

There sometimes occurs a senile and post-climacteric recrudescence of sex which is thoroughly morbid and sometimes leads to painful and most inconvenient effects. Some very unsuitable and even unnatural marriages of old men take place through this. It commonly does not last long. It is a mental rather than a physical phenomenon. Certain medical measures are sometimes helpful. The family distresses and disturbances thus caused are often most painful. It is well to understand its meaning and not to give a too exclusively moral aspect to the facts.

CHAPTER XVII

MENTAL HYGIENE OF ALCOHOL, TOBACCO, AND OTHER BRAIN STIMULANTS AND SEDATIVES

THERE are many physical agents in common or occasional use through which Mental Hygiene is improved or upset. Some of those act on the brain indirectly. There are others which act directly on the organ of the mind. Alcohol is the type of the latter. Through its common dietetic use in the form of wine in the countries where the grape is a natural product, it has there become virtually an article of diet of almost universal consumption. There are many other substances whose action on the brain is also direct and their effects somewhat similar, such as opium, which in the East is said to be used by more individuals than those who consume alcohol in the West. It is so little used here that I need scarcely refer to it in connection with hygiene. Except as a medicine, its use by Europeans may be condemned absolutely and without qualification. Still more does this condemnation hold good in regard to Indian hemp, which among the Malay people is a very common brain stimulant. Such powerful medical substances as chloral, sulphonal, trional, veronal, paraldehyde, and cocaine, are also nerve stimulants or sedatives that some of our people have got into the evil habit of using without sufficient medical reasons. Such use is to be most emphatically condemned. Cocaine is probably the most seductive and therefore dangerous of all the brain stimuli, and the most destructive to the great function of self-control. It is usually persons of a nervous temperament who take to the habitual use of such substances, and it is precisely to those persons they are most injurious and difficult to stop if a habit has once been formed. With alcohol the case is in many ways different. It is believed by many chemical physiologists to be a food, but it is admitted by them all to be a very inefficient and expensive one. To say that in the wine countries its use is always hurtful and to be deprecated would be to make a statement for which there is no definite scientific ground. To propose the entire disuse of wines in France and Italy would be to go against the universal and immemorial customs and traditions of the inhabitants of those countries. If such a recommendation were actually carried out in France it would upset and revolutionise one of the greatest agricultural industries of the country. No fact is more certain, looking to the history of mankind, than that it tried to obtain and largely use alcohol, or some such substance, from very early times as an adjunct and aid to feasting. Man was never satisfied with bread and butter only, and never will be. Substances that stimulate or soothe the brain and mind are craved for. Without going the length of Dr. Archdall Reid and saying that its use is an inherited " natural instinct," we must admit that its frequency is a strong argument for an exhaustive and impartial inquiry on the latest scientific and sociological methods before it is condemned.[1] There can be no doubt whatever that it often gives pleasure and accentuates the social instincts, and therefore adds to the happiness of the people where wine is an article of daily and dietetic consumption. In wines the alcohol is much diluted, and is

---

[1] Such an enquiry is embodied in a forthcoming volume of the *New Library of Medicine*. [Editor's Note.]

usually taken as a part of meals. Take Great Britain, Germany, Scandinavia, Russia, and a considerable part of America, the use of alcohol stands on a different basis from the wine countries. Beers, though essentially artificial products, may be dietetically used with pleasure and advantage to appetite and digestion, though they have undoubted dangers. Spirits undiluted cannot be said to have anything to do with any ordinary physiological diet. The tendency to excess in alcohol in most European countries has been so great, and when indulged in unduly has been so manifestly injurious to body, mind, and morals, that restrictions have been imposed by all civilised Governments on the making and selling of it. This was not for purposes of revenue only, but also to check undue use. Sweden and Norway are perhaps the best examples of the unhygienic and hurtful use of strong alcohol at one time—about sixty years ago, when there was no restriction on its manufacture and almost universal excess in its use—and of the enormous improvement in health and morals secured by very severe legislative measures restricting its production and sale in recent times. The use of alcohol has, in spite of those restrictions, been gradually increasing of late years in most of the European industrial nations. France stands at the head of European consumers of alcohol at the present time. It is estimated that from 15 to 16 gallons of pure alcohol is the average consumption per inhabitant of that country, most of this being in the form of wine. Unfortunately distilled liquors of a raw and very pernicious sort have come into general use by the French working people in addition to their wines. The universal testimony of physicians, statesmen, social reformers, and sociologists in that country is that a manifest deterioration in physique, in mind, and in morals has taken place in the workmen of the large cities through this excessive use of strong and bad alcohol. The democracy of France are gradually being educated to take this view, and the Government which represents it is devising measures for restricting the use of such liquors for the sake of the morals and hygiene of the people.

In Great Britain and Ireland the alcohol problem, in various aspects, has become a very acute one. We use about 14 gallons of absolute alcohol a year per inhabitant, the cost of which is worked out at £4 per person, or £160,000,000 of a total drink bill each year. That this is a huge excess is admitted by all who have looked into or thought about the question. It is admitted to be one of the chief sources of our poverty, crime, and disease mental and bodily. The latest returns, most fortunately, show a steady decrease of consumption, amounting to £33,000,000 for the past five years. There can be no doubt that when our industries are prosperous and our wage-earning population is receiving large wages a very undue amount of the money earned is spent on an excessive amount of alcohol. As yet they are not educated to spend their money rightly for their advantage. Few measures of hygiene, either bodily or mental, would produce so great an improvement in the Mental Hygiene of our population as the restriction of the use of alcohol to a moderate amount. There is no use talking at present of its total prohibition. No free people would tolerate that its wants, real or imaginary, should be so treated by Act of Parliament. There is, however, an enormous scope for teaching the bad effects of alcohol on the brain and mind, so that the moral sense of the people should be roused and a "health-conscience" created against this excess. In every school this should be done. In that way, not only would the bad effects of excess be diminished, but by the evolution of the moral sense in this direction a gain would be made to the higher life of the nation. The great faculty of inhibition thus strengthened and joined to a sense of right and wrong, would come in in other departments of life, and we should have a society not only better off through being more temperate, but more thoughtful, cleaner, sweeter, more moral, and in all probability more religious. Beyond any doubt, alcohol ministers to, and accentuates, the lower and the more animal part of man even though it may in many people also increase their happiness, transitorily at least, promote their social feelings, and rouse an ideal in the mind, of a sort. I cannot admit, because there is no proof of it, that alcohol makes the life of any people more effective by increasing its output of work done. No one who reads the accounts of the state of social life in England, and particularly in Scotland and Ireland in the early part of the nineteenth century, when alcoholic excess was habitual and respectable among the educated classes, can for a moment say that its present diminution in those classes has not resulted in a mental and moral improvement. This lessening of the use of alcohol among those classes was the result of an increase in their self-respect and moral tone. It did not come through legislation, and this is perhaps the most encouraging fact to make us hope that a similar social and moral education among the masses of our people will also have the effect of their voluntarily restricting its use to at least as moderate dimensions as now prevail among most of the educated classes.

Alcohol has a special affinity for the brain and affects its mental and bodily working at once after it has reached the organ through the blood. Recent experiments of a very careful nature have been made by Professor Kraepelin, of Munich, and others, to ascertain the real mental effect of alcohol in doses that would be called moderate. The results have unquestionably gone against even such moderate use. The reasoning power, the memory, and the will power were found to be all affected for the worse. Not so much mental work could be done with those moderate doses as without them, and it was less accurate. It was also found that a certain effect is left for a time in the brain cells, through which, after the alcohol has been completely stopped for a week or a fortnight and its use then resumed, the former effects recur sooner and under the use of smaller doses. The effect of such experiments has been that in Switzerland and Germany a very strong movement is going on among the medical profession against the use of alcohol in any shape and in any quantity. The craving for its continuous use which it creates in so many brains, especially those of the nervous types, the diminution of inhibition in every shape which is its direct result and the absolute destruction which it causes to the whole fabric of morals and conduct in many people who use it to excess, are indeed very strong arguments against its use. They are a tremendous set-off against the pleasurable effects and even the restorative and dietetic uses of this substance. As I have had occasion to point out strongly, in treating of the earlier periods of life, alcohol should certainly not then be used at all. Also it should not be used by those of a nervous temperament and with a predisposition to mental or nervous disease. Its effects in excess on such persons are entirely disastrous and destructive to the higher forms of mental life and conduct. I believe that the pessimism and nervousness which in many persons result from our modern city lives of excitement and unrest, are partly due to the use of alcohol. I am certain that its use accentuates and makes more dangerous those moral and mental characteristics of modern life. This I believe is more seen in America, where the pace of life is even faster than with us, where the climate is on the whole more stimulating and the type of man and woman is more nervous, though in America the consumption of alcohol is only about one-half per person of what it is in Great Britain. Few medical men or physiologists can doubt that America gains greatly through this smaller use of the beverage.

While it is certain that "men cannot be made sober by Act of Parliament," the proof is strong that the daily temptations to its excessive use on the part of certain of the more uneducated of our community, could be diminished by wise legislation. If that is true, then it is surely the duty of our representatives to try every reasonable experiment to this end, without crossing human nature entirely by attempting complete repression and prohibition. It is also the duty of every man and woman to try and create and foster a public opinion as to its great dangers and so to educate our people out of certain evil traditions that drinking is a good thing and goes with manliness and good fellowship. A Mental Hygiene that did not include a strict temperance in alcoholic drinks would be an incomplete benefactor to mankind.

The latest purely scientific study of alcohol in regard to its effect on "The Power of Attention" has just been published in the *British Journal of Psychology*, by Mr. W. McDougall. By means of an ingenious apparatus he was able to test his own power of attention and its relation to fine co-ordinated muscular action when in a normal condition, when under the influence of moderate doses of alcohol, when under the influence of tea, and when under the influence of fatigue. The experiments implied a testing of the sustained power of attention, and the use of his muscles in obedience to it. He found that under the influence of three ounces of whisky he made 54 per cent. more errors than when the brain was working in normal conditions. Under the influence of two breakfast cups of good tea he found that his errors were 28 per cent. less than when working under normal conditions. When

s

he took only one ounce of whisky his errors were 11 per cent. over the normal, while with one breakfast cup of good tea his errors were practically the same as normal. The condition of fatigue produced a large percentage of errors, while if he allowed himself half an hour's rest the power of attention in the brain and the muscular action in his fingers had been regained, and he could do his work with only the normal number of errors. Nothing could show more clearly the deteriorating effects of even a small quantity of alcohol on the mental and muscular working of the brain. It, of course, might be said that while alcohol may thus impair the intellectual faculty, it may at the same time have stimulated the faculty of imagination, social instinct, and the feeling of happiness. It might also be said that Mr. McDougall's three ounces of alcohol might have produced a soothing and restful condition if it had been taken, not before doing a bit of intellectual work, but after a hard day's work with food when brain rest was needed. As an example of this, a medical friend of mine, who usually takes little alcohol, on whose judgment I can depend, tells me that after any unusual mental and physical work in his profession, when he feels nearly played out, a few glasses of good wine with his dinner followed by sleep will act as a restorer of energy and a tonic. His wisdom and his safety no doubt lie in the very rare use he makes of this method of brain rest and restoration. His experience is that of many of us.

The injurious effects on the brain structure and functions of a steady habit of taking too much alcohol extending over years, is admitted by every physician and can be proved microscopically by any good modern pathologist. In the developmental stages of life this is very manifest. When guinea-pigs are subjected to the continuous use of alcohol during pregnancy, morbid changes are found in the brain of the offspring. There is also a marked general stunting and deficiency of growth and weight. There is a much greater tendency to disease and death. The litters of young are few and small. It is a well-known fact that the mortality among the children of drunkards is much higher than among those of the temperate. Alcoholic intoxication, if frequently repeated, has a very harmful action upon the natural defensive powers of the body against disease. Persons who so indulge are much more liable to consumption, to rheumatism, and to many other diseases. Pathologists say that " resistance " is weakened and that the "immunity" against the germs of disease is lessened. The brain cells when examined microscopically after death are found to have sustained marked damage. This injury is not confined to the cells. The packing tissue (neuroglia) is found to be seriously diseased and the blood-vessels are also markedly degenerated. Alcoholic excess is the cause of about 20 per cent. of all the insanity in Great Britain and Ireland. There are two common conditions of mental disease induced by chronic alcoholism, the one being a tendency to insane delusions, especially of suspicion. This is called " Alcoholic Delusional Insanity." It is apt to be an incurable condition because the changes in the brain cells on which it depends are incurable when they attain a certain degree of morbid change. The other form of mental disease to which all chronic alcoholics are liable in the end is called "Alcoholic Dementia." This consists of loss of memory, loss of intelligence, loss of will power—in fact, a general and incurable state of mindlessness, as compared with what had been the normal condition of the individual.

Tobacco, Tea, Coffee, and Cocoa.—There are certain substances whose action on the brain and mind is either stimulating or narcotic, which are not really foods and yet which are used most extensively and increasingly by men and women in all climates and of many races. Those are tobacco, tea, coffee, and cocoa. The use of tobacco has become the rule rather than the exception among the grown men of Europe and America and of some parts of Asia. If its use is restricted to the full-grown man, if only good tobacco is used not of too great strength, and if it is not used to excess, there are no scientific proofs that it has any injurious effects, if there is no idiosyncrasy against it. The evidence of the pleasure it gives is overwhelming. Speaking generally it exercises a soothing influence when the nervous system is in any way irritable. It tends to calm and continuous thinking, and in many men promotes the digestion of food. To those good results there are, however, exceptions. It sometimes sets up a very strong desire for its excessive use, this often passing into a morbid craving which leads to excess and hurt. Used in such excessive quantity tobacco acts injuriously on the heart, weakens digestion, and causes congestion of the throat as well as hindering mental action. In many people its use tends towards a desire for alcohol as well. I have repeatedly seen persons of a nervous temperament where the two excesses in tobacco and alcohol were linked together. A gentleman on whom I was lately impressing the injurious effects of an excessive use of alcohol said to me, "If you knock off my whisky then tobacco has to go too, because with me I can't take the one and stop the other." Tobacco properly used may, in some cases, undoubtedly be made a mental hygienic.

Tea and coffee are now used by a larger number of mankind than any other substance except food. It may be said indeed that the whole world that can attain them, the civilised and the uncivilised, male and female, white and brown, Buddhist, Mahometan, and Christian all take tea or coffee. This statement of fact completely exonerates me from any argument whatever as to any possible harm they may do. They are with us and certainly will not be displaced till a still more pleasant and subtle stimulant of the human brain is discovered. So far as scientific experiment goes, tea is proved not to weaken, but rather to stimulate the mental power of the brain cortex. Its use in moderate quantity is not followed by any injurious reaction and is not prejudicial to the working of any of the functions of the human body. Used in excess or by persons of a very nervous constitution it may cause insomnia, mental excitement, irritability, indigestion, and impaired nutrition of the body. No doubt, it should always be infused in a scientific manner, and I maintain there should always be taken along with tea some food, be it much or little. I do not think its use should be begun as a regular part of the diet till after 14, and from then till 20 its use should be in some degree restricted. Coffee and cocoa are less stimulating than tea, and are more strictly dietetic, as they are commonly taken with a good deal of milk. No mental hygienist can seriously object to their reasonable use. For women they, and tea, take the place of tobacco and alcohol, and thereby do a great service to the race.

CHAPTER XVIII

COUNTERACTIVE EFFECTS OF MENTAL HYGIENE ON THE TENDENCY TO MENTAL DEGENERATION IN OUR MODERN AND CITY LIFE

OF recent years, since our population has been moving from the more natural country life to take up its abode in cities, there has been a good deal of fear that not only a physical degeneration is taking place, especially among the very poor labouring classes, but that also a certain mental degeneracy is occurring in some of them. I do not refer to such decided mental changes as occur in insanity and idiocy. I understand that question is to be treated in a separate volume of this series. What I mean, is a certain narrowing of the mental horizon in the city-bred, a certain helplessness to cope with economic and social difficulties and a certain limitation of the general view of life which are seen in such persons. In childhood and youth they see little of Nature, with her many-sidedness, her infinite powers, her beauties and delights. They have not to look ahead and provide for the future and for seasonal changes as the countryman has. The weather and the sun and the moon have not to be watched and noted with a view to their practical effects on life. Things have not to be anticipated beforehand as the farmer and the gardener have to do. The unconsciously soothing effect of living in the midst of natural objects is not experienced.

The street, the shop, the electric car, the factory bell and the policeman keep life going for many dwellers in the city without any thinking on their part. Not having had access to Nature in childhood they cannot take her up afterwards. There may be sharpness of mind, cunning and activity, but without this nature-experience there is an undoubted arrestive effect, which, continued generation after generation, contracts the mental habit as well as the mental vision. The hygiene for all this is simply to introduce as much of Nature into our large cities as is possible, which fortunately is being largely done, or go frequently to playgrounds with grass and flowers and trees. Parks, excursions to the country, pet animals at home, geraniums grown in window-boxes are more needed. Above all things, the abolition of those enemies of mankind, high tenement houses with children living four stories above the ground, should be striven after. A week's camping out in the year for every city school with an education in providing their own bread and milk and cooking their own food would supplement as a hygienic and a preventive of mental degeneracy the school lessons of domestic economy.

I have a strong opinion that an Act, making it compulsory for all municipalities to provide a playground near their homes for every group of five hundred children of the industrial classes in our cities, would do more for our people in the long run than all the Acts passed in any average session of Parliament. Why should not the ground owner provide such playgrounds as much as he must now lay out streets of a certain width? The return for such an investment in mental health, efficiency, and happiness to future generations would far outweigh the money cost. The tendency to mental degeneration seen in our city life would thus be largely counteracted.

Two Commissions have lately reported on the subject of the possible deterioration produced by the conditions

of modern urban life, and most important, if not con-
clusive, facts have been ascertained, but they nearly all
related to the physique of our population, not to its
mental condition. The Annual Reports of the Lunacy
Commissions showing a steady annual increase in the
numbers of the registered insane, are the subjects of
yearly alarmist comments by the newspapers and
magazines, but are not really so alarming as they seem
—at least, so the experts say ; and I am with them in
that opinion.

I have always thought that Parliament would so modify
local taxation in country, and especially outlying districts,
as to encourage residence there, if the fact were more
realised that most of such districts are the real breeding-
places of the stable-minded, non-nervous element of our
population. If the cost of roads, piers, the poor, and
education, which press on them so heavily, were treated
as Imperial taxes, it would probably make a perceptible
difference in increasing the numbers of our country-bred
folks. Let the breeding of a good race, in short, become
an operative political motive.

CHAPTER XIX

HYGIENIC KNOWLEDGE AND PHYSIOLOGICAL CHARITY

I WOULD make a large moral claim on behalf of a right study and practice of the relation of mind to brain and of Mental Hygiene. I would place it near St. Paul's eulogium of charity in his Epistle to the Corinthians. We all know that many men and most women attribute the errors in life, the faults and the crimes of their fellow-creatures, to the foolishness and vice that could have been avoided had an effort been made to do so. Now the man or woman who fully realises the true action of mind in its relation to brain-working and to hereditary law, will always put a point of interrogation in the direction of charity, when discussing the conduct of his fellow-creatures. He does so, not because charity is enjoined by the Christian religion, or that it is the greatest of the virtues, but because he knows that human will, and therefore conduct, is strictly conditioned by the kind of vehicle through which it is exercised. The assertion that all men and all women are fully responsible at all times and in all conditions for all their speech and all their actions, he knows not to be true as a fact. If he is a physician he sees hundreds of people whose intentions are good, whose sense of right and wrong is keen and whose intellectual power is unimpaired, who behave in most absurd ways, say most irrational things, and frequently break the laws of conduct which they had laid down for themselves. He knows that those persons deserve sympathy rather than blame, kindly help rather than censure. Their conduct and speech should be judged by the facts of nature rather than by conventional rules, ideals, codes of morals, or by legal sanction. It is quite certain that there are in the world vast numbers of people who are foolish and weak. Carlyle's well-known saying was—"The population of England consists of thirty millions—mostly fools." Are all those "fools" to be judged by the high standard of moral wisdom and responsibility which really applies only to the strong-minded and the wise? They are fools by default. The two great guides of conduct are instinct and self-control, formed and modified by evolution, heredity, example, education, and experience. The want of the power of self-control is so very common amongst mankind that to some extent and in respect to some matters it may be regarded as the normal condition of the species. A perfect capacity of self-control in all directions and at all times is rather the ideal state at which we aim than the real condition of any of us. The men who have attained to a state of inhibitory perfection have been few and far between, and even in regard to them it may be said that they might have fallen if they had been exposed to sufficient temptation or irritation. The subject of mental inhibitory power, and following logically, that of conduct, should first be studied from the point of view of its gradual development in children. As we have already seen, self-control is developed as the brain develops and comes to maturity with the brain. There is no day or year in a child's life after which killing its little brother is murder and before which it was no crime at all. Do we scorn children's prattle, or blame their foolish acts? Do we scold them and call them "vicious" because their conduct is not up to our ideal standard? Why not, except that we instinctively know that their brains cannot always exhibit wisdom or virtue? For the good of society the law assumes as the basis of its enactments that all men have the inherent power to do certain things and avoid other things which would be inconsistent with the well-being of society. The assumption of complete responsibility may be so far necessary for an organised civilised society, even if not true as a fact, but the limitations and exceptions must be taken into account. Many persons never do acquire sufficient power of control to conform to either conventional, moral, or legal rules. In them this faculty has been arrested. We are bound to give credence to all such physiological facts and laws. There can be no doubt that there are many families in which nervousness, insanity, lawlessness, and drunkenness are hereditary, and that in consequence of this their members cannot conform to any very high standard of conduct and responsibility. In some the feeling of right and wrong, the conscience, never acquires sensitiveness. In others, again, it becomes hyper-sensitive, and often at early ages. I have seen many children of educated and nervous families who, by a kind of forcing-house treatment, had acquired strong moral ideas at too early ages. We doctors do not like this, because we find from experience that many such cases afterwards have a sort of moral reaction and are the worse for such early stimulation. As I have pointed out, the moral feelings were the last to be developed in human evolution, and in very many individuals we have a sort of return to the non-moral condition of our barbarian ancestors. It is a fact that the condition called irritability usually means a diminished power of control, and that it is apt to go with bodily and nervous weakness or with a state of fatigue. The best way to cure such irritability is usually by rest and good feeding, and not by moral lectures. As to crime, we should never have it at all in a physiologically sound—using the words in a large sense—society of men and women. A murder would naturally be attributed to disease, and the patient would be treated for it instead of being hanged. Sympathy and charity would take the place of blame and punishment for all social error and legal crime. The suddenness of the temptation or irritation makes a great difference to its being yielded to or resisted. If you suddenly strike most men they will automatically strike back again. Place cold water before a man dying of thirst and he will take and drink it if it was fifty times the property of another man. Not even a legal fool would blame him for this. Many persons have so small a reserve stock of brain power—that most valuable of all possessions—that it is soon used up, and they speak and act in unreasonable and foolish ways; they lose, in fact, their power of self-control and their full responsibility; they are angels or demons, just as they are fresh or tired. Nature, fortunately for humanity and society, does provide for most people a surplus stock of resistive force so that extra work and even extra dissipation does no great harm if not repeated too often. Some people have their inhibitory power developed, as it were, too strongly, and they can keep themselves at work or indulge in dissipation till all their reserves of brain energy are exhausted, when they become unresistive, callous, and wicked. Some people are "subject" to morbid impulses, imperative ideas and obsessions to which they must either yield, or the resistance to which implies so great an effort that they are exhausted thereby.

At the back of human nature, and no doubt existing as a survival of ancestral conditions, we often have obscure tendencies towards killing, torturing, destructiveness, appropriation, misrule, irritating and teasing others, "cussednesses" of every sort, which sometimes will come out in spite of Christianity and in defiance of morals. Such feelings and obsessions in those persons are always worse when health is bad, and can often be lessened or cured by improving the health. But they always call for charity, both on account of their essential nature and because evil and useless irritation result from their being misunderstood. No doubt, the great psychological difference between sanity and insanity consists in the existence or not of sufficient self-control, and there is no dividing line between the two conditions. Light and darkness are definite phenomena, but there is an undefinable twilight between.

There is no human faculty that is not subject in many persons to either explosion or partial paralysis. The instincts and the appetites are subject to the same rule. Gusts of uncontrollable emotion are common enough, especially in women. Orgies of work, of passion, or of dissipation many people are subject to. I should like to meet a dozen men or women who could truthfully say that they had not had at some time or other in their lives an intense desire to appropriate what was not theirs, to use bad language, or to eat and drink too much, or to slander their neighbours. Fortunately Nature throws a wonderful curtain of blessed forgetfulness in most people over such things after they have passed away. That also is a psychological law, and a very beneficent one. The man or the woman who begins to call up in too great vividness all the faults of thought, word, or deed of the past life should certainly go and consult the doctor. He or she needs hygienic and curative measures. The man or the woman who falls into the way of a universal censure of all their neighbour's faults and failings is not only devoid of Christian charity, but is probably in an unhealthy condition of brain, which accounts for this physiological uncharitableness. I knew a woman once who became greatly distressed at having taken advantage of a friend's good-nature, and had done her an injury in years gone by. About this she was a little nervous, sleepless and restless, and she went to her clergyman. Being a sensible man, he sent her to the country to have a rest from housekeeping and the care of a large family for a little, with absolutely good effect. I had a friend who once told me how badly some of his acquaintances were treating him, and what a bad lot he had discovered some of them to be. I said to him, "You need your holiday, and I believe when you come back your friends will behave much better to you," which turned out to be the case. How much family discord would be saved if physiological charity were exercised when the schoolboy, the adolescent, or the house-mother is fractious, cantankerous or irritable from ill-health or overstrain! How easily put right such things could be if properly understood! What alarm and distress could be saved if the irritability of indigestion, the fears of heart disease, the gloom of influenza, and the violence of temper of commencing brain disease were regarded with physiological charity and properly treated! What permanent estrangement between lads at 18 and fathers at the climacteric could not be saved if the psychology of those periods of life were taken into account! What difficulties the schoolmaster might not get over if he had this knowledge and exercised this charity! How much mental disease could be avoided if its causes were understood and its preliminary symptoms properly treated! How much blood was shed in France at the Revolution because men were hungry! How many repressive Acts of Parliament have been needed because our city workpeople and their wives and children had not fresh air enough and decent houses to live in! How many fewer policemen and judges should we need were the brains of our city people not poisoned with an excess of bad alcohol and their law-abidingness destroyed thereby! How much Russia might have saved in treasure, dragooning and blood in the past two years if its peasants had had their stomachs filled!

INDEX

UNWIN BROTHERS, LIMITED, THE GRESHAM PRESS, WOKING AND LONDON.

THE NEW LIBRARY OF MEDICINE
EDITED BY C. W. SALEEBY, M.D., F.R.S.Edin.

THESE Volumes, to be published by Messrs. Methuen, are planned upon the assumption that there are certain medical matters of the very gravest importance which urgently claim the attention and appreciation not only of the medical man, but also of the intelligent layman. It is the object of the editor to obtain the discussion of these subjects by the foremost authorities, and to have them so treated that the books are welcome alike to doctor and to patient, to statesman as well as to scientist. As to the authority with which the writers speak, that is so self-evident as to need no indication. The attempt is made to deal with the subjects that have a marked relation to life—personal and national, to insist less upon the purely technical aspects of the subjects than upon the practicability of applying our knowledge in practice,—so that matters like infantile mortality, consumption, and alcoholism may be duly exhibited to the public now that they have, in the main, been conquered by science and wait merely for the education of public opinion to be eliminated from human life.

INFANT MORTALITY. By GEORGE NEWMAN, M.D., D.P.H., F.R.S.E., Lecturer on Public Health at St. Bartholomew's Hospital, and Medical Officer of Health of the Metropolitan Borough of Finsbury. Demy 8vo, 7s. 6d. net.

A systematic treatise on one of the most pressing social questions of the time. Although the general death-rate has declined in recent years, the mortality of infants remains almost unaffected by sanitary advancement. Nor is the acuteness of the problem in any way lessened, but rather otherwise, by the declining birth-rate. Dr. Newman's book is concerned with the present distribution and chief causes of the mortality of infants in Great Britain. The chief fatal diseases of infancy, the relations of the occupation of women in factories, antenatal influences, infant feeding, and the effect of domestic and social habits upon infant mortality receive careful consideration. A chapter on practicable preventive methods is also added. The book is illustrated by a number of charts and maps.

THE HYGIENE OF MIND. By T. S. CLOUSTON, M.D., F.R.S.E., Lecturer on Mental Diseases in the University of Edinburgh. Demy 8vo.

A Treatise on Mental Health and Strength; its Genesis, Preservation and Risks from the Evolutionary, Hereditary, Physiological, Psychological, and Medical points of view; the dependence of Mind on Brain Development and Brain Care in childhood, the school age, adolescence, manhood, and old age; its connection with mental faculty and bodily function; its relation to manners, morals, religion, play, sex, temperament, education, and work; the dangers of the nervous temperament, disease, fatigue, strain, alcohol, and other brain stimulants and sedatives; mental effects of city life *v.* country life; the supreme importance for conduct of the *Mens Sana in Corpore Sano.*

THE CHILDREN OF THE NATION. By the Right Hon. Sir JOHN GORST. Demy 8vo.

This book calls attention to the national danger involved in neglecting the health of the nation's children. It discusses the political aspects of Infant Mortality, the overwork and underfeeding of children in the elementary schools, medical inspection of schools, the sanitary condition of schools, the mischief done in infant schools, hereditary diseases, child labour in factories and mines, and housing in town and country. It also deals with the question of finance.

THE CARE OF THE BODY. By F. Cavanagh, M.D.

Demy 8vo. *[Nearly ready.*

This book begins with a chapter on Sleep, since the body can only be cared for if this has been satisfactory. The value of Bathing and the different kinds of baths are discussed: then the questions affecting Exercise, including Training and Athletics. Proper Clothing, with the most suitable head and foot wear for the different ages, follow. The necessary attentions to the Skin, Hair, Teeth, Feet, and Hands, so that these may perform their various functions most efficiently, are described and explained. In conclusion, chapters are devoted to considering the need of attention to the Position of the body in its varying attitudes of work, and the importance, meaning, and gain to the individual acquired by an understanding of the formation of " Habit."

THE DRINK PROBLEM in its Medico-Sociological Aspects.

Edited by T. N. Kelynack, M.D., M.R.C.P., Hon. Secretary of the Society for the Study of Inebriety. Demy 8vo. *[Nearly ready.*

This is an authoritative work on the much discussed Alcohol Question. Each section is written by a medical expert. The subject is dealt with in a form appealing to the intelligent layman, as well as meeting the requirements of the medical practitioner. The drink problem is discussed in its biological bearings. The psychological, physiological, and pathological aspects are considered in their relation to sociological conditions and practical measures of temperance reform. The work appeals to all interested in the prevention, arrest, and amelioration of alcoholism, and is of service to those desirous of obtaining a scientific basis for efforts directed towards the care and control of the inebriate.

DISEASES OF OCCUPATION. By Professor Thomas Oliver,

M.A., M.D., LL.D., F.R.C.P., Physician, Royal Infirmary, Newcastle-upon-Tyne; late Medical Expert, Dangerous Trades Committee, etc., Home Office. Demy 8vo. *[Nearly ready.*

The work gives a succinct but comprehensive account of the aims of Factory Legislation and what it has accomplished. Among the subjects dealt with are Work and Fatigue; Women's Work; Diseases due to impure air in the factory and workshop; to dust, inorganic and organic; to working in compressed air (Caisson disease); to micro-organisms and parasites : and diseases the result of work in high temperatures, and consequent upon physical strain, electrical shock, etc.

CANCER AND THE PUBLIC. By Charles P. Childe, B.A.,

F.R.C.S. Demy 8vo. *[Nearly ready.*

The aim of this book is to acquaint the public with the favourable outlook which surgical operation to-day offers in the treatment of Cancer as compared with a quarter of a century ago. Further, its object is to show, both from a consideration of modern views of the nature of Cancer as well as from actual results obtained in its treatment, the improvement that might be anticipated, were it not for the deplorable ignorance that exists of its early signs and the dread of seeking advice at the only time when it is possible to cure it. It claims to establish that by improved education, and by this means alone, can the prospect be rendered generally hopeful.

THE HYGIENICS OF EDUCATION, MENTAL AND PHYSICAL. By W. Leslie Mackenzie, M.A., M.D., D.P.H., M.R.C.P.E., F.R.S.E., Medical Member of the Local Government Board for Scotland. Demy 8vo. *[In preparation.*

This book aims at presenting the problem of Education from the standpoint of the Physician. The child, as a growing mind in a growing body, is subjected to stresses. Education is conceived as at once the superintendence of growth and the "provision of an environment." The leading mental processes, the groundwork of acquisition, fatigue mental and physical, are discussed in the light of recent research. Consideration is also given to the signs and morbid results of overpressure, abnormalities of the organs of sense, diseases incident to the educational life from birth to adolescence, the health conditions of life at school, co-education, and other practical problems.

THE CAUSATION AND PREVENTION OF TUBERCULOSIS

(CONSUMPTION). By ARTHUR NEWSHOLME, M.D., F.R.C.P., Medical Officer of Health of Brighton; President of the Incorporated Society of Medical Officers of Health (1899-1900); Examiner in Public Health to the Universities of Cambridge and Victoria; late Examiner in State and Preventive Medicine to the Universities of London and Oxford. Demy 8vo.
[*In preparation.*

The main object of this book is practical. It is intended as a guide not only for medical officers of health, but for all engaged, whether on hospital committees or local governing bodies, in administrative measures for the control of tuberculosis and the advancement of the public health. A large part of the book therefore will consist of a discussion of measures of sanitary reform and of social improvement which are the chief indirect means; and of measures such as notification, visiting and advising patients, disinfection, sanatorium treatment and training of patients, and hospital segregation of advanced patients, which are the all-important direct means of controlling the disease. The relative importance of the above and allied measures can only be understood when the pathology and causation of tuberculosis are known. The prevention of Consumption must be based on a knowledge of its causation.

NUTRITION. By RALPH VINCENT, M.D., B.S., M.R.C.P.,

Physician to the Infants' Hospital; late Senior Resident Medical Officer, Queen Charlotte's Lying-in Hospital. Demy 8vo. [*In preparation.*

Nutrition, as the index of national power, is the leading feature of this work. The health and strength of a nation are primarily determined by its power of reproduction. The rearing of healthy infants and the prevention of defective structure arising from malnutrition are of cardinal economic importance. The present conditions, so seriously threatening the welfare of the country, and the practical remedies are discussed in detail. Diet, in relation to nutrition and structure, necessarily receives special attention.

DRUGS AND DRUG HABITS. By H. SAINSBURY, M.D.,

F.R.C.P. Demy 8vo. [*In preparation.*

On the subject of drugs, so called, very erroneous conceptions prevail. For some they are synonymous with poisons, yet many forget that this latter term has a significance which is relative only, and few, outside the ranks of those who practise medicine, realise how difficult it is to isolate drugs as a class, and to frame a definition which shall satisfactorily separate them from aliments. To draw attention to these misconceptions; to point out the more precise relations in which medicaments stand to disease, and the problems which disease puts before us for solution; to make prominent the fact that drug habits—including the use of tea, coffee, and tobacco—are but instances of a law which is fundamental, and in the manifestation of which temperament and education play primary parts,—these are the purposes of the present volume.

AIR AND HEALTH. By RONALD C. MACFIE, M.B. Demy 8vo.

[*In preparation.*

This book deals with the physical and chemical properties of air, particularly with reference to health and disease. The physiology of respiration will be considered in its practical bearings, and chapters will be devoted to the question of climate and to relevant questions of dust, fog, germs, air-borne epidemics, etc. Ventilation will be fully discussed, both in its private and public aspects.

FUNCTIONAL NERVE DISEASES. By A. T. SCHOFIELD,

M.D. Demy 8vo. [*In preparation.*

This book is called for, not only on account of the increasing importance of the subject, but because the treatment of these diseases is rapidly altering in character, and is taking more account of the psychic factors and laying less stress upon the physical. The present work seeks to present the newest view on this subject, and to be a practical handbook to medical psycho-therapeutics as far as they are applicable in these diseases. At the same time, various forms of quackery and pseudo-religious varieties of treatment will be described and their evils pointed out. Special allusion will also be made to functional nerve diseases in children.

ABNORMAL AND MENTALLY DEFECTIVE CHILDREN, THEIR EDUCATION AND TRAINING. By HENRY ASHBY, M.D., F.R.C.P., Lecturer on Diseases of Children, Victoria University. Illustrated. Demy 8vo. [*In preparation.*

Children differ from one another, in physical, mental, and moral characters. An attempt is made to describe those who are well below the normal line, and the effect which education and training has upon their defects. Neurotic children, the dull and backward, those with minor mental abnormalities, as well as the large and varied class who are feebly gifted as regards mental powers, come in for consideration. Reference is also made to "moral imbeciles," and those with convulsive disorders ; while deaf-mutes and those with speech defects are also dealt with. A good deal of space is given to testing the mental capacities of defective children and to their education and training.

THE PRINCIPLES OF VACCINATION AND SERUM THERAPY. By ALLAN MACFADYEN, M.D., B.Sc., F.I.C., Head of Bacteriological Department, Jenner Institute; Fullerian Professor of Physiology, Royal Institution. Demy 8vo. [*In preparation.*

The parasitic doctrine has revolutionised the conceptions of disease processes and the methods for their prevention and treatment. The knowledge that has been gained of the nature and mode of action of the living agents that invade the body and produce disease has led to the most notable advances in medicine, surgery, and hygiene. One of the most fascinating chapters of medical discovery is that relating to the evolution of a new therapy, based on scientific observation and experiment. The present volume relates, without undue technical detail, the facts and conceptions upon which the methods of Serum Therapy and Vaccination are based.

THE INSANE. By GEORGE R. WILSON, M.D., F.R.S.E., etc. Illustrated. Demy 8vo. [*In preparation.*

This book is intended to be an Introduction to the study of Insanity, and is specially designed for the medical student, the general practitioner, and the educated layman. It will deal with the nature and meaning of Insanity, and with the history of the subject ; with the causes of mental disease, its frequency, and its importance as a social factor ; and it will give a description of the varieties of Insanity now recognised by specialists, their pathology and their classification. But it will aim chiefly at practical rather than theoretical value, and will present cases of all varieties, especially in the early stages, and will discuss their management and treatment. The book will be illustrated by diagrams and photographs.

A TEXT-BOOK OF HEREDITY. By ARCHDALL REID, M.B., F.R.S.E. Demy 8vo. [*In preparation.*

This volume covers the whole field of heredity, but especial attention is paid to practical problems affecting human beings. Among the subjects dealt with are the method of the evolution of the race, the method of the development of the individual, the distinction between the different classes of traits of the individual, the function of sex, the various forms of inheritance, the development of mind and body in the human being, as well as the problems of heredity and evolution which arise in relation to disease, alcohol, civilisation, and education. Great care is taken to ensure lucidity. There is much original matter.

INFECTION. By SIMS WOODHEAD, M.D., F.R.S.E., etc., Professor of Pathology in the University of Cambridge. Demy 8vo. [*In preparation.*

IMPERIAL HYGIENE. By W. J. SIMPSON, M.D., etc., Professor of Hygiene in King's College, London. Demy 8vo. [*In preparation.*

METHUEN & CO., LONDON.

A CATALOGUE OF BOOKS PUBLISHED BY METHUEN AND COMPANY: LONDON 36 ESSEX STREET W.C.

CONTENTS

JULY 1906

A CATALOGUE OF

MESSRS. METHUEN'S
PUBLICATIONS

Colonial Editions are published of all Messrs. METHUEN's Novels issued at a price above 2s. 6d., and similar editions are published of some works of General Literature. These are marked in the Catalogue. Colonial editions are only for circulation in the British Colonies and India.

An asterisk denotes that a book is in the Press.
I.P.L. represents Illustrated Pocket Library.
S.Q.S. represents Social Questions Series.

PART I.—GENERAL LITERATURE

Abbot (Jacob). See Little Blue Books.
Abbott (J. H. M.). Author of 'Tommy Cornstalk.' AN OUTLANDER IN ENGLAND: BEING SOME IMPRESSIONS OF AN AUSTRALIAN ABROAD. *Second Edition. Cr. 8vo. 6s.*
A Colonial Edition is also published.
Acatos (M. J.). See Junior School Books.
Adams (Frank). JACK SPRATT. With 24 Coloured Pictures. *Super Royal 16mo. 2s.*
Adeney (W. F.), M.A. See Bennett and Adeney.
Æschylus. See Classical Translations.
Æsop. See I.P.L.
Ainsworth (W. Harrison). See I.P.L.
Alderson (J. P.). MR. ASQUITH. With Portraits and Illustrations. *Demy 8vo. 7s. 6d. net.*
A Colonial Edition is also published.
Aldis (Janet). MADAME GEOFFRIN, HER SALON, AND HER TIMES. With many Portraits and Illustrations. *Second Edition. Demy 8vo. 10s. 6d. net.*
A Colonial Edition is also published.
Alexander (William), D.D., Archbishop of Armagh. THOUGHTS AND COUNSELS OF MANY YEARS. *Demy 16mo. 2s. 6d.*
Aiken (Henry). THE NATIONAL SPORTS OF GREAT BRITAIN. With descriptions in English and French. With 51 Coloured Plates. *Royal Folio. Five Guineas net.* The Plates can be had separately in a Portfolio. *£3, 3s. net.*
See also I.P.L.
Allen (Jessie). See Little Books on Art.
Allen (J. Romilly), F.S.A. See Antiquary's Books.
Almack (E.). See Little Books on Art.
Amherst (Lady). A SKETCH OF EGYPTIAN HISTORY FROM THE EARLIEST TIMES TO THE PRESENT DAY. With many Illustrations. *Demy 8vo. 7s. 6d. net.*

Anderson (F. M.). THE STORY OF THE BRITISH EMPIRE FOR CHILDREN. With many Illustrations. *Cr. 8vo. 2s.*
Anderson (J. G.), B.A., Examiner to London University, NOUVELLE GRAMMAIRE FRANÇAISE. *Cr. 8vo. 2s.*
EXERCICES DE GRAMMAIRE FRANÇAISE. *Cr. 8vo. 1s. 6d.*
Andrewes (Bishop). PRECES PRIVATAE. Edited, with Notes, by F. E. BRIGHTMAN, M.A., of Pusey House, Oxford. *Cr. 8vo. 6s.*
Anglo-Australian. AFTER-GLOW MEMORIES. *Cr. 8vo. 6s.*
A Colonial Edition is also published.
Aristophanes. THE FROGS. Translated into English by E. W. HUNTINGFORD, M.A. *Cr. 8vo. 2s. 6d.*
Aristotle. THE NICOMACHEAN ETHICS. Edited, with an Introduction and Notes, by JOHN BURNET, M.A., Professor of Greek at St. Andrews. *Cheaper issue. Demy 8vo. 10s. 6d. net.*
Ashton (R.). See Little Blue Books.
Atkins (H. G.). See Oxford Biographies.
Atkinson (C. M.). JEREMY BENTHAM. *Demy 8vo. 5s. net.*
Atkinson (T. D.). A SHORT HISTORY OF ENGLISH ARCHITECTURE. With over 200 Illustrations. *Fcap. 8vo. 3s. 6d. net.*
A GLOSSARY OF TERMS USED IN ENGLISH ARCHITECTURE. Illustrated. *Fcap. 8vo. 3s. 6d. net.*
Auden (T.), M.A., F.S.A. See Ancient Cities.
Aurelius (Marcus). See Standard Library and W. H. D. Rouse.
Austen (Jane). See Little Library and Standard Library.
Aves (Ernest). See Books on Business.
Bacon (Francis). See Little Library and Standard Library.

Baden-Powell (R. S. S.), Major-General. THE DOWNFALL OF PREMPEH. A Diary of Life in Ashanti, 1895. Illustrated. *Third Edition. Large Cr. 8vo. 6s.*
A Colonial Edition is also published.
THE MATABELE CAMPAIGN, 1896. With nearly 100 Illustrations. *Fourth Edition. Large Cr. 8vo. 6s.*
A Colonial Edition is also published.
*Bagot (Richard). THE LAKE OF COMO. *Cr. 8vo. 3s. 6d. net.*
Bailey (J. C.), M.A. See Cowper.
Baker (W. G.), M.A. See Junior Examination Series.
Baker (Julian L.), F.I.C., F.C.S. See Books on Business.
Balfour (Graham). THE LIFE OF ROBERT LOUIS STEVENSON. *Second Edition. Two Volumes. Demy 8vo. 25s. net.*
A Colonial Edition is also published.
Bally (S. E.). See Commercial Series.
Banks (Elizabeth L.). THE AUTO-BIOGRAPHY OF A 'NEWSPAPER GIRL.' *Second Edition. Cr. 8vo. 6s.*
A Colonial Edition is also published.
Barham (R. H.). See Little Library.
Baring (The Hon. Maurice). WITH THE RUSSIANS IN MANCHURIA. *Third Edition. Demy 8vo. 7s. 6d. net.*
A Colonial Edition is also published.
Baring-Gould (S.). THE LIFE OF NAPOLEON BONAPARTE. With over 450 Illustrations in the Text, and 12 Photogravure Plates. *Gilt top. Large quarto. 36s.*
THE TRAGEDY OF THE CÆSARS. With numerous Illustrations from Busts, Gems, Cameos, etc. *Fifth Edition. Royal 8vo. 10s. 6d. net.*
A BOOK OF FAIRY TALES. With numerous Illustrations by A. J. GASKIN. *Second Edition. Cr. 8vo. Buckram. 6s.*
OLD ENGLISH FAIRY TALES. With numerous Illustrations by F. D. BEDFORD. *Second Edition. Cr. 8vo. Buckram. 6s.*
A Colonial Edition is also published.
THE VICAR OF MORWENSTOW. Revised Edition. With a Portrait. *Cr. 8vo. 3s. 6d.*
DARTMOOR: A Descriptive and Historical Sketch. With Plans and numerous Illustrations. *Cr. 8vo. 6s.*
A BOOK OF DEVON. Illustrated. *Second Edition. Cr. 8vo. 6s.*
A BOOK OF CORNWALL. Illustrated. *Second Edition. Cr. 8vo. 6s.*
A BOOK OF NORTH WALES. Illustrated. *Cr. 8vo. 6s.*
A BOOK OF SOUTH WALES. Illustrated. *Cr. 8vo. 6s.*
A BOOK OF BRITTANY. Illustrated. *Cr. 8vo. 6s.*
A BOOK OF THE RIVIERA. Illustrated. *Cr. 8vo. 6s.*
A Colonial Edition is also published.

*THE RHINE. Illustrated. *Cr. 8vo. 6s.*
A BOOK OF GHOSTS. With 8 Illustrations by D. MURRAY SMITH. *Second Edition. Cr. 8vo. 6s.*
A Colonial Edition is also published.
OLD COUNTRY LIFE. With 67 Illustrations. *Fifth Edition. Large Cr. 8vo. 6s.*
A GARLAND OF COUNTRY SONG: English Folk Songs with their Traditional Melodies. Collected and arranged by S. BARING-GOULD and H. F. SHEPPARD. *Demy 4to. 6s.*
SONGS OF THE WEST: Folk Songs of Devon and Cornwall. Collected from the Mouths of the People. By S. BARING-GOULD, M.A., and H. FLEETWOOD SHEPPARD, M.A. New and Revised Edition, under the musical editorship of CECIL J. SHARP, Principal of the Hampstead Conservatoire. *Large Imperial 8vo. 5s. net.*
See also Little Guides and Half-Crown Library.
Barker (Aldred F.). See Textbooks of Technology.
Barnes (W. E.), D.D. See Churchman's Bible.
Barnett (Mrs. P. A.). See Little Library.
Baron (R. R. N.), M.A. FRENCH PROSE COMPOSITION. *Second Edition. Cr. 8vo. 2s. 6d. Key, 3s. net.* See also Junior School Books.
Barron (H. M.), M.A., Wadham College, Oxford. TEXTS FOR SERMONS. With a Preface by Canon SCOTT HOLLAND. *Cr. 8vo. 3s. 6d.*
Bartholomew (J. G.), F.R.S.E. See C. G. Robertson.
Bastable (C. F.), M.A. See S.Q.S.
Batson (Mrs. Stephen). A BOOK OF THE COUNTRY AND THE GARDEN. Illustrated by F. CARRUTHERS GOULD and A. C. GOULD. *Demy 8vo. 10s. 6d.*
A CONCISE HANDBOOK OF GARDEN FLOWERS. *Fcap. 8vo. 3s. 6d.*
Batten (Loring W.), Ph.D., S.T.D. THE HEBREW PROPHET. *Cr. 8vo. 3s. 6d net.*
Beaman (A. Hulme). PONS ASINORUM; OR, A GUIDE TO BRIDGE. *Second Edition. Fcap. 8vo. 2s.*
Beard (W. S.). See Junior Examination Series and Beginner's Books.
Beckford (Peter). THOUGHTS ON HUNTING. Edited by J. OTHO PAGET, and Illustrated by G. H. JALLAND. *Second Edition. Demy 8vo. 6s.*
Beckford (William). See Little Library.
Beeching (H. C.), M.A., Canon of Westminster. See Library of Devotion.
Begbie (Harold). MASTER WORKERS. Illustrated. *Demy 8vo. 7s. 6d. net.*
Behmen (Jacob). DIALOGUES ON THE SUPERSENSUAL LIFE. Edited by BERNARD HOLLAND. *Fcap. 8vo. 3s. 6d.*

Belloc (Hillaire). PARIS. With Maps and Illustrations. *Cr. 8vo. 6s.*
*MARIE ANTOINETTE. With many Portraits and Illustrations. *Demy 8vo. 12s. 6d. net.*
A Colonial Edition is also published.
Bellot (H. H. L.), M.A. THE INNER AND MIDDLE TEMPLE. With numerous Illustrations. *Crown 8vo. 6s. net.*
See also L. A. A. Jones.
Bennett (W. H.), M.A. A PRIMER OF THE BIBLE. *Third Edition. Cr. 8vo. 2s. 6d.*
Bennett (W. H.) and Adeney (W. F.). A BIBLICAL INTRODUCTION. *Third Edition. Cr. 8vo. 7s. 6d.*
Benson (Archbishop) GOD'S BOARD: Communion Addresses. *Fcap. 8vo. 3s. 6d. net.*
Benson (A. C.), M.A. See Oxford Biographies.
Benson (R. M.). THE WAY OF HOLINESS: a Devotional Commentary on the 119th Psalm. *Cr. 8vo. 5s.*
Bernard (E. R.), M.A., Canon of Salisbury. THE ENGLISH SUNDAY. *Fcap. 8vo. 1s. 6d.*
Bertouch (Baroness de). THE LIFE OF FATHER IGNATIUS. Illustrated. *Demy 8vo. 10s. 6d. net.*
A Colonial Edition is also published.
Betham-Edwards (M.). HOME LIFE IN FRANCE. Illustrated. *Fourth Edition. Demy 8vo. 7s. 6d. net.*
A Colonial Edition is also published.
Bethune-Baker (J. F.), M.A. See Handbooks of Theology.
Bidez (M.). See Byzantine Texts.
Biggs (C. R. D.), D.D. See Churchman's Bible.
Bindley (T. Herbert), B.D. THE OECUMENICAL DOCUMENTS OF THE FAITH. With Introductions and Notes. *Cr. 8vo. 6s.*
Binns (H. B.). THE LIFE OF WALT WHITMAN. Illustrated. *Demy 8vo. 10s. 6d. net.*
A Colonial Edition is also published.
Binyon (Laurence). THE DEATH OF ADAM, AND OTHER POEMS. *Cr. 8vo. 3s. 6d. net.*
*WILLIAM BLAKE. In 2 volumes. *Super Royal Quarto. £1, 1s. each.*
Vol. I.—THE BOOK OF JOB.
Birnstingl (Ethel). See Little Books on Art.
Blackmantle (Bernard). See I.P.L.
Blair (Robert). See I.P.L.
Blake (William). See I.P.L. and Little Library.
Blaxland (B.), M.A. See Library of Devotion.
Bloom (T. Harvey), M.A. SHAKESPEARE'S GARDEN. Illustrated. *Fcap. 8vo. 3s. 6d. ; leather, 4s. 6d. net.*
See also Antiquary's Books

Blouet (Henri). See Beginner's Books.
Boardman (T. H.), M.A. See Textbooks of Science.
Bodley (J. E. C.), Author of 'France.' THE CORONATION OF EDWARD VII. *Demy 8vo. 21s. net.* By Command of the King.
Body (George), D.D. THE SOUL'S PILGRIMAGE : Devotional Readings from his writings. Selected by J. H. BURN, B.D., F.R.S.E. *Pott 8vo. 2s. 6d.*
Bona (Cardinal). See Library of Devotion.
Boon (F. C.). See Commercial Series.
Borrow (George). See Little Library.
Bos (J. Ritzema). AGRICULTURAL ZOOLOGY. Translated by J. R. AINSWORTH DAVIS, M.A. With 155 Illustrations. *Cr. 8vo. Third Edition. 3s. 6d.*
Botting (C. G.), B.A. EASY GREEK EXERCISES. *Cr. 8vo. 2s.* See also Junior Examination Series.
Boulton (E. S.), M.A. GEOMETRY ON MODERN LINES. *Cr. 8vo. 2s.*
Boulton (William B.). THOMAS GAINSBOROUGH With 40 Illustrations. *Second Ed. Demy 8vo. 7s. 6d. net.*
SIR JOSHUA REYNOLDS, P.R.A. With 49 Illustrations. *Demy 8vo. 7s. 6d. net.*
Bowden (E. M.). THE IMITATION OF BUDDHA : Being Quotations from Buddhist Literature for each Day in the Year. *Fifth Edition. Cr. 16mo. 2s. 6d.*
Boyle (W.). CHRISTMAS AT THE ZOO. With Verses by W. BOYLE and 24 Coloured Pictures by H. B. NEILSON. *Super Royal 16mo. 2s.*
Brabant (F. G.), M.A. See Little Guides.
Bradley (J. W.). See Little Books on Art.
Brailsford (H. N.). MACEDONIA. Illustrated. *Demy 8vo. 12s. 6d. net.*
Brodrick (Mary) and Morton (Anderson). A CONCISE HANDBOOK OF EGYPTIAN ARCHÆOLOGY. Illustrated. *Cr. 8vo. 3s. 6d.*
Brooke (A. S.), M.A. SLINGSBY AND SLINGSBY CASTLE. Illustrated. *Cr. 8vo. 7s. 6d.*
Brooks (E. W.). See Byzantine Texts.
Brown (P. H.), LL.D., Fraser Professor of Ancient (Scottish) History at the University of Edinburgh. SCOTLAND IN THE TIME OF QUEEN MARY. *Demy 8vo. 7s. 6d. net.*
Browne (Sir Thomas). See Standard Library.
Brownell (C. L.). THE HEART OF JAPAN. Illustrated. *Third Edition. Cr. 8vo. 6s. ; also Demy 8vo. 6d.*
A Colonial Edition is also published.
Browning (Robert). See Little Library.
Buckland (Francis T.). CURIOSITIES OF NATURAL HISTORY. Illustrated by H. B. NEILSON. *Cr. 8vo. 3s. 6d.*

Buckton (A. M.) THE BURDEN OF ENGELA: a Ballad-Epic. *Second Edition.* *Cr. 8vo.* 3s. 6d. net.
EAGER HEART: A Mystery Play. *Fourth Edition.* *Cr. 8vo.* 1s. net.
Budge (E. A. Wallis). THE GODS OF THE EGYPTIANS. With over 100 Coloured Plates and many Illustrations. *Two Volumes. Royal 8vo.* £3, 3s. net.
Bull (Paul), Army Chaplain. GOD AND OUR SOLDIERS. *Second Edition.* *Cr. 8vo.* 6s.
A Colonial Edition is also published.
Bulley (Miss). See S.Q.S.
Bunyan (John). THE PILGRIM'S PROGRESS. Edited, with an Introduction, by C. H. FIRTH, M.A. With 39 Illustrations by R. ANNING BELL. *Cr. 8vo.* 6s.
See also Library of Devotion and Standard Library.
Burch (G. J.), M.A., F.R.S. A MANUAL OF ELECTRICAL SCIENCE. Illustrated. *Cr. 8vo.* 3s.
Burgess (Gelett). GOOPS AND HOW TO BE THEM. Illustrated. *Small 4to.* 6s.
Burke (Edmund). See Standard Library.
Burn (A. E.), D.D., Rector of Handsworth and Prebendary of Lichfield.
See Handbooks of Theology.
Burn (J. H.), B.D. See Library of Devotion.
Burnand (Sir F. C.). RECORDS AND REMINISCENCES. With a Portrait by H. v. HERKOMER. *Cr. 8vo. Fourth and Cheaper Edition.* 6s.
A Colonial Edition is also published.
Burns (Robert), THE POEMS OF. Edited by ANDREW LANG and W. A. CRAIGIE. With Portrait. *Third Edition. Demy 8vo, gilt top.* 6s.
Burnside (W. F.), M.A. OLD TESTAMENT HISTORY FOR USE IN SCHOOLS. *Cr. 8vo.* 3s. 6d.
Burton (Alfred). See I.P.L.
Butler (Joseph). See Standard Library.
Caldecott (Alfred), D.D. See Handbooks of Theology.
Calderwood (D. S.), Headmaster of the Normal School, Edinburgh. TEST CARDS IN EUCLID AND ALGEBRA. In three packets of 40, with Answers. 1s. each. Or in three Books, price 2d., 2d., and 3d.
Cambridge (Ada) [Mrs. Cross]. THIRTY YEARS IN AUSTRALIA. *Demy 8vo.* 7s. 6d.
A Colonial Edition is also published.
Canning (George). See Little Library.
Capey (E. F. H.). See Oxford Biographies.
Careless (John). See I.P.L.
Carlyle (Thomas). THE FRENCH REVOLUTION. Edited by C. R. L. FLETCHER, Fellow of Magdalen College, Oxford. *Three Volumes. Cr. 8vo.* 18s.

THE LIFE AND LETTERS OF OLIVER CROMWELL. With an Introduction by C. H. FIRTH, M.A., and Notes and Appendices by Mrs. S. C. LOMAS. *Three Volumes. Demy 8vo.* 18s. net.
Carlyle (R. M. and A. J.), M.A. See Leaders of Religion.
***Carpenter (Margaret).** THE CHILD IN ART. Illustrated. *Cr. 8vo.* 6s.
Chamberlin (Wilbur B.). ORDERED TO CHINA. *Cr. 8vo.* 6s.
A Colonial Edition is also published.
Channer (C. C.) and Roberts (M. E.). LACEMAKING IN THE MIDLANDS, PAST AND PRESENT. With 16 full-page Illustrations. *Cr. 8vo.* 2s. 6d.
Chapman (S. J.). See Books on Business.
Chatterton (Thomas). See Standard Library.
Chesterfield (Lord), THE LETTERS OF, TO HIS SON. Edited, with an Introduction by C. STRACHEY, and Notes by A. CALTHROP. *Two Volumes. Cr. 8vo.* 12s.
***Chesterton (G. K.).** DICKENS. With Portraits and Illustrations. *Demy 8vo.* 7s. 6d. net.
A Colonial Edition is also published.
Christian (F. W.). THE CAROLINE ISLANDS. With many Illustrations and Maps. *Demy 8vo.* 12s. 6d. net.
Cicero. See Classical Translations.
Clarke (F. A.), M.A. See Leaders of Religion.
Cleather (A. L.) and Crump (B.). RICHARD WAGNER'S MUSIC DRAMAS: Interpretations, embodying Wagner's own explanations. *In Four Volumes. Fcap 8vo.* 2s. 6d. each.
VOL. I.—THE RING OF THE NIBELUNG. *Third Edition.*
VOL. II.—PARSIFAL, LOHENGRIN, and THE HOLY GRAIL.
VOL. III.—TRISTAN AND ISOLDE.
Clinch (G.). See Little Guides.
Clough (W. T.). See Junior School Books.
Coast (W. G.), B.A. EXAMINATION PAPERS IN VERGIL. *Cr. 8vo.* 2s.
Cobb (T.). See Little Blue Books.
Cobb (W. F.), M.A. THE BOOK OF PSALMS: with a Commentary. *Demy 8vo.* 10s. 6d. net.
Coleridge (S. T.), SELECTIONS FROM. Edited by ARTHUR SYMONS. *Fcap. 8vo.* 2s. 6d. net.
Collingwood (W. G.). See Half-Crown Library.
Collins (W. E.), M.A. See Churchman's Library.
Colonna. HYPNEROTOMACHIA POLIPHILI UBI HUMANA OMNIA NON NISI SOMNIUM ESSE DOCET ATQUE OBITER PLURIMA SCITU SANE QUAM DIGNA COMMEMORAT. An edition limited to 350 copies on handmade paper. *Folio. Three Guineas net.*
Combe (William). See I.P.L.

Cook (A. M.), M.A. See E. C. Marchant.
Cooke-Taylor (R. W.). See S.Q.S.
Corelli (Marie). THE PASSING OF THE GREAT QUEEN : *Fcap. 4to. 1s.*
A CHRISTMAS GREETING. *Cr. 4to. 1s.*
Corkran (Alice). See Little Books on Art.
Cotes (Rosemary). DANTE'S GARDEN. With a Frontispiece. *Second Edition. Fcap. 8vo. 2s. 6d.; leather, 3s. 6d. net.*
BIBLE FLOWERS. With a Frontispiece and Plan. *Fcap. 8vo. 2s. 6d. net.*
Cowley (Abraham). See Little Library.
Cowper (William), THE POEMS OF. Edited with an Introduction and Notes by J. C. BAILEY, M.A. Illustrated, including two unpublished designs by WILLIAM BLAKE. *Demy 8vo. 10s. 6d. net.*
Cox (J. Charles), LL.D., F.S.A. See Little Guides, The Antiquary's Books, and Ancient Cities.
Cox (Harold), B.A. See S.Q.S.
Crabbe (George). See Little Library.
Craigie (W. A.). A PRIMER OF BURNS. *Cr. 8vo. 2s. 6d.*
Craik (Mrs.). See Little Library.
Crashaw (Richard). See Little Library.
Crawford (F. G.). See Mary C. Danson.
Cross (J. A.). A LITTLE BOOK OF RELIGION. *Fcap. 8vo. 2s. 6d. net.*
Crouch (W.). BRYAN KING. With a Portrait. *Cr. 8vo. 3s. 6d. net.*
Cruikshank (G.). THE LOVING BALLAD OF LORD BATEMAN. With 11 Plates. *Cr. 16mo. 1s. 6d. net.*
Crump (B.). See A. L. Cleather.
Cunliffe (Sir F. H. E.), Fellow of All Souls' College, Oxford. THE HISTORY OF THE BOER WAR. With many Illustrations, Plans, and Portraits. *In 2 vols. Quarto. 15s. each.*
A Colonial Edition is also published.
Cunynghame (H.), C.B., See Connoisseur's Library.
Cutts (E. L.), D.D. See Leaders of Religion.
Daniell (G. W.), M.A. See Leaders of Religion.
Danson (Mary C.) and Crawford (F. G.). FATHERS IN THE FAITH. *Fcap. 8vo. 1s. 6d.*
Dante. LA COMMEDIA DI DANTE. The Italian Text edited by PAGET TOYNBEE, M.A., D.Litt. *Cr. 8vo. 6s.*
THE PURGATORIO OF DANTE. Translated into Spenserian Prose by C. GORDON WRIGHT. With the Italian text. *Fcap. 8vo. 2s. 6d. net.*
See also Paget Toynbee, Little Library and Standard Library.
Darley (George). See Little Library.
D'Arcy (R. F.), M.A. A NEW TRIGONOMETRY FOR BEGINNERS. *Cr. 8vo. 2s. 6d.*
Davenport (Cyril). See Connoisseur's Library and Little Books on Art.

Davey (Richard). THE PAGEANT OF LONDON With 40 Illustrations in Colour by JOHN FULLEYLOVE, R. I. *In Two Volumes. Demy 8vo. 7s. 6d. net.* Each volume may be purchased separately.
   VOL. I.—TO A.D. 1500.
   VOL. II.—A.D. 1500 TO 1900.
Davis (H. W. C.), M.A., Fellow and Tutor of Balliol College, Author of ' Charlemagne.' ENGLAND UNDER THE NORMANS AND ANGEVINS : 1066-1272. With Maps and Illustrations. *Demy 8vo. 10s. 6d. net.*
Dawson (A. J.). MOROCCO. Illustrated. *Demy 8vo. 10s. 6d. net.*
Deane (A. C.). See Little Library.
Delbos (Leon). THE METRIC SYSTEM. *Cr. 8vo. 2s.*
Demosthenes. THE OLYNTHIACS AND PHILIPPICS. Translated by OTHO HOLLAND. *Cr. 8vo. 2s. 6d.*
Demosthenes. AGAINST CONON AND CALLICLES. Edited by F. DARWIN SWIFT, M.A. *Fcap. 8vo. 2s.*
Dickens (Charles). See Little Library and I.P.L.
Dickinson (Emily). POEMS. *Cr. 8vo. 4s. 6d. net.*
Dickinson (G. L.), M.A., Fellow of King's College, Cambridge. THE GREEK VIEW OF LIFE. *Fourth Edition. Cr. 8vo. 2s. 6d.*
Dickson (H. N.). F.R.Met. Soc. METEOROLOGY. Illustrated. *Cr. 8vo. 2s. 6d.*
Dilke (Lady). See S.Q.S.
Dillon (Edward). See Connoisseur's Library and Little Books on Art.
Ditchfield (P. H.), M.A., F.S.A. THE STORY OF OUR ENGLISH TOWNS. With an Introduction by AUGUSTUS JESSOPP, D.D. *Second Edition. Cr. 8vo. 6s.*
OLD ENGLISH CUSTOMS : Extant at the Present Time. *Cr. 8vo. 6s.* See also Half-crown Library.
Dixon (W. M.), M.A. A PRIMER OF TENNYSON. *Second Edition. Cr. 8vo. 2s. 6d.*
ENGLISH POETRY FROM BLAKE TO BROWNING. *Second Edition. Cr. 8vo. 2s. 6d.*
Dole (N. H.). FAMOUS COMPOSERS. With Portraits. *Two Volumes. Demy 8vo. 12s. net.*
Doney (May). SONGS OF THE REAL. *Cr. 8vo. 3s. 6d. net.* A volume of poems.
Douglas (James). THE MAN IN THE PULPIT. *Cr. 8vo. 2s. 6d. net.*
Dowden (J.), D.D., Lord Bishop of Edinburgh. See Churchman's Library.
Drage (G.). See Books on Business.

Driver (S. R.), D.D., D.C.L., Canon of Christ Church, Regius Professor of Hebrew in the University of Oxford. SERMONS ON SUBJECTS CONNECTED WITH THE OLD TESTAMENT. *Cr. 8vo.* 6s. See also Westminster Commentaries.

Dry (Wakeling). See Little Guides.

Dryhurst (A. R.). See Little Books on Art.

Duguid (Charles). See Books on Business.

Dunn (J. T.), D.Sc., **and Mundella (V. A.).** GENERAL ELEMENTARY SCIENCE. With 114 Illustrations. *Second Edition. Cr. 8vo.* 3s. 6d.

Dunstan (A. E.), B.Sc. See Junior School Books and Textbooks of Science.

Durham (The Earl of). A REPORT ON CANADA. With an Introductory Note. *Demy 8vo.* 4s. 6d. net.

Dutt (W. A.). A POPULAR GUIDE TO NORFOLK. *Medium 8vo.* 6d. net. THE NORFOLK BROADS. With coloured Illustrations by FRANK SOUTH-GATE. *Cr. 8vo.* 6s. See also Little Guides.

Earle (John), Bishop of Salisbury. MICRO-COSMOGRAPHIE, OR A PIECE OF THE WORLD DISCOVERED. *Post 16mo.* 2s net.

Edmonds (Major J. E.), R.E.; D.A.Q.-M.G. See W. Birkbeck Wood.

Edwards (Clement). See S.Q.S.

Edwards (W. Douglas). See Commercial Series.

Egan (Pierce). See I.P.L.

Egerton (H. E.), M.A. A HISTORY OF BRITISH COLONIAL POLICY. New and Cheaper Issue. *Demy 8vo.* 7s. 6d. net. A Colonial Edition is also published.

Ellaby (C. G.). See The Little Guides.

Ellerton (F. G.). See S. J. Stone.

Ellwood (Thomas), THE HISTORY OF THE LIFE OF. Edited by C. G. CRUMP, M.A. *Cr. 8vo.* 6s.

Epictetus. See W. H. D. Rouse.

Erasmus. A Book called in Latin EN-CHIRIDION MILITIS CHRISTIANI, and in English the Manual of the Christian Knight.
From the edition printed by Wynken de Worde, 1533. *Fcap. 8vo* 3s. 6d. net.

Fairbrother (W. H.), M.A. THE PHILO-SOPHY OF T. H. GREEN. *Second Edition. Cr. 8vo.* 3s. 6d.

Farrer (Reginald). THE GARDEN OF ASIA. *Second Edition. Cr. 8vo.* 6s. A Colonial Edition is also published.

Fea (Allan). BEAUTIES OF THE SEVENTEENEH CENTURY. With 100 Illustrations. *Demy 8vo.* 12s. 6d. net.

FELISSA; OR, THE LIFE AND OPINIONS OF A KITTEN OF SENTI-MENT. With 12 Coloured Plates. *Post 16mo.* 2s. 6d. net.

Ferrier (Susan). See Little Library.

Fidler (T. Claxton), M.Inst. C.E. See Books on Business.

Fielding (Henry). See Standard Library.

Finn (S. W.), M.A. See Junior Examination Series.

Firth (C. H.), M.A. CROMWELL'S ARMY: A History of the English Soldier during the Civil Wars, the Commonwealth, and the Protectorate. *Cr. 8vo.* 6s.

Fisher (G. W.), M.A. ANNALS OF SHREWSBURY SCHOOL. Illustrated. *Demy 8vo.* 10s. 6d.

FitzGerald (Edward). THE RUBAIYAT OF OMAR KHAYYÁM. Printed from the Fifth and last Edition. With a Com-mentary by Mrs. STEPHEN BATSON, and a Biography of Omar by E. D. ROSS. *Cr. 8vo.* 6s. See also Miniature Library.

FitzGerald (H. P.). A CONCISE HAND-BOOK OF CLIMBERS, TWINERS, AND WALL SHRUBS. Illustrated. *Fcap. 8vo.* 3s. 6d. net.

Flecker (W. H.), M.A., D.C.L., Headmaster of the Dean Close School, Cheltenham. THE STUDENT'S PRAYER BOOK. THE TEXT OF MORNING AND EVENING PRAYER AND LITANY. With an Introduc-tion and Notes. *Cr. 8vo.* 2s. 6d.

Flux (A. W.), M.A., William Dow Professor of Political Economy in M'Gill University, Montreal. ECONOMIC PRINCIPLES. *Demy 8vo.* 7s. 6d. net.

Fortescue (Mrs. G.). See Little Books on Art.

Fraser (David). A MODERN CAM-PAIGN; OR, WAR AND WIRELESS TELEGRAPHY IN THE FAR EAST. Illustrated. *Cr. 8vo.* 6s. A Colonial Edition is also published.

Fraser (J. F.). ROUND THE WORLD ON A WHEEL. With 100 Illustrations. *Fourth Edition Cr. 8vo.* 6s. A Colonial Edition is also published.

French (W.), M.A. See Textbooks of Science.

Freudenreich (Ed. von). DAIRY BAC-TERIOLOGY. A Short Manual for the Use of Students. Translated by J. R. AINSWORTH DAVIS, M.A. *Second Edition. Revised. Cr. 8vo.* 2s. 6d.

Fulford (H. W.), M.A. See Churchman's Bible.

C. G., and F. C. G. JOHN BULL'S AD-VENTURES IN THE FISCAL WON-DERLAND. By CHARLES GEAKE. With 46 Illustrations by F. CARRUTHERS GOULD. *Second Edition. Cr. 8vo.* 1s. net.

*Gallaher (D.) and Stead (D. W.). THE COMPLETE RUGBY FOOTBALLER. With an Account of the Tour of the New Zealanders in England. With Illustra-tions. *Demy 8vo.* 10s. 6d. net.

Gallichan (W. M.). See Little Guides.

Gambado (Geoffrey, Esq.). See I.P.L.

Gaskell (Mrs.). See Little Library and Standard Library.

Gasquet, the Right Rev. Abbot, O.S.B. See Antiquary's Books.

George (H. B.), M.A., Fellow of New College, Oxford. BATTLES OF ENGLISH HISTORY. With numerous Plans. *Fourth Edition.* Revised, with a new Chapter including the South African War. *Cr. 8vo.* 3s. 6d.

A HISTORICAL GEOGRAPHY OF THE BRITISH EMPIRE. *Second Edition. Cr. 8vo.* 3s. 6d.

Gibbins (H. de B.), Litt.D., M.A. INDUSTRY IN ENGLAND : HISTORICAL OUTLINES. With 5 Maps. *Fourth Edition. Demy 8vo.* 10s. 6d.

A COMPANION GERMAN GRAMMAR. *Cr. 8vo.* 1s. 6d.

THE INDUSTRIAL HISTORY OF ENGLAND. *Eleventh Edition.* Revised. With Maps and Plans. *Cr. 8vo.* 3s.

ENGLISH SOCIAL REFORMERS. *Second Edition. Cr. 8vo.* 2s. 6d.

See also Commercial Series and S.Q.S.

Gibbon (Edward). THE DECLINE AND FALL OF THE ROMAN EMPIRE. A New Edition, edited with Notes, Appendices, and Maps, by J. B. BURY, M.A., Litt.D., Regius Professor of Greek at Cambridge. *In Seven Volumes. Demy 8vo. Gilt top,* 8s. 6d. each. *Also, Cr. 8vo.* 6s. *each.*

MEMOIRS OF MY LIFE AND WRITINGS. Edited by G. BIRKBECK HILL, LL.D. *Demy 8vo, Gilt top.* 8s. 6d. *Also Cr. 8vo.* 6s.

See also Standard Library.

Gibson (E. C. S.), D.D., Lord Bishop of Gloucester. See Westminster Commentaries, Handbooks of Theology, and Oxford Biographies.

Gilbert (A. R.). See Little Books on Art.

Gloag (M.). See K. Wyatt.

Godfrey (Elizabeth). A BOOK OF REMEMBRANCE. Edited by. *Fcap. 8vo.* 2s. 6d. net.

Godley (A. D.), M.A., Fellow of Magdalen College, Oxford. LYRA FRIVOLA. *Third Edition. Fcap. 8vo.* 2s. 6d.

VERSES TO ORDER. *Second Edition. Fcap. 8vo.* 2s. 6d.

SECOND STRINGS. *Fcap. 8vo.* 2s. 6d.

Goldsmith (Oliver). THE VICAR OF WAKEFIELD. *Fcap. 32mo.* With 10 Plates in Photogravure by Tony Johannot. *Leather,* 2s. 6d. *net.* See also I.P.L. and Standard Library.

Goodrich-Freer (A.). IN A SYRIAN SADDLE. *Demy 8vo.* 7s. 6d. *net.* A Colonial Edition is also published.

Goudge (H. L.), M.A., Principal of Wells Theological College. See Westminster Commentaries.

Graham (P. Anderson). See S.Q.S.

Granger (F. S.), M.A., Litt.D. PSYCHOLOGY. *Third Edition. Cr. 8vo.* 2s. 6d.

THE SOUL OF A CHRISTIAN. *Cr. 8vo.* 6s.

Gray (E. M'Queen). GERMAN PASSAGES FOR UNSEEN TRANSLATION. *Cr. 8vo.* 2s. 6d.

Gray (P. L.), B.Sc. THE PRINCIPLES OF MAGNETISM AND ELECTRICITY : an Elementary Text-Book. With 181 Diagrams. *Cr. 8vo.* 3s. 6d.

Green (G. Buckland), M.A., late Fellow of St. John's College, Oxon. NOTES ON GREEK AND LATIN SYNTAX. *Cr. 8vo.* 3s. 6d.

Green (E. T.), M.A. See Churchman's Library.

Greenidge (A. H. J.), M.A. A HISTORY OF ROME : During the Later Republic and the Early Principate. *In Six Volumes. Demy 8vo.* Vol. I. (133-104 B.C.). 10s. 6d. *net.*

Greenwell (Dora). See Miniature Library.

Gregory (R. A.). THE VAULT OF HEAVEN. A Popular Introduction to Astronomy. Illustrated. *Cr. 8vo.* 2s. 6d.

Gregory (Miss E. C.). See Library of Devotion.

Greville Minor. A MODERN JOURNAL. Edited by J. A. SPENDER. *Cr. 8vo.* 3s. 6d. net.

Grubb (H. C.). See Textbooks of Technology.

Guiney (Louisa I.). HURRELL FROUDE : Memoranda and Comments. Illustrated. *Demy 8vo.* 10s. 6d. net.

Gwynn (M. L.). A BIRTHDAY BOOK. New and cheaper issue. *Royal 8vo.* 5s. net.

Hackett (John), B.D. A HISTORY OF THE ORTHODOX CHURCH OF CYPRUS. With Maps and Illustrations. *Demy 8vo.* 15s. net.

Haddon (A. C.), Sc.D., F.R.S. HEADHUNTERS BLACK, WHITE, AND BROWN. With many Illustrations and a Map. *Demy 8vo.* 15s.

Hadfield (R. A.). See S.Q.S.

Hall (R. N.) and Neal (W. G.). THE ANCIENT RUINS OF RHODESIA. Illustrated. *Second Edition, revised. Demy 8vo.* 10s. 6d. net. A Colonial Edition is also published.

Hall (R. N.). GREAT ZIMBABWE. With numerous Plans and Illustrations. *Second Edition. Royal 8vo.* 21s. net.

Hamilton (F. J.), D.D. See Byzantine Texts.

Hammond (J. L.). CHARLES JAMES FOX. *Demy 8vo.* 10s. 6d.

Hannay (D.). A SHORT HISTORY OF THE ROYAL NAVY, Illustrated. Two Volumes. *Demy 8vo.* 7s. 6d. each. Vol. I. 1200-1688.

Hannay (James O.), M.A. THE SPIRIT AND ORIGIN OF CHRISTIAN MONASTICISM. *Cr. 8vo.* 6s.

THE WISDOM OF THE DESERT. *Fcap. 8vo.* 3s. 6d. net.

Hare (A. T.), M.A. THE CONSTRUCTION OF LARGE INDUCTION COILS. With numerous Diagrams. *Demy 8vo.* 6s.

Harrison (Clifford). READING AND READERS. *Fcap. 8vo.* 2s. 6d.

Hawthorne (Nathaniel). See Little Library. HEALTH, WEALTH AND WISDOM. *Cr. 8vo.* 1s. net.

Heath (Frank R.). See Little Guides.

Heath (Dudley). See Connoisseur's Library.

Hello (Ernest). STUDIES IN SAINT-SHIP. Translated from the French by V. M. CRAWFORD. *Fcap 8vo.* 3s. 6d.

Henderson (B. W.), Fellow of Exeter College, Oxford. THE LIFE AND PRINCIPATE OF THE EMPEROR NERO. Illustrated. *New and cheaper issue. Demy 8vo.* 7s. 6d. net. AT INTERVALS. *Fcap 8vo.* 2s. 6d. net.

Henderson (T. F.). See Little Library and Oxford Biographies.

Henley (W. E.). See Half-Crown Library.

Henson (H. H.), B.D., Canon of Westminster. APOSTOLIC CHRISTIANITY: As Illustrated by the Epistles of St. Paul to the Corinthians. *Cr. 8vo.* 6s.
LIGHT AND LEAVEN : HISTORICAL AND SOCIAL SERMONS. *Cr. 8vo.* 6s.
DISCIPLINE AND LAW. *Fcap. 8vo.* 2s. 6d.

Herbert (George). See Library of Devotion.

Herbert of Cherbury (Lord). See Miniature Library.

Hewins (W. A. S.), B.A. ENGLISH TRADE AND FINANCE IN THE SEVENTEENTH CENTURY. *Cr. 8vo.* 2s. 6d.

Hewitt (Ethel M.) A GOLDEN DIAL. A Day Book of Prose and Verse. *Fcap. 8vo.* 2s. 6d. net.

Heywood (W.). PALIO AND PONTE : A Book of Tuscan Games. Illustrated. *Royal 8vo.* 21s. net.

Hilbert (T.). See Little Blue Books.

Hill (Clare). See Textbooks of Technology.

Hill (Henry), B.A., Headmaster of the Boy's High School, Worcester, Cape Colony. A SOUTH AFRICAN ARITHMETIC. *Cr. 8vo.* 3s. 6d.

Hillegas (Howard C.). WITH THE BOER FORCES. With 24 Illustrations. *Second Edition. Cr. 8vo.* 6s.
A Colonial Edition is also published.

Hirst (F. W.) See Books on Business.

Hobhouse (Emily). THE BRUNT OF THE WAR. With Map and Illustrations. *Cr. 8vo.* 6s.
A Colonial Edition is also published.

Hobhouse (L. T.), Fellow of C.C.C., Oxford. THE THEORY OF KNOWLEDGE. *Demy 8vo.* 10s. 6d. net.

Hobson (J. A.), M.A. INTERNATIONAL TRADE : A Study of Economic Principles. *Cr. 8vo.* 2s. 6d. net.
PROBLEMS OF POVERTY. *Fifth Edition. Cr. 8vo.* 2s. 6d.

Hodgkin (T.), D.C.L. See Leaders of Religion.

Hodgson (Mrs. W.) HOW TO IDENTIFY OLD CHINESE PORCELAIN. *Second Edition. Post 8vo.* 6s.

Hogg (Thomas Jefferson). SHELLEY AT OXFORD. With an Introduction by R. A. STREATFEILD. *Fcap. 8vo.* 2s. net.

Holden-Stone (G. de). See Books on Business.

Holdich (Sir T. H.), K.C.I.E. THE INDIAN BORDERLAND : being a Personal Record of Twenty Years. Illustrated. *Demy 8vo.* 10s. 6d. net.
A Colonial Edition is also published.

Holdsworth (W. S.), M.A. A HISTORY OF ENGLISH LAW. *In Two Volumes. Vol. I. Demy 8vo.* 10s. 6d. net.

Holland (Canon Scott). See Library of Devotion.

Holt (Emily). THE SECRET OF POPULARITY : How to Achieve Social Success. *Cr. 8vo.* 3s. 6d. net.
A Colonial Edition is also published.

Holyoake (G. J.). THE CO-OPERATIVE MOVEMENT TO-DAY. *Fourth Edition. Cr. 8vo.* 2s. 6d.

Hone (Nathaniel J.). See Antiquary's Books.

Hoppner. See Little Galleries.

Horace. See Classical Translations.

Horsburgh (E. L. S.), M.A. WATERLOO : A Narrative and Criticism. With Plans. *Second Edition. Cr. 8vo.* 5s. See also Oxford Biographies.

Horth (A. C.). See Textbooks of Technology.

Horton (R. F.), D.D. See Leaders of Religion.

Hosie (Alexander). MANCHURIA. With Illustrations and a Map. *Second Edition. Demy 8vo.* 7s. 6d. net.
A Colonial Edition is also published.

How (F. D.). SIX GREAT SCHOOL-MASTERS. With Portraits and Illustrations. *Second Edition. Demy 8vo.* 7s. 6d.

Howell (G.). See S. Q. S.

Hudson (Robert). MEMORIALS OF A WARWICKSHIRE PARISH. Illustrated. *Demy 8vo.* 15s. net.

Hughes (C. E.). THE PRAISE OF SHAKESPEARE. An English Anthology. With a Preface by SIDNEY LEE. *Demy 8vo.* 3s. 6d. net.

Hughes (Thomas). TOM BROWN'S SCHOOLDAYS. With an Introduction and Notes by VERNON RENDALL. *Leather. Royal 32mo.* 2s. 6d. net.

Hutchinson (Horace G.) THE NEW FOREST. Illustrated in colour with 50 Pictures by WALTER TYNDALE and 4 by Miss LUCY KEMP WELCH. *Large Demy 8vo.* 21s. net.

Hutton (A. W.), M.A. See Leaders of Religion and Library of Devotion.

Hutton (Edward). THE CITIES OF UMBRIA. With many Illustrations, of which 20 are in Colour, by A. PISA. *Second Edition. Cr. 8vo.* 6s.
A Colonial Edition is also published.

ENGLISH LOVE POEMS. Edited with an Introduction. *Fcap. 8vo. 3s. 6d. net.*

Hutton (R. H.). See Leaders of Religion.

Hutton (W. H.), M.A. THE LIFE OF SIR THOMAS MORE. With Portraits. *Second Edition. Cr. 8vo. 5s.* See also Leaders of Religion.

Hyett (F. A.). A SHORT HISTORY OF FLORENCE. *Demy 8vo. 7s. 6d. net.*

Ibsen (Henrik). BRAND. A Drama. Translated by WILLIAM WILSON. *Third Edition. Cr. 8vo. 3s. 6d.*

Inge (W. R.), M.A., Fellow and Tutor of Hertford College, Oxford. CHRISTIAN MYSTICISM. The Bampton Lectures for 1899. *Demy 8vo. 12s. 6d. net.* See also Library of Devotion.

Innes (A. D.), M.A. A HISTORY OF THE BRITISH IN INDIA. With Maps and Plans. *Cr. 8vo. 6s.*
ENGLAND UNDER THE TUDORS. With Maps. *Demy 8vo. 10s. 6d. net.*

Jackson (C. E.), B.A. See Textbooks of Science.

Jackson (S.), M.A. See Commercial Series.

Jackson (F. Hamilton). See Little Guides.

Jacob (F.), M.A. See Junior Examination Series.

Jeans (J. Stephen). See S. Q. S. and Business Books.

Jeffreys (D. Gwyn). DOLLY'S THEATRI-CALS. Described and Illustrated with 24 Coloured Pictures. *Super Royal 16mo. 2s.6d.*

Jenks (E.), M.A., Reader of Law in the University of Oxford. ENGLISH LOCAL GOVERNMENT. *Cr. 8vo. 2s. 6d.*

Jenner (Mrs. H.). See Little Books on Art.

Jessopp (Augustus), D.D. See Leaders of Religion.

Jevons (F. B.), M.A., Litt.D., Principal of Bishop Hatfield's Hall, Durham. RE-LIGION IN EVOLUTION. *Cr. 8vo. 3s. 6d. net.*
See also Churchman's Library and Handbooks of Theology.

Johnson (Mrs. Barham). WILLIAM BOD-HAM DONNE AND HIS FRIENDS. Illustrated. *Demy 8vo. 10s. 6d. net.*

Johnston (Sir H. H.), K.C.B. BRITISH CENTRAL AFRICA. With nearly 200 Illustrations and Six Maps. *Third Edition. Cr. 4to. 18s. net.*
A Colonial Edition is also published.

Jones (R. Crompton), M.A. POEMS OF THE INNER LIFE. Selected by. *Eleventh Edition. Fcap. 8vo. 2s. 6d. net.*

Jones (H.). See Commercial Series.

Jones (L. A. Atherley), K.C., M.P., and **Bellot (Hugh H. L.).** THE MINERS' GUIDE TO THE COAL MINES REGULATION ACTS. *Cr.8vo. 2s. 6d. net.*
*COMMERCE IN WAR. *Demy 8vo. 21s. net.*

Jonson (Ben). See Standard Library.

Julian (Lady) of Norwich. REVELA-TIONS OF DIVINE LOVE. Edited by GRACE WARRACK. *Cr. 8vo. 3s. 6d.*

Juvenal. See Classical Translations.

'Kappa.' LET YOUTH BUT KNOW : A Plea for Reason in Education. *Cr. 8vo. 3s. 6d. net.*

Kaufmann (M.). See S. Q. S.

Keating (J. F.), D.D. THE AGAPE AND THE EUCHARIST. *Cr. 8vo. 3s. 6d.*

Keats (John). THE POEMS OF. Edited with Introduction and Notes by E. de Selincourt, M.A. *Demy 8vo. 7s. 6d. net.* See also Little Library, Standard Library, and E. de Selincourt.

Keble (John). THE CHRISTIAN YEAR. With an Introduction and Notes by W. LOCK, D.D., Warden of Keble College. Illustrated by R. ANNING BELL. *Third Edition. Fcap. 8vo. 3s. 6d. ; padded morocco, 5s.* See also Library of Devotion.

Kempis (Thomas à). THE IMITATION OF CHRIST. With an Introduction by DEAN FARRAR. Illustrated by C. M. GERE. *Third Edition. Fcap. 8vo. 3s. 6d.; padded morocco. 5s.*
Also Translated by C. BIGG, D.D. *Cr. 8vo. 3s. 6d.* See also Library of Devotion and Standard Library.

Kennedy (Bart.). THE GREEN SPHINX. *Cr. 8vo. 3s. 6d. net.*
A Colonial Edition is also published.

Kennedy (James Houghton), D.D., Assistant Lecturer in Divinity in the University of Dublin. ST. PAUL'S SECOND AND THIRD EPISTLES TO THE CORIN-THIANS. With Introduction, Dissertations and Notes. *Cr. 8vo. 6s.*

Kestell (J. D.). THROUGH SHOT AND FLAME : Being the Adventures and Experiences of J. D. KESTELL, Chaplain to General Christian de Wet. *Cr. 8vo. 6s.*
A Colonial Edition is also published.

Kimmins (C. W.), M.A. THE CHEMIS-TRY OF LIFE AND HEALTH. Illustrated. *Cr. 8vo. 2s. 6d.*

Kinglake (A. W.). See Little Library.

Kipling (Rudyard). BARRACK-ROOM BALLADS. *73rd Thousand. Twenty-first Edition. Cr. 8vo. 6s.*
A Colonial Edition is also published.
THE SEVEN SEAS. *62nd Thousand. Tenth Edition. Cr. 8vo. 6s.*
A Colonial Edition is also published.
THE FIVE NATIONS. *41st Thousand. Second Edition. Cr. 8vo. 6s.*
A Colonial Edition is also published.
DEPARTMENTAL DITTIES. *Sixteenth Edition. Cr. 8vo. 6s.*
A Colonial Edition is also published.

Knight (Albert E.). THE COMPLETE CRICKETER. Illustrated. *Demy 8vo. 7s. 6d. net.*
A Colonial Edition is also published.

Knowling (R. J.), M.A., Professor of New Testament Exegesis at King's College, London. See Westminster Commentaries.

Lamb (Charles and Mary), THE WORKS OF. Edited by E. V. LUCAS. Illustrated. *In Seven Volumes. Demy 8vo. 7s. 6d. each.*
THE LIFE OF. See E. V. Lucas.
See also Little Library.

Lambert (F. A. H.). See Little Guides.

Lambros (Professor). See Byzantine Texts.

Lane-Poole (Stanley). A HISTORY OF EGYPT IN THE MIDDLE AGES. Fully Illustrated. *Cr. 8vo. 6s.*

Langbridge (F.), M.A. BALLADS OF THE BRAVE: Poems of Chivalry, Enterprise, Courage, and Constancy. *Second Edition. Cr. 8vo. 2s. 6d.*

Law (William). See Library of Devotion and Standard Library.

Leach (Henry). THE DUKE OF DEVON-SHIRE. A Biography. With 12 Illustrations. *Demy 8vo. 12s. 6d.*
A Colonial Edition is also published.

Le Braz (Anatole). THE LAND OF PARDONS. Translated by FRANCES M. GOSTLING. Illustrated in colour. *Crown 8vo. 6s.*

Lee (Captain L. Melville). A HISTORY OF POLICE IN ENGLAND. *Cr. 8vo. 3s. 6d. net.*

Leigh (Percival). THE COMIC ENGLISH GRAMMAR. Embellished with upwards of 50 characteristic Illustrations by JOHN LEECH. *Post 16mo. 2s. 6d. net.*

Lewes (V. B.), M.A. AIR AND WATER. Illustrated. *Cr. 8vo. 2s. 6d.*

Lewis (Mrs. Gwyn). A CONCISE HANDBOOK OF GARDEN SHRUBS. Illustrated. *Fcap. 8vo. 3s. 6d. net.*

Lisle (Fortunéede). See Little Books on Art.

Littlehales (H.). See Antiquary's Books.

Lock (Walter), D.D., Warden of Keble College. ST. PAUL, THE MASTER-BUILDER. *Second Edition. Cr. 8vo. 3s. 6d.*
THE BIBLE AND CHRISTIAN LIFE. *Cr. 8vo. 6s.*
See also Leaders of Religion and Library of Devotion.

Locker (F.). See Little Library.

Longfellow (H. W.). See Little Library.

Lorimer (George Horace). LETTERS FROM A SELF-MADE MERCHANT TO HIS SON. *Fourteenth Edition. Cr. 8vo. 6s.*
A Colonial Edition is also published.
OLD GORGON GRAHAM. *Second Edition. Cr. 8vo. 6s.*
A Colonial Edition is also published.

Lover (Samuel). See I. P. L.

E. V. L. and C. L. 'G. ENGLAND DAY BY DAY: Or, The Englishman's Handbook to Efficiency. Illustrated by GEORGE MORROW. *Fourth Edition. Fcap. 4to. 1s. net.*

Lucas (E. V.). THE LIFE OF CHARLES LAMB. With numerous Portraits and Illustrations. *Third Edition. Two Vols. Demy 8vo. 21s. net.*
A Colonial Edition is also published.
A WANDERER IN HOLLAND. With many Illustrations, of which 20 are in Colour by HERBERT MARSHALL. *Fifth Edition. Cr. 8vo. 6s.*
A Colonial Edition is also published.
THE OPEN ROAD: a Little Book for Wayfarers. *Ninth Edition. Fcap. 8vo. 5s.; India Paper, 7s. 6d.*
THE FRIENDLY TOWN: a Little Book for the Urbane. *Second Edition. Fcap. 8vo. 5s.; India Paper, 7s. 6d.*

Lucian. See Classical Translations.

Lyde (L. W.), M.A. See Commercial Series.

Lydon (Noel S.). See Junior School Books.

Lyttelton (Hon. Mrs. A.). WOMEN AND THEIR WORK. *Cr. 8vo. 2s. 6d.*

M. M. HOW TO DRESS AND WHAT TO WEAR. *Cr. 8vo. 1s. net.*

Macaulay (Lord). CRITICAL AND HISTORICAL ESSAYS. Edited by F. C. MONTAGUE, M.A. *Three Volumes. Cr. 8vo. 18s.* The only edition of this book completely annotated.

M'Allen (J. E. B.), M.A. See Commercial Series.

MacCulloch (J. A.). See Churchman's Library.

MacCunn (Florence A.). MARY STUART. With over 60 Illustrations, including a Frontispiece in Photogravure. *Demy 8vo. 10s. 6d. net.*
A Colonial Edition is also published. See also Leaders of Religion.

McDermott (E. R.). See Books on Business.

M'Dowall (A. S.). See Oxford Biographies.

Mackay (A. M.). See Churchman's Library.

Magnus (Laurie), M.A. A PRIMER OF WORDSWORTH. *Cr. 8vo. 2s. 6d.*

Mahaffy (J. P.), Litt.D. A HISTORY OF THE EGYPT OF THE PTOLEMIES. Fully Illustrated. *Cr. 8vo. 6s.*

Maitland (F. W.), LL.D., Downing Professor of the Laws of England in the University of Cambridge. CANON LAW IN ENGLAND. *Royal 8vo. 7s. 6d.*

Malden (H. E.), M.A. ENGLISH RECORDS. A Companion to the History of England. *Cr. 8vo. 3s. 6d.*
THE ENGLISH CITIZEN: HIS RIGHTS AND DUTIES. *Fifth Edition. Cr. 8vo. 1s. 6d.*
A SCHOOL HISTORY OF SURREY Illustrated. *Cr. 8vo. 1s. 6d.*

Marchant (E. C.), M.A., Fellow of Peterhouse, Cambridge. A GREEK ANTHOLOGY *Second Edition. Cr. 8vo. 3s. 6d.*

Marchant (C. E.)), M.A., and Cook (A. M.), M.A. PASSAGES FOR UNSEEN TRANSLATION. *Third Edition. Cr. 8vo. 3s. 6d.*

Marlowe (Christopher). See Standard Library.

Marr (J. E.), F.R.S., F llow of St John's College, Cambridge. THE SCIENTIFIC STUDY OF SCENERY. *Second Edition.* Illustrated. *Cr. 8vo. 6s.*

AGRICULTURAL GEOLOGY. Illustrated. *Cr. 8vo. 6s.*

Marvell (Andrew). See Little Library.

Masefield (John). SEA LIFE IN NELSON'S TIME. Illustrated. *Cr. 8vo. 3s. 6d. net.*

ON THE SPANISH MAIN. With Portraits and Illustrations. *Demy 8vo. 10s. 6d. net.*
A Colonial Edition is also published.

Maskell (A.). See Connoisseur's Library.

Mason (A. J.), D.D. See Leaders of Religion.

Massee (George). THE EVOLUTION OF PLANT LIFE : Lower Forms. Illustrated. *Cr. 8vo. 2s. 6d.*

Massinger (P.). See Standard Library.

Masterman (C. F. G.), M.A. TENNYSON AS A RELIGIOUS TEACHER. *Cr. 8vo. 6s.*

Matheson (Mrs. E. F.). COUNSELS OF LIFE. *Fcap. 8vo. 2s. 6d. net.*

May (Phil). THE PHIL MAY ALBUM. *Second Edition.* 4to. 1s. net.

Mellows (Emma S.). A SHORT STORY OF ENGLISH LITERATURE. *Cr. 8vo. 3s. 6d.*

Methuen (A. M. S.). THE TRAGEDY OF SOUTH AFRICA. *Cr. 8vo. 2s. net. Also Cr. 8vo. 3d. net.*
A revised and enlarged edition of the author's 'Peace or War in South Africa.'

ENGLAND'S RUIN : DISCUSSED IN SIXTEEN LETTERS TO THE RIGHT HON. JOSEPH CHAMBERLAIN, M.P. *Seventh Edition. Cr. 8vo. 3d. net.*

Michell (E. B.). THE ART AND PRACTICE OF HAWKING. With 3 Photogravures by G. E. LODGE, and other Illustrations. *Demy 8vo. 10s. 6d.*

Millais (J. G.). THE LIFE AND LETTERS OF SIR JOHN EVERETT MILLAIS, President of the Royal Academy. With many Illustrations, of which 2 are in Photogravure. *New Edition. Demy 8vo. 7s. 6d. net.*
A Colonial Edition is also published.

Millin (G. F.). PICTORIAL GARDENING. Illustrated. *Cr. 8vo. 3s. 6d. net.*

Millis (C. T.), M.I.M.E. See Textbooks of Technology.

Milne (J. G.), M.A. A HISTORY OF ROMAN EGYPT. Fully Illustrated. *Cr. 8vo. 6s.*

Milton (John), THE POEMS OF, BOTH ENGLISH AND LATIN, Compos'd at several times. Printed by his true Copies.
The Songs were set in Musick by Mr. HENRY LAWES, Gentleman of the Kings Chappel, and one of His Majesties Private Musick.
Printed and publish'd according to Order.
Printed by RUTH RAWORTH for HUMPHREY MOSELEY, and are to be sold at the signe of the Princes Armes in Pauls Churchyard, 1645,
See also Little Library, Standard Library, and R. F. Towndrow.

Minchin (H. C.), M.A. See R. Peel.

Mitchell (P. Chalmers), M.A. OUTLINES OF BIOLOGY. Illustrated. *Second Edition. Cr. 8vo. 6s.*

Mitton (G. E.). JANE AUSTEN AND HER TIMES. With many Portraits and Illustrations. *Second Edition. Demy 8vo. 10s. 6d. net.*
A Colonial Edition is also published.

'Moil (A.).' See Books on Business.

Moir (D. M.). See Little Library.

Money (L. G. Chiozza). RICHES AND POVERTY. *Second Edition Demy 8vo. 5s. net.*

Montaigne. See C. F. Pond.

Moore (H. E.). See S. Q. S.

Moran (Clarence G.). See Books on Business.

More (Sir Thomas). See Standard Library.

Morfill (W. R.), Oriel College, Oxford. A HISTORY OF RUSSIA FROM PETER THE GREAT TO ALEXANDER II. With Maps and Plans. *Cr. 8vo. 3s. 6d.*

Morich (R. J.), late of Clifton College. See School Examination Series.

Morris (J.). THE MAKERS OF JAPAN. With many portraits and Illustrations. *Demy 8vo. 12s. 6d. net.*
A Colonial Edition is also published.

Morris (J. E.). See Little Guides.

Morton (Miss Anderson). See Miss Brodrick.

THE MOTOR YEAR-BOOK FOR 1906. With many Illustrations and Diagrams. *Demy 8vo. 7s. 6d. net.*

Moule (H. C. G.), D.D., Lord Bishop of Durham. See Leaders of Religion.

Muir (M. M. Pattison), M.A. THE CHEMISTRY OF FIRE. Illustrated. *Cr. 8vo. 2s. 6d.*

Mundella (V. A.), M.A. See J. T. Dunn.

Munro (R.), LL.D. See Antiquary's Books.

Naval Officer (A). See I. P. L.

Neal (W. G.). See R. N. Hall.

Newman (J. H.) and others. See Library of Devotion.

Nichols (J. B. B.). See Little Library.

Nicklin (T.), M.A. EXAMINATION PAPERS IN THUCYDIDES. *Cr. 8vo. 2s.*

Nimrod. See I. P. L.

Norgate (G. Le G.). SIR WALTER SCOTT. Illustrated. *Demy 8vo. 7s. 6d. net.*

Norregaard (B. W.). THE GREAT SIEGE: The Investment and Fall of Port Arthur. Illustrated. *Demy 8vo.* 10s. 6d. net.

Northcote (James), R.A. THE CONVERSATIONS OF JAMES NORTHCOTE, R.A., AND JAMES WARD. Edited by ERNEST FLETCHER. With many Portraits. *Demy 8vo.* 10s. 6d.

Norway (A. H.). NAPLES. With 25 Coloured Illustrations by MAURICE GREIFFENHAGEN. A New Edition. *Cr. 8vo.* 6s.

Novalis. THE DISCIPLES AT SAÏS AND OTHER FRAGMENTS. Edited by Miss UNA BIRCH. *Fcap. 8vo.* 3s. 6d.

Oldfield (W. J.), Canon of Lincoln. A PRIMER OF RELIGION. *Fcap 8vo.* 2s. 6d.

Oliphant (Mrs.). See Leaders of Religion.

Oman (C. W. C.), M.A., Fellow of All Souls', Oxford. A HISTORY OF THE ART OF WAR. Vol. II.: The Middle Ages, from the Fourth to the Fourteenth Century. Illustrated. *Demy 8vo.* 10s. 6d. net.

Ottley (R. L.), D.D. See Handbooks of Theology and Leaders of Religion.

Overton (J. H.). See Leaders of Religion.

Owen (Douglas). See Books on Business.

Oxford (M. N.), of Guy's Hospital. A HANDBOOK OF NURSING. *Third Edition. Cr. 8vo.* 3s. 6d.

Pakes (W. C. C.). THE SCIENCE OF HYGIENE. Illustrated. *Demy 8vo.* 15s.

Palmer (Frederick). WITH KUROKI IN MANCHURIA. Illustrated. *Third Edition. Demy 8vo.* 7s. 6d. net. A Colonial Edition is also published.

Parker (Gilbert). A LOVER'S DIARY. *Fcap. 8vo.* 5s.

Parkes (A. K.). SMALL LESSONS ON GREAT TRUTHS. *Fcap. 8vo.* 1s. 6d.

Parkinson (John). PARADISI IN SOLE PARADISUS TERRESTRIS, OR A GARDEN OF ALL SORTS OF PLEASANT FLOWERS. *Folio.* £4, 4s. net.

Parmenter (John). HELIO-TROPES, OR NEW POSIES FOR SUNDIALS, 1625. Edited by PERCIVAL LANDON. *Quarto.* 3s. 6d. net.

Parmentier (Prof. Leon). See Byzantine Texts.

Pascal. See Library of Devotion.

Paston (George). SOCIAL CARICATURES IN THE EIGHTEENTH CENTURY. *Imperial Quarto.* £2, 12s. 6d. net. See also Little Books on Art and I.P.L.

Paterson (W. R.) (Benjamin Swift). LIFE'S QUESTIONINGS. *Cr. 8vo.* 3s. 6d. net.

Patterson (A. H.). NOTES OF AN EAST COAST NATURALIST. Illustrated in Colour by F. SOUTHGATE. *Second Edition. Cr. 8vo.* 6s.

NATURE IN EASTERN NORFOLK. A series of observations on the Birds, Fishes, Mammals, Reptiles, and stalk-eyed Crustaceans found in that neighbourhood, with a list of the species. With 12 Illustrations in colour, by FRANK SOUTHGATE. *Second Edition. Cr. 8vo.* 6s.

Peacock (N.). See Little Books on Art.

Pearce (E. H.), M.A. ANNALS OF CHRIST'S HOSPITAL. Illustrated. *Demy 8vo.* 7s. 6d.

Peel (Robert), and **Minchin (H. C.),** M.A. OXFORD. With 100 Illustrations in Colour. *Cr. 8vo.* 6s.

Peel (Sidney), late Fellow of Trinity College, Oxford, and Secretary to the Royal Commission on the Licensing Laws. PRACTICAL LICENSING REFORM. *Second Edition. Cr. 8vo.* 1s. 6d.

Peters (J. P.), D.D. See Churchman's Library.

Petrie (W. M. Flinders), D.C.L., LL.D., Professor of Egyptology at University College. A HISTORY OF EGYPT, FROM THE EARLIEST TIMES TO THE PRESENT DAY. Fully Illustrated. *In six volumes. Cr. 8vo.* 6s. each.

VOL. I. PREHISTORIC TIMES TO XVITH DYNASTY. *Fifth Edition.*

VOL. II. THE XVIITH AND XVIIITH DYNASTIES. *Fourth Edition.*

VOL. III. XIXTH TO XXXTH DYNASTIES.

VOL. IV. THE EGYPT OF THE PTOLEMIES. J. P. MAHAFFY, Litt.D.

VOL. V. ROMAN EGYPT. J. G. MILNE, M.A.

VOL. VI. EGYPT IN THE MIDDLE AGES. STANLEY LANE-POOLE, M.A.

RELIGION AND CONSCIENCE IN ANCIENT EGYPT. Illustrated. *Cr. 8vo.* 2s. 6d.

SYRIA AND EGYPT, FROM THE TELL EL AMARNA TABLETS. *Cr. 8vo.* 2s. 6d.

EGYPTIAN TALES. Illustrated by TRISTRAM ELLIS. *In Two Volumes. Cr. 8vo.* 3s. 6d. each.

EGYPTIAN DECORATIVE ART. With 120 Illustrations. *Cr. 8vo.* 3s. 6d.

Phillips (W. A.). See Oxford Biographies.

Phillpotts (Eden). MY DEVON YEAR. With 38 Illustrations by J. LEY PETHYBRIDGE. *Second and Cheaper Edition. Large Cr. 8vo.* 6s.

UP ALONG AND DOWN ALONG. Illustrated by CLAUDE SHEPPERSON. *Cr. 4to.* 5s. net. A volume of poems.

Pienaar (Philip). WITH STEYN AND DE WET. *Second Edition. Cr. 8vo.* 3s. 6d. A Colonial Edition is also published.

Plarr (Victor G.) and Walton (F. W.). A SCHOOL HISTORY OF MIDDLESEX. Illustrated. *Cr. 8vo.* 1s. 6d.

Plato. See Standard Library.

Plautus. THE CAPTIVI. Edited, with an Introduction, Textual Notes, and a Commentary, by W. M. LINDSAY, Fellow of Jesus College, Oxford. *Demy 8vo.* 10s. 6d. *net.*

Plowden-Wardlaw (J. T.), B.A., King's College, Cambridge. See School Examination Series.

Podmore (Frank). MODERN SPIRITUALISM. *Two Volumes. Demy 8vo.* 21s. *net.*
A History and a Criticism.

Poer (J. Patrick Le). A MODERN LEGIONARY. *Cr. 8vo.* 6s.
A Colonial Edition is also published.

Pollard (Alice). See Little Books on Art.

Pollard (A. W.). OLD PICTURE BOOKS. Illustrated. *Demy 8vo.* 7s. 6d. *net.*

Pollard (Eliza F.). See Little Books on Art.

Pollock (David), M.I.N.A. See Books on Business.

Pond (C. F.). A DAY BOOK OF MONTAIGNE. Edited by. *Fcap. 8vo.* 3s. 6d. *net.*

Potter (M. C.), M.A., F.L.S. A TEXTBOOK OF AGRICULTURAL BOTANY. Illustrated. *Second Edition. Cr. 8vo.* 4s. 6d.

Power (J. O'Connor). THE MAKING OF AN ORATOR. *Cr. 8vo.* 6s.

Pradeau (G.). A KEY TO THE TIME ALLUSIONS IN THE DIVINE COMEDY. With a Dial. *Small quarto.* 3s. 6d.

Prance (G.). See Half-Crown Library.

Prescott (O. L.). ABOUT MUSIC, AND WHAT IT IS MADE OF. *Cr. 8vo.* 3s. 6d. *net.*

Price (L. L.), M.A., Fellow of Oriel College, Oxon. A HISTORY OF ENGLISH POLITICAL ECONOMY. *Fourth Edition. Cr. 8vo.* 2s. 6d.

Primrose (Deborah). A MODERN BŒOTIA. *Cr. 8vo.* 6s.

Pugin and Rowlandson. THE MICROCOSM OF LONDON, OR LONDON IN MINIATURE. With 104 Illustrations in colour. *In Three Volumes. Small 4to.* £3, 3s. *net.*

'Q' (A. T. Quiller Couch). See Half-Crown Library.

Quevedo Villegas. See Miniature Library.

G. R. and E. S. THE WOODHOUSE CORRESPONDENCE. *Cr. 8vo.* 6s.
A Colonial Edition is also published.

Rackham (R. B.), M.A. See Westminster Commentaries.

Randolph (B. W.), D.D. See Library of Devotion.

Rannie (D. W.), M.A. A STUDENT'S HISTORY OF SCOTLAND. *Cr. 8vo.* 3s. 6d.

Rashdall (Hastings), M.A., Fellow and Tutor of New College, Oxford. DOCTRINE AND DEVELOPMENT. *Cr. 8vo.* 6s.

Rawstorne (Lawrence, Esq.). See I.P.L.

Raymond (Walter). A SCHOOL HISTORY OF SOMERSETSHIRE. Illustrated. *Cr. 8vo.* 1s. 6d.

A Real Paddy. See I.P-L.

Reason (W.), M.A. See S.Q.S.

Redfern (W. B.), Author of 'Ancient Wood and Iron Work in Cambridge,' etc. ROYAL AND HISTORIC GLOVES AND ANCIENT SHOES. Profusely Illustrated in colour and half-tone. *Quarto,* £2, 2s. *net.*

Reynolds. See Little Galleries.

*Rhodes (W. E.). A SCHOOL HISTORY OF LANCASHIRE. Illustrated. *Cr. 8vo.* 1s. 6d.

Roberts (M. E.). See C. C. Channer.

Robertson (A.), D.D., Lord Bishop of Exeter. REGNUM DEI. The Bampton Lectures of 1901. *Demy 8vo.* 12s. 6d. *net.*

Robertson (C. Grant), M.A., Fellow of All Souls' College, Oxford, Examiner in the Honours School of Modern History, Oxford, 1901-1904. SELECT STATUTES, CASES, AND CONSTITUTIONAL DOCUMENTS, 1660-1832. *Demy 8vo.* 10s. 6d. *net.*

Robertson (C. Grant) and **Bartholomew (J. G.),** F.R.S.E., F.R.G.S. A HISTORICAL AND MODERN ATLAS OF THE BRITISH EMPIRE. *Demy Quarto.* 4s. 6d. *net.*

Robertson (Sir G. S.), K.C.S.I. See Half-Crown Library.

Robinson (A. W.), M.A. See Churchman's Bible.

Robinson (Cecilia). THE MINISTRY OF DEACONESSES. With an Introduction by the late Archbishop of Canterbury. *Cr. 8vo.* 3s. 6d.

Robinson (F. S.). See Connoisseur's Library.

Rochefoucauld (La). See Little Library.

Rodwell (G.), B.A. NEW TESTAMENT GREEK. A Course for Beginners. With a Preface by WALTER LOCK, D.D., Warden of Keble College. *Fcap. 8vo.* 3s. 6d.

Roe (Fred). ANCIENT COFFERS AND CUPBOARDS: Their History and Description. Illustrated. *Quarto.* £3, 3s. *net.*
OLD OAK FURNITURE. With many Illustrations by the Author, including a frontispiece in colour. *Demy 8vo.* 10s. 6d. *net.*

Rogers (A. G. L.), M.A. See Books on Business.

Roscoe (E. S.). ROBERT HARLEY, EARL OF OXFORD. Illustrated. *Demy 8vo.* 7s. 6d.
This is the only life of Harley in existence.
See also Little Guides.

Rose (Edward). THE ROSE READER. Illustrated. *Cr. 8vo. 2s. 6d. Also in 4 Parts. Parts I. and II. 6d. each; Part III. 8d.; Part IV. 10d.*

Rouse (W. H. D.). WORDS OF THE ANCIENT WISE: Thoughts from Epictetus and Marcus Aurelius. Edited by. *Fcap. 8vo. 3s. 6d. net.*

Rowntree (Joshua). THE IMPERIAL DRUG TRADE. *Second and Cheaper Edition. Cr. 8vo. 2s. net.*

Rubie (A. E.), D.D. See Junior School Books.

Russell (W. Clark). THE LIFE OF ADMIRAL LORD COLLINGWOOD. With Illustrations by F. BRANGWYN. *Fourth Edition. Cr. 8vo. 6s.* A Colonial Edition is also published.

St. Anslem. See Library of Devotion.

St. Augustine. See Library of Devotion.

St. Cyres (Viscount). See Oxford Biographies.

St. Francis of Assisi. See Standard Library.

'Saki' (H. Munro). REGINALD. *Second Edition. Fcap. 8vo. 2s. 6d. net.*

Sales (St. Francis de). See Library of Devotion.

Salmon (A. L.). A POPULAR GUIDE TO DEVON. *Medium 8vo. 6d. net.* See also Little Guides.

Sargeant (J.), M.A. ANNALS OF WESTMINSTER SCHOOL. Illustrated. *Demy 8vo. 7s. 6d.*

Sathas (C.). See Byzantine Texts.

Schmitt (John). See Byzantine Texts.

Scott (A. M.). WINSTON SPENCER CHURCHILL. With Portraits and Illustrations. *Cr. 8vo. 3s. 6d.* A Colonial Edition is also published.

Seeley (H. G.), F.R.S. DRAGONS OF THE AIR. Illustrated. *Cr. 8vo. 6s.*

Sells (V. P.), M.A. THE MECHANICS OF DAILY LIFE. Illustrated. *Cr. 8vo. 2s. 6d.*

Selous (Edmund). TOMMY SMITH'S ANIMALS. Illustrated by G. W. ORD. *Fifth Edition. Fcap. 8vo. 2s. 6d.*

Settle (J. H.). ANECDOTES OF SOLDIERS. *Cr. 8vo. 3s. 6d. net.* A Colonial Edition is also published.

Shakespeare (William).
THE FOUR FOLIOS, 1623; 1632; 1664; 1685. Each *Four Guineas net*, or a complete set, *Twelve Guineas net.*
Folios 3 and 4 are ready.
Folio 2 is nearly ready.

The Arden Shakespeare.
Demy 8vo. 2s. 6d. net each volume.
General Editor, W. J. CRAIG. An Edition of Shakespeare in single Plays. Edited with a full Introduction, Textual Notes, and a Commentary at the foot of the page.

HAMLET. Edited by EDWARD DOWDEN, Litt.D.
ROMEO AND JULIET. Edited by EDWARD DOWDEN, Litt.D.
KING LEAR. Edited by W. J. CRAIG.
JULIUS CAESAR. Edited by M. MACMILLAN, M.A.
THE TEMPEST. Edited by MORETON LUCE.
OTHELLO. Edited by H. C. HART.
TITUS ANDRONICUS. Edited by H. B. BAILDON.
CYMBELINE. Edited by EDWARD DOWDEN.
THE MERRY WIVES OF WINDSOR. Edited by H. C. HART.
A MIDSUMMER NIGHT'S DREAM. Edited by H. CUNINGHAM.
KING HENRY V. Edited by H. A. EVANS.
ALL'S WELL THAT ENDS WELL. Edited by W. O. BRIGSTOCKE.
THE TAMING OF THE SHREW. Edited by R. WARWICK BOND.
TIMON OF ATHENS. Edited by K. DEIGHTON.
MEASURE FOR MEASURE. Edited by H. C. HART.
TWELFTH NIGHT. Edited by MORETON LUCE.
THE MERCHANT OF VENICE. Edited by C. KNOX POOLER.
TROILUS AND CRESSIDA. Edited by K. DEIGHTON.

The Little Quarto Shakespeare. Edited by W. J. CRAIG. With Introductions and Notes. *Pott 16mo. In 40 Volumes. Leather, price 1s. net each volume.* Mahogany Revolving Book Case. *10s. net.* See also Standard Library.

Sharp (A.). VICTORIAN POETS. *Cr. 8vo. 2s. 6d.*

Sharp (Cecil). See S. Baring-Gould.

Sharp (Mrs. E. A.). See Little Books on Art.

Shedlock (J. S.) THE PIANOFORTE SONATA. *Cr. 8vo. 5s.*

Shelley (Percy B.). ADONAIS; an Elegy on the death of John Keats, Author of 'Endymion,' etc. Pisa. From the types of Didot, 1821. *2s. net.*

Sheppard (H. F.), M.A. See S. Baring-Gould.

Sherwell (Arthur), M.A. See S.Q.S.

Shipley (Mary E.). AN ENGLISH CHURCH HISTORY FOR CHILDREN. With a Preface by the Bishop of Gibraltar. With Maps and Illustrations. Part I. *Cr. 8vo. 2s. 6d. net.*

Sichel (Walter). DISRAELI: A Study in Personality and Ideas. With 3 Portraits. *Demy 8vo. 12s. 6d. net.* A Colonial Edition is also published. See also Oxford Biographies.

Sime (J.). See Little Books on Art.

Simonson (G. A.). FRANCESCO GUARDI. With 41 Plates. *Imperial 4to. £2, 2s. net.*

Sketchley (R. E. D.). See Little Books on Art.

Skipton (H. P. K.). See Little Books on Art.

Sladen (Douglas). SICILY: The New Winter Resort. With over 200 Illustrations. *Second Edition. Cr. 8vo. 5s. net.*

Small (Evan), M.A. THE EARTH. An Introduction to Physiography. Illustrated. *Cr. 8vo. 2s. 6d.*

Smallwood (M. G.). See Little Books on Art.

Smedley (F. E.). See I.P.L.

Smith (Adam). THE WEALTH OF NATIONS. Edited with an Introduction and numerous Notes by EDWIN CANNAN, M.A. *Two volumes. Demy 8vo. 21s. net.*
See also English Library.

Smith (Horace and James). See Little Library.

Smith (H. Bompas), M.A. A NEW JUNIOR ARITHMETIC. *Crown 8vo. 2s. 6d.*

Smith (R. Mudie). THOUGHTS FOR THE DAY. Edited by. *Fcap. 8vo. 3s. 6d. net.*

Smith (Nowell C.). See W. Wordsworth.

Smith (John Thomas). A BOOK FOR A RAINY DAY : Or Recollections of the Events of the Years 1766-1833. Edited by WILFRED WHITTEN. Illustrated. *Demy 8vo. 12s. 6d. net.*

Snell (F. J.). A BOOK OF EXMOOR. Illustrated. *Cr. 8vo. 6s.*

Snowden (C. E.). A HANDY DIGEST OF BRITISH HISTORY. *Demy 8vo. 4s. 6d.*

Sophocles. See Classical Translations.

Sornet (L. A.). See Junior School Books.

South (Wilton E.), M.A. See Junior School Books.

Southey (R.). ENGLISH SEAMEN. Edited by DAVID HANNAY.
Vol. I. (Howard, Clifford, Hawkins, Drake, Cavendish). *Second Edition. Cr. 8vo. 6s.*
Vol. II. (Richard Hawkins, Grenville, Essex, and Raleigh). *Cr. 8vo. 6s.*
See also Standard Library.

Spence (C. H.), M.A. See School Examination Series.

Spooner (W. A.), M.A. See Leaders of Religion.

Staley (Edgcumbe). THE GUILDS OF FLORENCE. Illustrated. *Royal 8vo. 16s. net.*

Stanbridge (J. W.), B.D. See Library of Devotion.

'Stancliffe.' GOLF DO'S AND DONT'S. *Second Edition. Fcap. 8vo. 1s.*

Stead (D. W.). See D. Gallaher.

Stedman (A. M. M.), M.A.

INITIA LATINA : Easy Lessons on Elementary Accidence. *Ninth Edition. Fcap. 8vo. 1s.*

FIRST LATIN LESSONS. *Ninth Edition. Cr. 8vo. 2s.*

FIRST LATIN READER. With Notes adapted to the Shorter Latin Primer and Vocabulary. *Sixth Edition revised. 18mo. 1s. 6d.*

EASY SELECTIONS FROM CÆSAR. The Helvetian War. *Second Edition 18mo. 1s.*

EASY SELECTIONS FROM LIVY. The Kings of Rome. *18mo. Second Edition. 1s. 6d.*

EASY LATIN PASSAGES FOR UNSEEN TRANSLATION. *Tenth Edition Fcap. 8vo. 1s. 6d.*

EXEMPLA LATINA. First Exercises in Latin Accidence. With Vocabulary. *Third Edition. Cr. 8vo. 1s.*

EASY LATIN EXERCISES ON THE SYNTAX OF THE SHORTER AND REVISED LATIN PRIMER. With Vocabulary. *Tenth and Cheaper Edition, re-written. Cr. 8vo. 1s. 6d. Original Edition. 2s. 6d.* KEY, 3s. net.

THE LATIN COMPOUND SENTENCE : Rules and Exercises. *Second Edition. Cr. 8vo. 1s. 6d.* With Vocabulary. 2s.

NOTANDA QUAEDAM : Miscellaneous Latin Exercises on Common Rules and Idioms. *Fourth Edition. Fcap. 8vo. 1s. 6d.* With Vocabulary. 2s. Key, 2s. net.

LATIN VOCABULARIES FOR REPETITION : Arranged according to Subjects. *Thirteenth Edition. Fcap. 8vo. 1s. 6d.*

A VOCABULARY OF LATIN IDIOMS. *18mo. Second Edition. 1s.*

STEPS TO GREEK. *Second Edition, revised. 18mo. 1s.*

A SHORTER GREEK PRIMER. *Cr. 8vo. 1s. 6d.*

EASY GREEK PASSAGES FOR UNSEEN TRANSLATION. *Third Edition, revised. Fcap. 8vo. 1s. 6d.*

GREEK VOCABULARIES FOR REPETITION. Arranged according to Subjects. *Fourth Edition. Fcap. 8vo. 1s. 6d.*

GREEK TESTAMENT SELECTIONS. For the use of Schools. With Introduction, Notes, and Vocabulary. *Fourth Edition. Fcap. 8vo. 2s. 6d.*

STEPS TO FRENCH. *Seventh Edition. 18mo. 8d.*

FIRST FRENCH LESSONS. *Seventh Edition, revised. Cr. 8vo. 1s.*

EASY FRENCH PASSAGES FOR UNSEEN TRANSLATION. *Fifth Edition, revised. Fcap. 8vo. 1s. 6d.*

EASY FRENCH EXERCISES ON ELE-
MENTARY SYNTAX. With Vocabu-
lary. *Fourth Edition. Cr. 8vo. 2s. 6d.*
KEY. *3s. net.*
FRENCH VOCABULARIES FOR RE-
PETITION : Arranged according to Sub-
jects. *Twelfth Edition. Fcap. 8vo. 1s.*
See also School Examination Series.
Steel (R. Elliott), M.A., F.C.S. THE
WORLD OF SCIENCE. With 147
Illustrations. *Second Edition. Cr. 8vo. 2s. 6d.*
See also School Examination Series.
Stephenson (C.), of the Technical College,
Bradford, and **Suddards (F.)** of the
Yorkshire College, Leeds. ORNAMEN-
TAL DESIGN FOR WOVEN FABRICS.
Illustrated. *Demy 8vo. Third Edition.
7s. 6d.*
Stephenson (J.), M.A. THE CHIEF
TRUTHS OF THE CHRISTIAN
FAITH. *Cr. 8vo. 3s. 6d.*
Sterne (Laurence). See Little Library.
Sterry (W.). M.A. ANNALS OF ETON
COLLEGE. Illustrated. *Demy 8vo. 7s. 6d.*
Steuart (Katherine). BY ALLAN
WATER. *Second Edition. Cr. 8vo. 6s.*
Stevenson (R. L.) THE LETTERS OF
ROBERT LOUIS STEVENSON TO
HIS FAMILY AND FRIENDS.
Selected and Edited by SIDNEY COLVIN.
Sixth Edition. Cr. 8vo. 12s.
LIBRARY EDITION. *Demy 8vo. 2 vols. 25s. net.*
A Colonial Edition is also published.
VAILIMA LETTERS. With an Etched
Portrait by WILLIAM STRANG. *Fifth
Edition. Cr. 8vo. Buckram. 6s.*
A Colonial Edition is also published.
THE LIFE OF R. L. STEVENSON. See
G. Balfour.
Stevenson (M. I.). FROM SARANAC
TO THE MARQUESAS. Being Letters
written by Mrs. M. I. STEVENSON during
1887-8. *Cr. 8vo. 6s. net.*
A Colonial Edition is also published.
LETTERS FROM SAMOA. Edited and
arranged by M. C. BALFOUR. With many
Illustrations. *Second Ed. Cr. 8vo. 6s. net.*
Stoddart (Anna M.). See Oxford Bio-
graphies.
Stokes (F. G.), B.A. HOURS WITH
RABELAIS. From the translation of SIR
T. URQUHART and P. A. MOTTEUX. With
a Portrait in Photogravure. *Cr. 8vo. 3s. 6d.
net.*
Stone (S. J.). POEMS AND HYMNS.
With a Memoir by F. G. ELLERTON,
M.A. With Portrait. *Cr. 8vo. 6s.*
Storr (Vernon F.), M.A., Lecturer in
the Philosophy of Religion in Cambridge
University ; Examining Chaplain to the
Archbishop of Canterbury; formerly Fellow
of University College, Oxford. DEVELOP-
MENT AND DIVINE PURPOSE *Cr.
8vo. 5s. net.*
Straker (F.). See Books on Business.

Streane (A. W.), D.D. See Churchman's
Bible.
Stroud (H.), D.Sc., M.A. See Textbooks of
Science.
Strutt (Joseph). THE SPORTS AND
PASTIMES OF THE PEOPLE OF
ENGLAND. Illustrated by many engrav-
ings. Revised by J. CHARLES COX, LL.D.,
F.S.A. *Quarto. 21s. net.*
Stuart (Capt. Donald). THE STRUGGLE
FOR PERSIA. With a Map. *Cr. 8vo. 6s.*
Sturch (F.), Staff Instructor to the Surrey
County Council. MANUAL TRAINING,
DRAWING (WOODWORK). Its Prin-
ciples and Application, with Solutions to
Examination Questions, 1892-1905. Ortho-
graphic, Isometric and Oblique Projection.
With 50 Plates and 140 Figures. *Foolscap.
5s. net.*
Suckling (Sir John). FRAGMENTA
AUREA : a Collection of all the Incom-
parable Peeces, written by. And published
by a friend to perpetuate his memory.
Printed by his own copies.
Printed for HUMPHREY MOSELEY, and
are to be sold at his shop, at the sign of the
Princes Arms in St. Paul's Churchyard, 1646.
Suddards (F.). See C. Stephenson.
Surtees (R. S.). See I.P.L.
Swift (Jonathan). THE JOURNAL TO
STELLA. Edited by G. A. AITKEN. *Cr.
8vo. 6s.*
Symes (J. E.), M.A. THE FRENCH
REVOLUTION. *Second Edition. Cr. 8vo.
2s. 6d.*
Sympson (E. M.), M.A., M.D. See Ancient
Cities.
Syrett (Netta). See Little Blue Books.
Tacitus. AGRICOLA. With Introduction
Notes, Map, etc. By R. F. DAVIS, M.A.,
Fcap. 8vo. 2s.
GERMANIA. By the same Editor. *Fcap.
8vo. 2s.* See also Classical Translations.
Tallack (W.). HOWARD LETTERS AND
MEMORIES. *Demy 8vo. 10s. 6d. net.*
Tauler (J.). See Library of Devotion.
Taunton (E. L.). A HISTORY OF THE
JESUITS IN ENGLAND. Illustrated.
Demy 8vo. 21s. net.
Taylor (A. E.). THE ELEMENTS OF
METAPHYSICS. *Demy 8vo. 10s. 6d. net.*
Taylor (F. G.), M.A. See Commercial Series.
Taylor (I. A.). See Oxford Biographies.
Taylor (T. M.), M.A., Fellow of Gonville
and Caius College, Cambridge. A CON-
STITUTIONAL AND POLITICAL
HISTORY OF ROME. *Cr. 8vo. 7s. 6d.*
Tennyson (Alfred, Lord). THE EARLY
POEMS OF. Edited, with Notes and
an Introduction, by J. CHURTON COLLINS,
M.A. *Cr. 8vo. 6s.*
IN MEMORIAM, MAUD, AND THE
PRINCESS. Edited by J. CHURTON
COLLINS, M.A. *Cr. 8vo. 6s.* See also
Little Library.

A 3

Terry (C. S.). See Oxford Biographies.

Terton (Alice). LIGHTS AND SHADOWS IN A HOSPITAL. *Cr. 8vo.* 3s. 6d.

Thackeray (W. M.). See Little Library.

Theobald (F. V.), M.A. INSECT LIFE. Illustrated. *Second Ed. Revised. Cr. 8vo.* 2s. 6d.

Thompson (A. H.). See Little Guides.

Tileston (Mary W.). DAILY STRENGTH FOR DAILY NEEDS. *Twelfth Edition. Medium 16mo.* 2s. 6d. net. Also an edition in superior binding, 6s.

Tompkins (H. W.), F.R.H.S. See Little Guides.

Towndrow (R. F.). A DAY BOOK OF MILTON. Edited by. *Fcap. 8vo.* 3s. 6d. net.

Townley (Lady Susan). MY CHINESE NOTE-BOOK With 16 Illustrations and 2 Maps. *Third Edition. Demy 8vo.* 10s. 6d. net.
A Colonial Edition is also published.

*Toynbee (Paget), M.A., D.Litt. DANTE IN ENGLISH LITERATURE. *Demy 8vo.* 12s. 6d. net.
See also Oxford Biographies.

Trench (Herbert). DEIRDRE WED and Other Poems. *Cr. 8vo.* 5s.

Trevelyan (G. M.), Fellow of Trinity College, Cambridge. ENGLAND UNDER THE STUARTS. With Maps and Plans. *Second Edition. Demy 8vo.* 10s. 6d. net.

Troutbeck (G. E.). See Little Guides.

Tyler (E. A.), B.A., F.C.S. See Junior School Books.

Tyrell-Gill (Frances). See Little Books on Art.

Vardon (Harry). THE COMPLETE GOLFER. Illustrated. *Seventh Edition. Demy 8vo.* 10s. 6d. net.
A Colonial Edition is also published.

Vaughan (Henry). See Little Library.

Voegelin (A.), M.A. See Junior Examination Series.

Waddell (Col. L. A.), LL.D., C.B. LHASA AND ITS MYSTERIES. With a Record of the Expedition of 1903-1904. With 2000 Illustrations and Maps. *Demy 8vo.* 21s. net.
Also Third and Cheaper Edition. With 155 Illustrations and Maps. *Demy 8vo.* 7s. 6d. net.

Wade (G. W.), D.D. OLD TESTAMENT HISTORY. With Maps. *Third Edition. Cr. 8vo.* 6s.

Wagner (Richard). See A. L. Cleather.

Wall (J. C.). DEVILS. Illustrated by the Author and from photographs. *Demy 8vo.* 4s. 6d. net. See also Antiquary's Books.

Walters (H. B.). See Little Books on Art.

Walton (F. W.). See Victor G. Plarr.

Walton (Izaac) and **Cotton (Charles).** See I.P.L., Standard Library, and Little Library.

Warmelo (D. S. Van). ON COMMANDO. With Portrait. *Cr. 8vo.* 3s. 6d.
A Colonial Edition is also published.

Warren-Vernon (Hon. William), M.A. READINGS ON THE INFERNO OF DANTE, chiefly based on the Commentary of BENVENUTO DA IMOLA. With an Introduction by the Rev. Dr. MOORE. In Two Volumes. *Second Edition. Cr. 8vo.* 15s. net.

Waterhouse (Mrs. Alfred). WITH THE SIMPLE-HEARTED: Little Homilies to Women in Country Places. *Second Edition. Small Pott 8vo.* 2s. net. See also Little Library.

Weatherhead (T. C.), M.A. EXAMINATION PAPERS IN HORACE. *Cr. 8vo.* 2s. See also Junior Examination Series.

Webb (W. T.). See Little Blue Books.

Webber (F. C.). See Textbooks of Technology.

Wells (Sidney H.). See Textbooks of Science.

Wells (J.), M.A., Fellow and Tutor of Wadham College. OXFORD AND OXFORD LIFE. *Third Edition. Cr. 8vo.* 3s. 6d.
A SHORT HISTORY OF ROME. *Sixth Edition.* With 3 Maps. *Cr. 8vo.* 3s. 6d.
See also Little Guides.

'Westminster Gazette' Office Boy (Francis Brown). THE DOINGS OF ARTHUR. *Cr. 4to.* 2s. 6d. net.

Wetmore (Helen C.). THE LAST OF THE GREAT SCOUTS ('Buffalo Bill'). Illustrated. *Second Edition. Demy 8vo.* 6s.
A Colonial Edition is also published.

Whibley (C.). See Half-crown Library.

Whibley (L.), M.A., Fellow of Pembroke College, Cambridge. GREEK OLIGARCHIES: THEIR ORGANISATION AND CHARACTER. *Cr. 8vo.* 6s.

Whitaker (G. H.), M.A. See Churchman's Bible.

White (Gilbert). THE NATURAL HISTORY OF SELBORNE. Edited by L. C. MIALL, F.R.S., assisted by W. WARDE FOWLER, M.A. *Cr. 8vo.* 6s. See also Standard Library.

Whitfield (E. E.). See Commercial Series.

Whitehead (A. W.). GASPARD DE COLIGNY. Illustrated. *Demy 8vo.* 12s. 6d. net.

Whiteley (R. Lloyd), F.I.C., Principal of the Municipal Science School, West Bromwich. AN ELEMENTARY TEXTBOOK OF INORGANIC CHEMISTRY. *Cr. 8vo.* 2s. 6d.

Whitley (Miss). See S.Q.S.

Whitten (W.). See John Thomas Smith.

Whyte (A. G.), B.Sc. See Books on Business.

Wilberforce (Wilfrid). See Little Books on Art.

Wilde (Oscar). DE PROFUNDIS. *Sixth Edition. Cr. 8vo.* 5s. net.
A Colonial Edition is also published.

GENERAL LITERATURE 19

Wilkins (W. H.), B.A. See S.Q.S.

Wilkinson (J. Frome). See S.Q.S.

***Williams (A.).** PETROL PETER: or Mirth for Motorists. Illustrated in Colour by A. W. MILLS. *Demy 4to.* *3s. 6d. net.*

Williamson (M. G.). See Ancient Cities.

Williamson (W.). THE BRITISH GARDENER. Illustrated. *Demy 8vo.* *10s. 6d.*

Williamson (W.), B.A. See Junior Examination Series, Junior School Books, and Beginner's Books.

Willson (Beckles). LORD STRATHCONA: the Story of his Life. Illustrated. *Demy 8vo.* *7s. 6d.*
A Colonial Edition is also published.

Wilmot-Buxton (E. M.). MAKERS OF EUROPE. *Cr. 8vo.* *Fifth Ed.* *3s. 6d.*
A Text-book of European History for Middle Forms.

THE ANCIENT WORLD. With Maps and Illustrations. *Cr. 8vo.* *3s. 6d.*
See also Beginner's Books.

Wilson (Bishop.). See Library of Devotion.

Wilson (A. J.). See Books on Business.

Wilson (H. A.). See Books on Business.

Wilton (Richard), M.A. LYRA PASTORALIS: Songs of Nature, Church, and Home. *Pott 8vo.* *2s. 6d.*

Winbolt (S. E.), M.A. EXERCISES IN LATIN ACCIDENCE. *Cr. 8vo.* *1s. 6d.*
LATIN HEXAMETER VERSE: An Aid to Composition. *Cr. 8vo.* *3s. 6d.* KEY, *5s. net.*

Windle (B. C. A.), D.Sc., F.R.S. See Antiquary's Books, Little Guides and Ancient Cities.

Winterbotham (Canon), M.A., B.Sc., LL.B. See Churchman's Library.

Wood (J. A. E.). See Textbooks of Technology.

Wood (J. Hickory). DAN LENO. Illustrated. *Third Edition.* *Cr. 8vo.* *6s.*
A Colonial Edition is also published.

Wood (W. Birkbeck), M.A., late Scholar of Worcester College, Oxford, and **Edmonds (Major J. E.)**, R.E., D.A.Q.-M.G. A HISTORY OF THE CIVIL WAR IN THE UNITED STATES. With an Introduction by H. SPENSER WILKINSON. With 24 Maps and Plans. *Demy 8vo.* *12s. 6d. net.*

Wordsworth (Christopher). See Antiquary's Books.

***Wordsworth (W.).** THE POEMS OF. With Introduction and Notes by NOWELL C. SMITH, Fellow of New College, Oxford. *In Four Volumes.* *Demy 8vo.* *5s. net each.* See also Little Library.

Wordsworth (W.) and Coleridge (S. T.). See Little Library.

Wright (Arthur), M.A., Fellow of Queen's College, Cambridge. See Churchman's Library.

Wright (C. Gordon). See Dante.

Wright (J. C.). TO-DAY. *Fcap. 16mo.* *1s. net.*

Wright (Sophie). GERMAN VOCABULARIES FOR REPETITION. *Fcap. 8vo.* *1s. 6d.*

Wrong (George M.), Professor of History in the University of Toronto. THE EARL OF ELGIN. Illustrated. *Demy 8vo.* *7s. 6d. net.*
A Colonial Edition is also published.

Wyatt (Kate) and Gloag (M.). A BOOK OF ENGLISH GARDENS. With 24 Illustrations in Colour. *Demy 8vo.* *10s. 6s. net.*

Wylde (A. B.). MODERN ABYSSINIA. With a Map and a Portrait. *Demy 8vo.* *15s. net.*
A Colonial Edition s also published

Wyndham (George). THE POEMS OF WILLIAM SHAKESPEARE. With an Introduction and Notes. *Demy 8vo.* *Buckram, gilt top.* *10s. 6d.*

Wyon (R.). See Half-crown Library.

Yeats (W. B.). AN ANTHOLOGY OF IRISH VERSE. *Revised and Enlarged Edition.* *Cr. 8vo.* *3s. 6d.*

Young (Filson). THE COMPLETE MOTORIST. With 138 Illustrations. *Sixth Edition.* *Demy 8vo.* *12s. 6d. net.*
A Colonial Edition is also published.

Young (T. M.). THE AMERICAN COTTON INDUSTRY: A Study of Work and Workers. *Cr. 8vo.* *Cloth, 2s. 6d.; paper boards, 1s. 6d.*

Zimmern (Antonia). WHAT DO WE KNOW CONCERNING ELECTRICITY? *Fcap. 8vo.* *1s. 6d. net.*

Ancient Cities

General Editor, B. C. A. WINDLE, D.Sc., F.R.S.

Cr. 8vo. *4s. 6d. net.*

CHESTER. By B. C. A. Windle, D.Sc. F.R.S. Illustrated by E. H. New.

SHREWSBURY. By T. Auden, M.A., F.S.A. Illustrated.

CANTERBURY. By J. C. Cox, LL.D., F.S.A. Illustrated.

EDINBURGH. By M. G. Williamson. Illustrated by Herbert Railton.

LINCOLN. By E. Mansel Sympson, M.A., M.D. Illustrated by E. H. New.

BRISTOL. By Alfred Harvey. Illustrated by E. H. New.

Antiquary's Books, The

General Editor, J. CHARLES COX, LL.D., F.S.A.

A series of volumes dealing with various branches of English Antiquities; comprehensive and popular, as well as accurate and scholarly.

Demy 8vo.   7s. 6d. net.

ENGLISH MONASTIC LIFE. By the Right Rev. Abbot Gasquet, O.S B. Illustrated. *Third Edition.*

REMAINS OF THE PREHISTORIC AGE IN ENGLAND. By B. C. A. Windle, D.Sc., F.R.S. With numerous Illustrations and Plans.

OLD SERVICE BOOKS OF THE ENGLISH CHURCH. By Christopher Wordsworth, M.A., and Henry Littlehales. With Coloured and other Illustrations.

CELTIC ART. By J. Romilly Allen, F.S.A. With numerous Illustrations and Plans.

ARCHÆOLOGY AND FALSE ANTIQUITIES. By R. Munro, LL.D. Illustrated.

SHRINES OF BRITISH SAINTS. By J. C. Wall. With numerous Illustrations and Plans.

THE ROYAL FORESTS OF ENGLAND. By J. C. Cox, LL.D., F.S.A. Illustrated.

THE MANOR AND MANORIAL RECORDS. By Nathaniel J. Hone. Illustrated.

SEALS. By J. Harvey Bloom. Illustrated.

Beginner's Books, The

Edited by W. WILLIAMSON, B.A.

EASY FRENCH RHYMES. By Henri Blouet. Illustrated. *Fcap. 8vo.* 1s.

EASY STORIES FROM ENGLISH HISTORY. By E. M. Wilmot-Buxton, Author of 'Makers of Europe.' *Cr. 8vo.* 1s.

EASY EXERCISES IN ARITHMETIC. Arranged by W. S. Beard. *Fcap. 8vo.* Without Answers, 1s. With Answers, 1s. 3d.

EASY DICTATION AND SPELLING. By W. Williamson, B.A. *Fifth Edition. Fcap. 8vo.* 1s.

Business, Books on

Cr. 8vo.   2s. 6d. net.

A series of volumes dealing with all the most important aspects of commercial and financial activity. The volumes are intended to treat separately all the considerable industries and forms of business, and to explain accurately and clearly what they do and how they do it. Some are Illustrated. The first volumes are—

PORTS AND DOCKS. By Douglas Owen.

RAILWAYS. By E. R. McDermott.

THE STOCK EXCHANGE. By Chas. Duguid. *Second Edition.*

THE BUSINESS OF INSURANCE. By A. J. Wilson.

THE ELECTRICAL INDUSTRY : LIGHTING, TRACTION, AND POWER. By A. G. Whyte, B.Sc.

THE SHIPBUILDING INDUSTRY : Its History, Science, Practice, and Finance. By David Pollock, M.I.N.A.

THE MONEY MARKET. By F. Straker.

THE BUSINESS SIDE OF AGRICULTURE. By A. G. L. Rogers, M.A.

LAW IN BUSINESS. By H. A. Wilson.

THE BREWING INDUSTRY. By Julian L. Baker, F.I.C., F.C.S.

THE AUTOMOBILE INDUSTRY. By G. de H. Stone.

MINING AND MINING INVESTMENTS. By 'A. Moil.'

THE BUSINESS OF ADVERTISING. By Clarence G. Moran, Barrister-at-Law. Illustrated.

TRADE UNIONS. By G. Drage.

CIVIL ENGINEERING. By T. Claxton Fidler, M. Inst. C.E. Illustrated.

THE IRON TRADE. By J. Stephen Jeans. Illustrated.

MONOPOLIES, TRUSTS, AND KARTELLS. By F. W. Hirst.

THE COTTON INDUSTRY AND TRADE. By Prof. S. J. Chapman, Dean of the Faculty of Commerce in the University of Manchester. Illustrated.

Byzantine Texts
Edited by J. B. BURY, M.A., Litt.D.
A series of texts of Byzantine Historians, edited by English and foreign scholars.

ZACHARIAH OF MITYLENE. Translated by F. J. Hamilton, D.D., and E. W. Brooks. *Demy 8vo.* 12s. 6d. net.

EVAGRIUS. Edited by Léon Parmentier and M. Bidez. *Demy 8vo.* 10s. 6d. net.

THE HISTORY OF PSELLUS. Edited by C. Sathas. *Demy 8vo.* 15s. net.

ECTHESIS CHRONICA. Edited by Professor Lambros. *Demy 8vo.* 7s. 6d. net.

THE CHRONICLE OF MOREA. Edited by John Schmitt. *Dem⁴ 8vo.* 15s. net.

Churchman's Bible, The
General Editor, J. H. BURN, B.D., F.R.S.E.
A series of Expositions on the Books of the Bible, which will be of service to the general reader in the practical and devotional study of the Sacred Text.

Each Book is provided with a full and clear Introductory Section, in which is stated what is known or conjectured respecting the date and occasion of the composition of the Book, and any other particulars that may help to elucidate its meaning as a whole. The Exposition is divided into sections of a convenient length, corresponding as far as possible with the divisions of the Church Lectionary. The Translation of the Authorised Version is printed in full, such corrections as are deemed necessary being placed in footnotes.

THE EPISTLE OF ST. PAUL THE APOSTLE TO THE GALATIANS. Edited by A. W. Robinson, M.A. *Second Edition. Fcap. 8vo.* 1s. 6d. net.

ECCLESIASTES. Edited by A. W. Streane, D.D. *Fcap. 8vo.* 1s. 6d. net.

THE EPISTLE OF ST. PAUL THE APOSTLE TO THE PHILIPPIANS. Edited by C. R. D. Biggs, D.D. *Second Edition. Fcap 8vo.* 1s. 6d. net.

THE EPISTLE OF ST. JAMES. Edited by H. W. Fulford, M.A. *Fcap. 8vo.* 1s. 6d. net.

ISAIAH. Edited by W. E. Barnes, D.D. *Two Volumes. Fcap. 8vo.* 2s. net each. With Map.

THE EPISTLE OF ST. PAUL THE APOSTLE TO THE EPHESIANS. Edited by G. H. Whitaker, M.A. *Fcap. 8vo.* 1s. 6d. net.

Churchman's Library, The
General Editor, J. H. BURN, B.D., F.R.S.E.

THE BEGINNINGS OF ENGLISH CHRISTIANITY. By W. E. Collins, M.A. With Map. *Cr. 8vo.* 3s. 6d.

SOME NEW TESTAMENT PROBLEMS. By Arthur Wright, M.A. *Cr. 8vo.* 6s.

THE KINGDOM OF HEAVEN HERE AND HEREAFTER. By Canon Winterbotham, M.A., B.Sc., LL.B. *Cr. 8vo.* 3s. 6d.

THE WORKMANSHIP OF THE PRAYER BOOK: Its Literary and Liturgical Aspects. By J. Dowden, D.D. *Second Edition. Cr. 8vo.* 3s. 6d.

EVOLUTION. By F. B. Jevons, M.A., Litt.D *Cr. 8vo.* 3s. 6d.

THE OLD TESTAMENT AND THE NEW SCHOLARSHIP. By J. W. Peters, D.D. *Cr. 8vo.* 6s.

THE CHURCHMAN'S INTRODUCTION TO THE OLD TESTAMENT. By A. M. Mackay, B.A. *Cr. 8vo.* 3s. 6d.

THE CHURCH OF CHRIST. By E. T. Green, M.A. *Cr. 8vo.* 6s.

COMPARATIVE THEOLOGY. By J. A. MacCulloch. *Cr. 8vo.* 6s.

Classical Translations
Edited by H. F. FOX, M.A., Fellow and Tutor of Brasenose College, Oxford.
Crown 8vo.
A series of Translations from the Greek and Latin Classics, distinguished by literary excellence as well as by scholarly accuracy.

ÆSCHYLUS — Agamemnon, Choephoroe, Eumenides. Translated by Lewis Campbell, LL.D. 5s.

CICERO—De Oratore I. Translated by E. N. P. Moor, M.A. 3s. 6d.

CICERO—Select Orations (Pro Milone, Pro Mureno, Philippic II., in Catilinam). Translated by H. E. D. Blakiston, M.A. 5s.

CICERO—De Natura Deorum. Translated by F. Brooks, M.A. 3s. 6d.

[*Continued.*

CLASSICAL TRANSLATIONS—*continued.*

CICERO—De Officiis. Translated by G. B. Gardiner, M.A. 2*s.* 6*d.*
HORACE—The Odes and Epodes. Translated by A. D. Godley, M.A. 2*s.*
LUCIAN—Six Dialogues (Nigrinus, Icaro-Menippus, The Cock, The Ship, The Parasite, The Lover of Falsehood) Translated by S.

T. Irwin, M.A. 3*s.* 6*d.*
SOPHOCLES—Electra and Ajax. Translated by E. D. A. Morshead, M.A. 2*s.* 6*d.*
TACITUS—Agricola and Germania. Translated by R. B. Townshend. 2*s.* 6*d.*
THE SATIRES OF JUVENAL. Translated by S. G. Owen. 2*s.* 6*d.*

Commercial Series

Edited by H. DE B. GIBBINS, Litt.D., M.A.

Crown 8vo.

A series intended to assist students and young men preparing for a commercial career, by supplying useful handbooks of a clear and practical character, dealing with those subjects which are absolutely essential in the business life.

COMMERCIAL EDUCATION IN THEORY AND PRACTICE. By E. E. Whitfield, M.A. 5*s.*
   An introduction to Methuen's Commercial Series treating the question of Commercial Education fully from both the point of view of the teacher and of the parent.
BRITISH COMMERCE AND COLONIES FROM ELIZABETH TO VICTORIA. By H. de B. Gibbins, Litt.D., M.A. *Third Edition.* 2*s.*
COMMERCIAL EXAMINATION PAPERS. By H. de B. Gibbins, Litt.D., M.A. 1*s.* 6*d.*
THE ECONOMICS OF COMMERCE, By H. de B. Gibbins, Litt.D., M.A. *Second Edition.* 1*s.* 6*d.*
A GERMAN COMMERCIAL READER. By S. E. Bally. With Vocabulary. 2*s.*
A COMMERCIAL GEOGRAPHY OF THE BRITISH EMPIRE. By L. W. Lyde, M.A. *Fourth Edition.* 2*s.*
A COMMERCIAL GEOGRAPHY OF FOREIGN NATIONS. By F. C. Boon, B.A. 2*s.*

A PRIMER OF BUSINESS. By S. Jackson, M.A. *Third Edition.* 1*s.* 6*d.*
COMMERCIAL ARITHMETIC. By F. G. Taylor, M.A. *Fourth Edition.* 1*s.* 6*d.*
FRENCH COMMERCIAL CORRESPONDENCE. By S. E. Bally. With Vocabulary. *Third Edition.* 2*s.*
GERMAN COMMERCIAL CORRESPONDENCE. By S. E. Bally. With Vocabulary. *Second Edition.* 2*s.* 6*d.*
A FRENCH COMMERCIAL READER. By S. E. Bally. With Vocabulary. *Second Edition.* 2*s.*
PRECIS WRITING AND OFFICE CORRESPONDENCE. By E. E. Whitfield, M.A. *Second Edition.* 2*s.*
A GUIDE TO PROFESSIONS AND BUSINESS. By H. Jones. 1*s.* 6*d.*
THE PRINCIPLES OF BOOK-KEEPING BY DOUBLE ENTRY. By J. E. B. M'Allen, M.A. 2*s.*
COMMERCIAL LAW. By W. Douglas Edwards. *Second Edition.* 2*s.*

Connoisseur's Library, The

Wide Royal 8vo. 25*s. net.*

A sumptuous series of 20 books on art, written by experts for collectors, superbly illustrated in photogravure, collotype, and colour. The technical side of the art is duly treated. The first volumes are—

MEZZOTINTS. By Cyril Davenport. With 40 Plates in Photogravure.
PORCELAIN. By Edward Dillon. With 19 Plates in Colour, 20 in Collotype, and 5 in Photogravure.
MINIATURES. By Dudley Heath. With 9 Plates in Colour, 15 in Collotype, and 15 in Photogravure.

IVORIES. By A. Maskell. With 80 Plates in Collotype and Photogravure.
ENGLISH FURNITURE. By F. S. Robinson. With 160 Plates in Collotype and one in Photogravure. *Second Edition.*
EUROPEAN ENAMELS. By H. CUNYNGHAME, C.B. With many Plates in Collotype and a Frontispiece in Photogravure.

Devotion, The Library of

With Introductions and (where necessary) Notes.

Small Pott 8vo, cloth, 2s. ; leather, 2s. 6d. net.

These masterpieces of devotional literature are furnished with such Introductions and Notes as may be necessary to explain the standpoint of the author and the obvious difficulties of the text, without unnecessary intrusion between the author and the devout mind.

THE CONFESSIONS OF ST. AUGUSTINE. Edited by C. Bigg, D.D. *Fifth Edition.*
THE CHRISTIAN YEAR. Edited by Walter Lock, D.D. *Third Edition.*
THE IMITATION OF CHRIST. Edited by C. Bigg, D.D. *Fourth Edition.*
A BOOK OF DEVOTIONS. Edited by J. W. Stanbridge. B.D. *Second Edition.*
LYRA INNOCENTIUM. Edited by Walter Lock, D.D.
A SERIOUS CALL TO A DEVOUT AND HOLY LIFE. Edited by C. Bigg, D.D. *Second Edition*
THE TEMPLE. Edited by E. C. S. Gibson, D.D. *Second Edition.*
A GUIDE TO ETERNITY. Edited by J. W. Stanbridge, B.D.
THE PSALMS OF DAVID. Edited by B. W. Randolph, D.D.
LYRA APOSTOLICA. By Cardinal Newman and others. Edited by Canon Scott Holland and Canon H. C. Beeching, M.A.
THE INNER WAY. By J. Tauler. Edited by A. W. Hutton, M.A.
THE THOUGHTS OF PASCAL. Edited by C. S. Jerram, M.A.

ON THE LOVE OF GOD. By St. Francis de Sales. Edited by W. J. Knox-Little, M.A.
A MANUAL OF CONSOLATION FROM THE SAINTS AND FATHERS. Edited by J. H. Burn, B.D.
THE SONG OF SONGS. Edited by B. Blaxland, M.A.
THE DEVOTIONS OF ST. ANSELM. Edited by C. C. J. Webb, M.A.
GRACE ABOUNDING. By John Bunyan. Edited by S. C. Freer, M.A.
BISHOP WILSON'S SACRA PRIVATA. Edited by A. E. Burn, B.D.
LYRA SACRA : A Book of Sacred Verse. Edited by H. C. Beeching, M.A., Canon of Westminster.
A DAY BOOK FROM THE SAINTS AND FATHERS. Edited by J. H. Burn, B.D.
HEAVENLY WISDOM. A Selection from the English Mystics. Edited by E. C. Gregory.
LIGHT, LIFE, and LOVE. A Selection from the German Mystics. Edited by W. R. Inge, M.A.
AN INTRODUCTION TO THE DEVOUT LIFE. By St. Francis de Sales. Translated and Edited by T. Barns, M.A.

Methuen's Standard Library

In Sixpenny Volumes.

THE STANDARD LIBRARY is a new series of volumes containing the great classics of the world, and particularly the finest works of English literature. All the great masters will be represented, either in complete works or in selections. It is the ambition of the publishers to place the best books of the Anglo-Saxon race within the reach of every reader, so that the series may represent something of the diversity and splendour of our English tongue. The characteristics of THE STANDARD LIBRARY are four :—1. SOUNDNESS OF TEXT. 2. CHEAPNESS. 3. CLEARNESS OF TYPE. 4. SIMPLICITY. The books are well printed on good paper at a price which on the whole is without parallel in the history of publishing. Each volume contains from 100 to 250 pages, and is issued in paper covers, Crown 8vo, at Sixpence net, or in cloth gilt at One Shilling net. In a few cases long books are issued as Double Volumes or as Treble Volumes.

The following books are ready with the exception of those marked with a †, which denotes that the book is nearly ready :—

THE MEDITATIONS OF MARCUS AURELIUS. The translation is by R. Graves.
THE NOVELS OF JANE AUSTEN. In 5 volumes. VOL. I.—Sense and Sensibility.
ESSAYS AND COUNSELS and THE NEW ATLANTIS. By Francis Bacon, Lord Verulam.

RELIGIO MEDICI and URN BURIAL. By Sir Thomas Browne. The text has been collated by A. R. Waller.
THE PILGRIM'S PROGRESS. By John Bunyan.
REFLECTIONS ON THE FRENCH REVOLUTION. By Edmund Burke.
THE ANALOGY OF RELIGION, NATURAL AND REVEALED. By Joseph Butler, D.D.

[Continued.]

THE STANDARD LIBRARY—*continued.*

THE POEMS OF THOMAS CHATTERTON. In 2 volumes.
Vol. I.—Miscellaneous Poems.
†Vol. II.—The Rowley Poems.

†VITA NUOVA. By Dante. Translated into English by D. G. Rossetti.

TOM JONES. By Henry Fielding. Treble Vol.

CRANFORD. By Mrs. Gaskell.

THE HISTORY OF THE DECLINE AND FALL OF THE ROMAN EMPIRE. By Edward Gibbon. In 7 double volumes.
Vol. V. is nearly ready.
The Text and Notes have been revised by J. B. Bury, Litt. D., but the Appendices of the more expensive edition are not given.

†THE VICAR OF WAKEFIELD. By Oliver Goldsmith.

THE POEMS AND PLAYS OF OLIVER GOLDSMITH.

THE WORKS OF BEN JONSON.
†Vol. I.—The Case is Altered. Every Man in His Humour. Every Man out of His Humour.
The text has been collated by H. C. Hart.

THE POEMS OF JOHN KEATS. Double volume. The Text has been collated by E. de Selincourt.

ON THE IMITATION OF CHRIST. By Thomas à Kempis.
The translation is by C. Bigg, DD., Canon of Christ Church.

A SERIOUS CALL TO A DEVOUT AND HOLY LIFE. By William Law.

THE PLAYS OF CHRISTOPHER MARLOWE.
†Vol. I.—Tamburlane the Great. The Tragical History of Dr. Faustus.

THE PLAYS OF PHILIP MASSINGER.
†Vol. I.—The Duke of Milan.

THE POEMS OF JOHN MILTON. In 2 volumes.
Vol. I.—Paradise Lost.

THE PROSE WORKS OF JOHN MILTON.
VOL. I.—Eikonoklastes and The Tenure of Kings and Magistrates.

SELECT WORKS OF SIR THOMAS MORE.
Vol. I.—Utopia and Poems.

THE REPUBLIC OF PLATO. Translated by Sydenham and Taylor. Double Volume. The translation has been revised by W. H. D. Rouse.

THE LITTLE FLOWERS OF ST. FRANCIS. Translated by W. Heywood.

THE WORKS OF WILLIAM SHAKESPEARE. In 10 volumes.
VOL. I.—The Tempest; The Two Gentlemen of Verona; The Merry Wives of Windsor; Measure for Measure; The Comedy of Errors.
VOL. II.—Much Ado About Nothing; Love's Labour's Lost; A Midsummer Night's Dream; The Merchant of Venice; As You Like It.
VOL. III.—The Taming of the Shrew; All's Well that Ends Well; Twelfth Night; The Winter's Tale.
Vol. IV.—The Life and Death of King John; The Tragedy of King Richard the Second; The First Part of King Henry IV.; The Second Part of King Henry IV.
Vol. V.—The Life of King Henry V.; The First Part of King Henry VI.; The Second Part of King Henry VI.

THE LIFE OF NELSON. By Robert Southey.

THE NATURAL HISTORY AND ANTIQUITIES OF SELBORNE. By Gilbert White.

Half-Crown Library

Crown 8vo.   2s. 6d. net.

THE LIFE OF JOHN RUSKIN. By W. G. Collingwood, M.A. With Portraits. *Sixth Edition.*

ENGLISH LYRICS. By W. E. Henley. *Second Edition.*

THE GOLDEN POMP. A Procession of English Lyrics. Arranged by A. T. Quiller Couch. *Second Edition.*

CHITRAL: The Story of a Minor Siege. By Sir G. S. Robertson, K.C.S.I. *Third Edition.* Illustrated.

STRANGE SURVIVALS AND SUPERSTITIONS. By S. Baring-Gould. *Third Edition.*

YORKSHIRE ODDITIES AND STRANGE EVENTS. By S. Baring-Gould. *Fourth Edition.*

ENGLISH VILLAGES. By P. H. Ditchfield, M.A., F.S.A. Illustrated.

A BOOK OF ENGLISH PROSE. By W. E. Henley and C. Whibley.

THE LAND OF THE BLACK MOUNTAIN. Being a Description of Montenegro. By R. Wyon and G. Prance. With 40 Illustrations.

Illustrated Pocket Library of Plain and Coloured Books, The

Fcap 8vo.   3s. 6d. net each volume.

A series, in small form, of some of the famous illustrated books of fiction and general literature. These are faithfully reprinted from the first or best editions without introduction or notes. The Illustrations are chiefly in colour.

COLOURED BOOKS

OLD COLOURED BOOKS. By George Paston. With 16 Coloured Plates. *Fcap. 8vo. 2s. net.*

THE LIFE AND DEATH OF JOHN MYTTON, ESQ.

By Nimrod. With 18 Coloured Plates by Henry Alken and T. J. Rawlins. *Third Edition.*

[*Continued.*

ILLUSTRATED POCKET LIBRARY OF PLAIN AND COLOURED BOOKS—*continued.*

THE LIFE OF A SPORTSMAN. By Nimrod. With 35 Coloured Plates by Henry Alken.

HANDLEY CROSS. By R. S. Surtees. With 17 Coloured Plates and 100 Woodcuts in the Text by John Leech. *Second Edition.*

MR. SPONGE'S SPORTING TOUR. By R. S. Surtees. With 13 Coloured Plates and 90 Woodcuts in the Text by John Leech.

JORROCKS' JAUNTS AND JOLLITIES. By R. S. Surtees. With 15 Coloured Plates by H. Alken. *Second Edition.*

This volume is reprinted from the extremely rare and costly edition of 1843, which contains Alken's very fine illustrations instead of the usual ones by Phiz.

ASK MAMMA. By R. S. Surtees. With 13 Coloured Plates and 70 Woodcuts in the Text by John Leech.

THE ANALYSIS OF THE HUNTING FIELD. By R. S. Surtees. With 7 Coloured Plates by Henry Alken, and 43 Illustrations on Wood.

THE TOUR OF DR. SYNTAX IN SEARCH OF THE PICTURESQUE. By William Combe. With 30 Coloured Plates by T. Rowlandson.

THE TOUR OF DOCTOR SYNTAX IN SEARCH OF CONSOLATION. By William Combe. With 24 Coloured Plates by T. Rowlandson.

THE THIRD TOUR OF DOCTOR SYNTAX IN SEARCH OF A WIFE. By William Combe. With 24 Coloured Plates by T. Rowlandson.

THE HISTORY OF JOHNNY QUAE GENUS: the Little Foundling of the late Dr. Syntax. By the Author of 'The Three Tours.' With 24 Coloured Plates by Rowlandson.

THE ENGLISH DANCE OF DEATH, from the Designs of T. Rowlandson, with Metrical Illustrations by the Author of 'Doctor Syntax.' *Two Volumes.*

This book contains 76 Coloured Plates.

THE DANCE OF LIFE: A Poem. By the Author of 'Doctor Syntax.' Illustrated with 26 Coloured Engravings by T. Rowlandson.

LIFE IN LONDON: or, the Day and Night Scenes of Jerry Hawthorn, Esq., and his Elegant Friend, Corinthian Tom. By Pierce Egan. With 36 Coloured Plates by I. R. and G. Cruikshank. With numerous Designs on Wood.

REAL LIFE IN LONDON: or, the Rambles and Adventures of Bob Tallyho, Esq., and his Cousin, The Hon. Tom Dashall. By an Amateur (Pierce Egan). With 31 Coloured Plates by Alken and Rowlandson, etc. *Two Volumes.*

THE LIFE OF AN ACTOR. By Pierce Egan. With 27 Coloured Plates by Theodore Lane, and several Designs on Wood.

THE VICAR OF WAKEFIELD. By Oliver Goldsmith. With 24 Coloured Plates by T. Rowlandson.

THE MILITARY ADVENTURES OF JOHNNY NEWCOME. By an Officer. With 15 Coloured Plates by T. Rowlandson.

THE NATIONAL SPORTS OF GREAT BRITAIN. With Descriptions and 51 Coloured Plates by Henry Alken.

This book is completely different from the large folio edition of 'National Sports' by the same artist, and none of the plates are similar.

THE ADVENTURES OF A POST CAPTAIN. By A Naval Officer. With 24 Coloured Plates by Mr. Williams.

GAMONIA : or, the Art of Preserving Game ; and an Improved Method of making Plantations and Covers, explained and illustrated by Lawrence Rawstorne, Esq. With 15 Coloured Plates by T. Rawlins.

AN ACADEMY FOR GROWN HORSEMEN : Containing the completest Instructions for Walking, Trotting, Cantering, Galloping, Stumbling, and Tumbling. Illustrated with 27 Coloured Plates, and adorned with a Portrait of the Author. By Geoffrey Gambado, Esq.

REAL LIFE IN IRELAND, or, the Day and Night Scenes of Brian Boru, Esq., and his Elegant Friend, Sir Shawn O'Dogherty. By a Real Paddy. With 19 Coloured Plates by Heath, Marks, etc.

THE ADVENTURES OF JOHNNY NEWCOME IN THE NAVY. By Alfred Burton. With 16 Coloured Plates by T. Rowlandson.

THE OLD ENGLISH SQUIRE: A Poem. By John Careless, Esq. With 20 Coloured Plates after the style of T. Rowlandson.

*THE ENGLISH SPY. By Bernard Blackmantle. With 72 Coloured Plates by R. Cruikshank, and many Illustrations on wood. *Two Volumes.*

PLAIN BOOKS

THE GRAVE: A Poem. By Robert Blair. Illustrated by 12 Etchings executed by Louis Schiavonetti from the original Inventions of William Blake. With an Engraved Title Page and a Portrait of Blake by T. Phillips, R.A.

The illustrations are reproduced in photogravure.

ILLUSTRATIONS OF THE BOOK OF JOB. Invented and engraved by William Blake. These famous Illustrations—21 in number —are reproduced in photogravure.

ÆSOP'S FABLES. With 380 Woodcuts by Thomas Bewick.

[*Continued.*

ILLUSTRATED POCKET LIBRARY OF PLAIN AND COLOURED BOOKS—*continued.*

WINDSOR CASTLE. By W. Harrison Ainsworth. With 22 Plates and 87 Woodcuts in the Text by George Cruikshank.

THE TOWER OF LONDON. By W. Harrison Ainsworth. With 40 Plates and 58 Woodcuts in the Text by George Cruikshank.

FRANK FAIRLEGH. By F. E. Smedley. With 30 Plates by George Cruikshank.

HANDY ANDY. By Samuel Lover. With 24 Illustrations by the Author.

THE COMPLEAT ANGLER. By Izaak Walton and Charles Cotton. With 14 Plates and 77 Woodcuts in the Text. This volume is reproduced from the beautiful edition of John Major of 1824.

THE PICKWICK PAPERS. By Charles Dickens. With the 43 Illustrations by Seymour and Phiz, the two Buss Plates, and the 32 Contemporary Onwhyn Plates.

Junior Examination Series

Edited by A. M. M. STEDMAN, M.A.   *Fcap. 8vo.   1s.*

This series is intended to lead up to the School Examination Series, and is intended for the use of teachers and students, to supply material for the former and practice for the latter. The papers are carefully graduated, cover the whole of the subject usually taught, and are intended to form part of the ordinary class work. They may be used *vivâ voce* or as a written examination.

JUNIOR FRENCH EXAMINATION PAPERS. By F. Jacob, M.A.

JUNIOR LATIN EXAMINATION PAPERS. By C. G. Botting, B.A. *Fourth Edition.*

JUNIOR ENGLISH EXAMINATION PAPERS. By W. Williamson, B.A.

JUNIOR ARITHMETIC EXAMINATION PAPERS. By W. S. Beard. *Second Edition.*

JUNIOR ALGEBRA EXAMINATION PAPERS. By S. W. Finn, M.A.

JUNIOR GREEK EXAMINATION PAPERS. By T. C. Weatherhead, M.A.

JUNIOR GENERAL INFORMATION EXAMINATION PAPERS. By W. S. Beard.

A KEY TO THE ABOVE. *Crown 8vo.   3s. 6d. net.*

JUNIOR GEOGRAPHY EXAMINATION PAPERS. By W. G. Baker, M.A.

JUNIOR GERMAN EXAMINATION PAPERS. By A. Voegelin, M.A.

Junior School-Books

Edited by O. D. INSKIP, LL.D., and W. WILLIAMSON, B.A.

A series of elementary books for pupils in lower forms, simply written by teachers of experience.

A CLASS-BOOK OF DICTATION PASSAGES. By W. Williamson, B.A. *Eleventh Edition. Cr. 8vo.   1s. 6d.*

THE GOSPEL ACCORDING TO ST. MATTHEW. Edited by E. Wilton South, M.A. With Three Maps. *Cr. 8vo.   1s. 6d.*

THE GOSPEL ACCORDING TO ST. MARK. Edited by A. E. Rubie, D.D. With Three Maps. *Cr. 8vo.   1s. 6d.*

A JUNIOR ENGLISH GRAMMAR. By W. Williamson, B.A. With numerous passages for parsing and analysis, and a chapter on Essay Writing. *Third Edition. Cr. 8vo.   2s.*

A JUNIOR CHEMISTRY. By E. A. Tyler, B.A., F.C.S. With 78 Illustrations. *Second Edition. Cr. 8vo.   2s. 6d.*

THE ACTS OF THE APOSTLES. Edited by A. E. Rubie, D.D. *Cr. 8vo.   2s.*

A JUNIOR FRENCH GRAMMAR. By L. A. Sornet and M. J. Acatos. *Cr. 8vo.   2s.*

ELEMENTARY EXPERIMENTAL SCIENCE. PHYSICS by W. T. Clough, A.R.C.S. CHEMISTRY by A. E. Dunstan, B.Sc. With 2 Plates and 154 Diagrams. *Third Edition. Cr. 8vo.   2s. 6d.*

A JUNIOR GEOMETRY. By Noel S. Lydon. With 276 Diagrams. *Second Edition. Cr. 8vo.   2s.*

A JUNIOR MAGNETISM AND ELECTRICITY. By W. T. Clough. Illustrated. *Cr. 8vo.   2s. 6d.*

ELEMENTARY EXPERIMENTAL CHEMISTRY. By A. E. Dunstan, B.Sc. With 4 Plates and 109 Diagrams. *Cr. 8vo.   2s.*

A JUNIOR FRENCH PROSE COMPOSITION. By R. R. N. Baron, M.A. *Cr. 8vo.   2s.*

THE GOSPEL ACCORDING TO ST. LUKE. With an Introduction and Notes by William Williamson, B.A. With Three Maps. *Cr. 8vo.   2s.*

Leaders of Religion

Edited by H. C. BEECHING, M.A., Canon of Westminster. *With Portraits.*
Cr. 8vo. 2s. net.

A series of short biographies of the most prominent leaders of religious life and thought of all ages and countries.

CARDINAL NEWMAN. By R. H. Hutton.
JOHN WESLEY. By J. H. Overton, M.A.
BISHOP WILBERFORCE. By G. W. Daniell, M.A.
CARDINAL MANNING. By A. W. Hutton, M.A.
CHARLES SIMEON. By H. C. G. Moule, D.D.
JOHN KEBLE. By Walter Lock, D.D.
THOMAS CHALMERS. By Mrs. Oliphant.
LANCELOT ANDREWES. By R. L. Ottley, D.D. *Second Edition.*
AUGUSTINE OF CANTERBURY. By E. L. Cutts, D.D.

WILLIAM LAUD. By W. H. Hutton, M.A. *Third Edition.*
JOHN KNOX. By F. MacCunn. *Second Edition.*
JOHN HOWE. By R. F. Horton, D.D.
BISHOP KEN. By F. A. Clarke, M.A.
GEORGE FOX, THE QUAKER. By T. Hodgkin, D.C.L. *Third Edition.*
JOHN DONNE. By Augustus Jessopp, D.D.
THOMAS CRANMER. By A. J. Mason, D.D.
BISHOP LATIMER. By R. M. Carlyle and A. J. Carlyle, M.A.
BISHOP BUTLER. By W. A. Spooner, M.A.

Little Blue Books, The

General Editor, E. V. LUCAS.

Illustrated. Demy 16mo. 2s. 6d.

A series of books for children. The aim of the editor is to get entertaining or exciting stories about normal children, the moral of which is implied rather than expressed.

1. THE CASTAWAYS OF MEADOWBANK. By Thomas Cobb.
2. THE BEECHNUT BOOK. By Jacob Abbott. Edited by E. V. Lucas.
3. THE AIR GUN. By T. Hilbert.
4. A SCHOOL YEAR. By Netta Syrett.
5. THE PEELES AT THE CAPITAL. By Roger Ashton.
6. THE TREASURE OF PRINCEGATE PRIORY. By T. Cobb.
7. MRS. BARBERRY'S GENERAL SHOP. By Roger Ashton.
8. A BOOK OF BAD CHILDREN. By W. T. Webb.
9. THE LOST BALL. By Thomas Cobb.

Little Books on Art

With many Illustrations. Demy 16mo. 2s. 6d. net.

A series of monographs in miniature, containing the complete outline of the subject under treatment and rejecting minute details. These books are produced with the greatest care. Each volume consists of about 200 pages, and contains from 30 to 40 illustrations, including a frontispiece in photogravure.

GREEK ART. H. B. Walters. *Second Edition.*
BOOKPLATES. E. Almack.
REYNOLDS. J. Sime. *Second Edition.*
ROMNEY. George Paston.
WATTS. R. E. D. Sketchley.
LEIGHTON. Alice Corkran.
VELASQUEZ. Wilfrid Wilberforce and A. R. Gilbert.
GREUZE AND BOUCHER. Eliza F. Pollard.
VANDYCK. M. G. Smallwood.
TURNER. Frances Tyrell-Gill.
DÜRER. Jessie Allen.
HOPPNER. H. P. K. Skipton.

HOLBEIN. Mrs. G. Fortescue.
BURNE-JONES. Fortunée de Lisle. *Second Edition.*
REMBRANDT. Mrs. E. A. Sharp.
COROT. Alice Pollard and Ethel Birnstingl.
RAPHAEL. A. R. Dryhurst.
MILLET. Netta Peacock.
ILLUMINATED MSS. J. W. Bradley.
CHRIST IN ART. Mrs. Henry Jenner.
JEWELLERY. Cyril Davenport.
CLAUDE. Edward Dillon.
THE ARTS OF JAPAN. Edward Dillon.

Little Galleries, The

Demy 16mo.   2s. 6d. net.

A series of little books containing examples of the best work of the great painters. Each volume contains 20 plates in photogravure, together with a short outline of the life and work of the master to whom the book is devoted.

A LITTLE GALLERY OF REYNOLDS.
A LITTLE GALLERY OF ROMNEY.
A LITTLE GALLERY OF HOPPNER.

A LITTLE GALLERY OF MILLAIS.
A LITTLE GALLERY OF ENGLISH POETS.

Little Guides, The

Small Pott 8vo, cloth, 2s. 6d. net.; leather, 3s. 6d. net.

OXFORD AND ITS COLLEGES. By J. Wells, M.A. Illustrated by E. H. New. *Sixth Edition.*

CAMBRIDGE AND ITS COLLEGES. By A. Hamilton Thompson. Illustrated by E. H. New. *Second Edition.*

THE MALVERN COUNTRY. By B. C. A. Windle, D.Sc., F.R.S. Illustrated by E. H. New.

SHAKESPEARE'S COUNTRY. By B. C. A. Windle, D.Sc., F.R.S. Illustrated by E. H. New. *Second Edition.*

SUSSEX. By F. G. Brabant, M.A. Illustrated by E. H. New. *Second Edition.*

WESTMINSTER ABBEY. By G. E. Troutbeck. Illustrated by F. D. Bedford.

NORFOLK. By W. A. Dutt. Illustrated by B. C. Boulter.

CORNWALL. By A. L. Salmon. Illustrated by B. C. Boulter.

BRITTANY. By S. Baring-Gould. Illustrated by J. Wylie.

HERTFORDSHIRE. By H. W. Tompkins, F.R.H.S. Illustrated by E. H. New.

THE ENGLISH LAKES. By F. G. Brabant, M.A. Illustrated by E. H. New.

KENT. By G. Clinch. Illustrated by F. D. Bedford.

ROME By C. G. Ellaby. Illustrated by B. C. Boulter.

THE ISLE OF WIGHT. By G. Clinch. Illustrated by F. D. Bedford.

SURREY. By F. A. H. Lambert. Illustrated by E. H. New.

BUCKINGHAMSHIRE. By E. S. Roscoe. Illustrated by F. D. Bedford.

SUFFOLK. By W. A. Dutt. Illustrated by J. Wylie.

DERBYSHIRE. By J. C. Cox, LL.D., F.S.A. Illustrated by J. C. Wall.

THE NORTH RIDING OF YORKSHIRE. By J. E. Morris. Illustrated by R. J. S. Bertram.

HAMPSHIRE. By J. C. Cox. Illustrated by M. E. Purser.

SICILY. By F. H. Jackson. With many Illustrations by the Author.

DORSET. By Frank R. Heath. Illustrated.

CHESHIRE. By W. M. Gallichan. Illustrated by Elizabeth Hartley.

NORTHAMPTONSHIRE. By Wakeling Dry. Illustrated.

THE EAST RIDING OF YORKSHIRE. By J. E. Morris. Illustrated.

OXFORDSHIRE. By F. G. Brabant. Illustrated by E. H. New.

ST. PAUL'S CATHEDRAL. By George Clinch. Illustrated by Beatrice Alcock.

Little Library, The

With Introductions, Notes, and Photogravure Frontispieces.

Small Pott 8vo.   Each Volume, cloth, 1s. 6d. net ; leather, 2s. 6d. net.

A series of small books under the above title, containing some of the famous works in English and other literatures, in the domains of fiction, poetry, and belles lettres. The series also contains volumes of selections in prose and verse. The books are edited with the most scholarly care. Each one contains an introduction which gives (1) a short biography of the author ; (2) a critical estimate of the book. Where they are necessary, short notes are added at the foot of the page.

Each volume has a photogravure frontispiece, and the books are produced with great care.

Anon. ENGLISH LYRICS, A LITTLE BOOK OF.

Austen (Jane). PRIDE AND PREJUDICE. Edited by E. V. LUCAS. *Two Volumes.*

NORTHANGER ABBEY. Edited by E. V. LUCAS.

Bacon (Francis). THE ESSAYS OF LORD BACON. Edited by EDWARD WRIGHT.

Barham (R. H.). THE INGOLDSBY LEGENDS. Edited by J. B. ATLAY. *Two Volumes.*

Barnett (Mrs. P. A.). A LITTLE BOOK OF ENGLISH PROSE.

Beckford (William). THE HISTORY OF THE CALIPH VATHEK. Edited by E. DENISON ROSS.

Blake (William). SELECTIONS FROM WILLIAM BLAKE. Edited by M. PERUGINI.

Borrow (George). LAVENGRO. Edited by F. HINDES GROOME. *Two Volumes.* THE ROMANY RYE. Edited by JOHN SAMPSON.

Browning (Robert). SELECTIONS FROM THE EARLY POEMS OF ROBERT BROWNING. Edited by W. HALL GRIFFIN, M.A.

Canning (George). SELECTIONS FROM THE ANTI-JACOBIN: with GEORGE CANNING's additional Poems. Edited by LLOYD SANDERS.

Cowley (Abraham). THE ESSAYS OF ABRAHAM COWLEY. Edited by H. C. MINCHIN.

Crabbe (George). SELECTIONS FROM GEORGE CRABBE. Edited by A. C. DEANE.

Craik (Mrs.). JOHN HALIFAX, GENTLEMAN. Edited by ANNE MATHESON. *Two Volumes.*

Crashaw (Richard). THE ENGLISH POEMS OF RICHARD CRASHAW. Edited by EDWARD HUTTON.

Dante (Alighieri). THE INFERNO OF DANTE. Translated by H. F. CARY. Edited by PAGET TOYNBEE, M.A., D.Litt. THE PURGATORIO OF DANTE. Translated by H. F. CARY. Edited by PAGET TOYNBEE, M.A., D.Litt. THE PARADISO OF DANTE. Translated by H. F. CARY. Edited by PAGET TOYNBEE, M.A., D.Litt.

Darley (George). SELECTIONS FROM THE POEMS OF GEORGE DARLEY. Edited by R. A. STREATFEILD.

Deane (A. C.). A LITTLE BOOK OF LIGHT VERSE.

Dickens (Charles). CHRISTMAS BOOKS. *Two Volumes.*

Ferrier (Susan). MARRIAGE. Edited by A. GOODRICH - FREER and LORD IDDESLEIGH. *Two Volumes.* THE INHERITANCE. *Two Volumes.*

Gaskell (Mrs.). CRANFORD. Edited by E. V. LUCAS. *Second Edition.*

Hawthorne (Nathaniel). THE SCARLET LETTER. Edited by PERCY DEARMER.

Henderson (T. F.). A LITTLE BOOK OF SCOTTISH VERSE.

Keats (John). POEMS. With an Introduction by L. BINYON, and Notes by J. MASEFIELD.

Kinglake (A. W.). EOTHEN. With an Introduction and Notes. *Second Edition.*

Lamb (Charles). ELIA, AND THE LAST ESSAYS OF ELIA. Edited by E. V. LUCAS.

Locker (F.). LONDON LYRICS. Edited by A. D. GODLEY, M.A. A reprint of the First Edition.

Longfellow (H. W.). SELECTIONS FROM LONGFELLOW. Edited by L. M. FAITHFULL.

Marvell (Andrew). THE POEMS OF ANDREW MARVELL. Edited by E. WRIGHT.

Milton (John). THE MINOR POEMS OF JOHN MILTON. Edited by H. C. BEECHING, M.A., Canon of Westminster.

Moir (D. M.). MANSIE WAUCH. Edited by T. F. HENDERSON.

Nichols (J. B. B.). A LITTLE BOOK OF ENGLISH SONNETS.

Rochefoucauld (La). THE MAXIMS OF LA ROCHEFOUCAULD. Translated by Dean STANHOPE. Edited by G. H. POWELL.

Smith (Horace and James). REJECTED ADDRESSES. Edited by A. D. GODLEY, M.A.

Sterne (Laurence). A SENTIMENTAL JOURNEY. Edited by H. W. PAUL.

Tennyson (Alfred, Lord). THE EARLY POEMS OF ALFRED, LORD TENNYSON. Edited by J. CHURTON COLLINS, M.A.

IN MEMORIAM. Edited by H. C. BEECHING, M.A.

THE PRINCESS. Edited by ELIZABETH WORDSWORTH.

MAUD. Edited by ELIZABETH WORDSWORTH.

Thackeray (W. M.). VANITY FAIR. Edited by S. GWYNN. *Three Volumes.*

PENDENNIS. Edited by S. GWYNN. *Three Volumes.*

ESMOND. Edited by S. GWYNN.

CHRISTMAS BOOKS. Edited by S. GWYNN.

Vaughan (Henry). THE POEMS OF HENRY VAUGHAN. Edited by EDWARD HUTTON.

Walton (Izaak). THE COMPLEAT ANGLER. Edited by J. BUCHAN.

Waterhouse (Mrs. Alfred). A LITTLE BOOK OF LIFE AND DEATH. Edited by. *Eighth Edition.*

Wordsworth (W.). SELECTIONS FROM WORDSWORTH. Edited by NOWELL C. SMITH.

Wordsworth (W.) and Coleridge (S. T.). LYRICAL BALLADS. Edited by GEORGE SAMPSON.

Miniature Library

Reprints in miniature of a few interesting books which have qualities of
humanity, devotion, or literary genius.

EUPHRANOR: A Dialogue on Youth. By
Edward FitzGerald. From the edition published by W. Pickering in 1851. *Demy
32mo. Leather, 2s. net.*

POLONIUS: or Wise Saws and Modern Instances. By Edward FitzGerald. From
the edition published by W. Pickering in
1852. *Demy 32mo. Leather, 2s. net.*

THE RUBÁIYÁT OF OMAR KHAYYÁM. By
Edward FitzGerald. From the 1st edition
of 1859, *Third Edition. Leather, 1s. net.*

THE LIFE OF EDWARD, LORD HERBERT OF
CHERBURY. Written by himself. From
the edition printed at Strawberry Hill in
the year 1764. *Medium 32mo. Leather,
2s. net.*

THE VISIONS OF DOM FRANCISCO QUEVEDO
VILLEGAS, Knight of the Order of St.
James. Made English by R. L. From the
edition printed for H. Herringman, 1668.
Leather. 2s. net.

POEMS. By Dora Greenwell. From the edition of 1848. *Leather, 2s. net.*

Oxford Biographies

Fcap. 8vo.   Each volume, cloth, 2s. 6d. net ; leather, 3s. 6d. net.

These books are written by scholars of repute, who combine knowledge and
literary skill with the power of popular presentation. They are illustrated from
authentic material.

DANTE ALIGHIERI. By Paget Toynbee, M.A.,
D.Litt. With 12 Illustrations. *Second
Edition.*

SAVONAROLA. By E. L. S. Horsburgh, M.A.
With 12 Illustrations. *Second Edition.*

JOHN HOWARD. By E. C. S. Gibson, D.D.,
Bishop of Gloucester. With 12 Illustrations.

TENNYSON. By A. C. BENSON, M.A. With
9 Illustrations.

WALTER RALEIGH. By I. A. Taylor. With
12 Illustrations.

ERASMUS. By E. F. H. Capey. With 12
Illustrations.

THE YOUNG PRETENDER. By C. S. Terry.
With 12 Illustrations.

ROBERT BURNS. By T. F. Henderson.
With 12 Illustrations.

CHATHAM. By A. S. M'Dowall. With 12
Illustrations.

ST. FRANCIS OF ASSISI. By Anna M. Stoddart. With 16 Illustrations.

CANNING. By W. Alison Phillips. With 12
Illustrations.

BEACONSFIELD. By Walter Sichel. With 12
Illustrations.

GOETHE. By H. G. Atkins. With 12 Illustrations.

FENELON. By Viscount St. Cyres. With
12 Illustrations.

School Examination Series

Edited by A. M. M. STEDMAN, M.A.   *Cr. 8vo.   2s. 6d.*

FRENCH EXAMINATION PAPERS. By A. M.
M. Stedman, M.A. *Thirteenth Edition.*
A KEY, issued to Tutors and Private
Students only to be had on application
to the Publishers. *Fifth Edition.
Crown 8vo. 6s. net.*

LATIN EXAMINATION PAPERS. By A. M. M.
Stedman, M.A. *Thirteenth Edition.*
KEY (*Fourth Edition*) issued as above.
6s. net.

GREEK EXAMINATION PAPERS. By A. M. M.
Stedman, M.A. *Eighth Edition.*
KEY (*Third Edition*) issued as above.
6s. net.

GERMAN EXAMINATION PAPERS. By R. J.
Morich. *Sixth Edition.*

KEY (*Third Edition*) issued as above.
6s. net.

HISTORY AND GEOGRAPHY EXAMINATION
PAPERS. By C. H. Spence, M.A. *Second
Edition.*

PHYSICS EXAMINATION PAPERS. By R. E.
Steel, M.A., F.C.S.

GENERAL KNOWLEDGE EXAMINATION
PAPERS. By A. M. M. Stedman, M.A.
Fifth Edition.
KEY (*Third Edition*) issued as above.
7s. net.

EXAMINATION PAPERS IN ENGLISH HISTORY.
By J. Tait Plowden-Wardlaw, B.A.

Science, Textbooks of

Edited by G. F. GOODCHILD, B.A., B.Sc., and G. R. MILLS, M.A.

PRACTICAL MECHANICS. By Sidney H. Wells. *Third Edition.* Cr. 8vo. 3s. 6d.
PRACTICAL PHYSICS. By H. Stroud, D.Sc., M.A. Cr. 8vo. 3s. 6d.
PRACTICAL CHEMISTRY. Part I. By W. French, M.A. Cr. 8vo. Fourth Edition. 1s. 6d. Part II. By W. French, M.A., and T. H. Boardman, M.A. Cr. 8vo. 1s. 6d.

TECHNICAL ARITHMETIC AND GEOMETRY. By C. T. Millis, M.I.M.E. Cr. 8vo. 3s. 6d.
EXAMPLES IN PHYSICS. By C. E. Jackson, B.A. Cr. 8vo. 2s. 6d.
*ELEMENTARY ORGANIC CHEMISTRY. By A. E. Dunstan, B.Sc. Illustrated. Cr. 8vo.

Social Questions of To-day

Edited by H. DE B. GIBBINS, Litt.D., M.A. Crown 8vo. 2s. 6d.

A series of volumes upon those topics of social, economic, and industrial interest that are foremost in the public mind.

TRADE UNIONISM—NEW AND OLD. By G. Howell. *Third Edition.*
THE COMMERCE OF NATIONS. By C. F. Bastable, M.A. *Third Edition.*
THE ALIEN INVASION. By W. H. Wilkins, B.A.
THE RURAL EXODUS. By P. Anderson Graham.
LAND NATIONALIZATION. By Harold Cox, B.A. *Second Edition.*
A SHORTER WORKING DAY. By H. de B. Gibbins and R. A. Hadfield.
BACK TO THE LAND. An Inquiry into Rural Depopulation. By H. E. Moore.
TRUSTS, POOLS, AND CORNERS. By J. Stephen Jeans.

THE FACTORY SYSTEM. By R. W. Cooke Taylor.
WOMEN'S WORK. By Lady Dilke, Miss Bulley, and Miss Whitley.
SOCIALISM AND MODERN THOUGHT. By M. Kauffmann.
THE PROBLEM OF THE UNEMPLOYED. By J. A. Hobson, M.A.
LIFE IN WEST LONDON By Arthur Sherwell, M.A. *Third Edition.*
RAILWAY NATIONALIZATION. By Clement Edwards.
UNIVERSITY AND SOCIAL SETTLEMENTS. By W. Reason, M.A.

Technology, Textbooks of

Edited by G. F. GOODCHILD, B.A., B.Sc., and G. R. MILLS, M.A.
Fully Illustrated.

HOW TO MAKE A DRESS. By J. A. E. Wood. *Third Edition.* Cr. 8vo. 1s. 6d.
CARPENTRY AND JOINERY. By F. C. Webber. *Fourth Edition.* Cr. 8vo. 3s. 6d.
MILLINERY, THEORETICAL AND PRACTICAL. By Clare Hill. *Second Edition.* Cr. 8vo. 2s.

AN INTRODUCTION TO THE STUDY OF TEXTILE DESIGN. By Aldred F. Barker. *Demy 8vo. 7s. 6d.*
BUILDERS' QUANTITIES. By H. C. Grubb. Cr. 8vo. 4s. 6d.
RÉPOUSSÉ METAL WORK. By A. C. Horth. Cr. 8vo. 2s. 6d.

Theology, Handbooks of

Edited by R. L. OTTLEY, D.D., Professor of Pastoral Theology at Oxford, and Canon of Christ Church, Oxford.

The series is intended, in part, to furnish the clergy and teachers or students of Theology with trustworthy Textbooks, adequately representing the present position of the questions dealt with; in part, to make accessible to the reading public an accurate and concise statement of facts and principles in all questions bearing on Theology and Religion.

THE XXXIX. ARTICLES OF THE CHURCH OF ENGLAND. Edited by E. C. S. Gibson, D.D. *Fifth and Cheaper Edition in one Volume. Demy 8vo. 12s. 6d.*
AN INTRODUCTION TO THE HISTORY OF RELIGION. By F. B. Jevons. M.A., Litt.D. *Third Edition. Demy 8vo. 10s. 6d.*
THE DOCTRINE OF THE INCARNATION. By R. L. Ottley, D.D. *Second and Cheaper Edition. Demy 8vo. 12s. 6d.*

AN INTRODUCTION TO THE HISTORY OF THE CREEDS. By A. E. Burn, .D.D *Demy 8vo. 10s. 6d.*
THE PHILOSOPHY OF RELIGION IN ENGLAND AND AMERICA. By Alfred Caldecott, D.D. *Demy 8vo. 10s. 6d.*
A HISTORY OF EARLY CHRISTIAN DOCTRINE. By J. F. Bethune Baker, M.A. *Demy 8vo. 10s. 6d.*

Westminster Commentaries, The

General Editor, WALTER LOCK, D.D., Warden of Keble College,
Dean Ireland's Professor of Exegesis in the University of Oxford.

The object of each commentary is primarily exegetical, to interpret the author's
meaning to the present generation. The editors will not deal, except very subor-
dinately, with questions of textual criticism or philology ; but, taking the English
text in the Revised Version as their basis, they will try to combine a hearty accept-
ance of critical principles with loyalty to the Catholic Faith.

THE BOOK OF GENESIS. Edited with Intro-
duction and Notes by S. R. Driver, D.D.
Fifth Edition Demy 8vo. 10s. 6d.
THE BOOK OF JOB. Edited by E. C. S. Gibson,
D.D. *Second Edition. Demy 8vo. 6s.*
THE ACTS OF THE APOSTLES. Edited by R.
B. Rackham, M.A. *Demy 8vo. Second and
Cheaper Edition. 10s. 6d.*

THE FIRST EPISTLE OF PAUL THE APOSTLE
TO THE CORINTHIANS. Edited by H. L.
Goudge, M.A. *Demy 8vo. 6s.*

THE EPISTLE OF ST. JAMES. Edited with Introduction and Notes by R. J. Knowling,
M.A. *Demy 8vo. 6s.*

PART II.—FICTION

Albanesi (E. Maria). SUSANNAH AND
ONE OTHER. *Fourth Edition. Cr.
8vo. 6s.*
THE BLUNDER OF AN INNOCENT.
Second Edition. Cr. 8vo. 6s.
CAPRICIOUS CAROLINE. *Second Edi-
tion. Cr. 8vo. 6s.*
LOVE AND LOUISA. *Second Edition.
Cr. 8vo. 6s.*
PETER, A PARASITE. *Cr. 8vo. 6s.*
THE BROWN EYES OF MARY. *Third
Edition. Cr. 8vo. 6s.*
Anstey (F.). Author of 'Vice Versâ.' A
BAYARD FROM BENGAL. Illustrated
by BERNARD PARTRIDGE. *Third Edition.
Cr. 8vo. 3s. 6d.*
Bacheller (Irving), Author of 'Eben Holden.'
DARREL OF THE BLESSED ISLES.
Third Edition. Cr. 8vo. 6s.
Bagot (Richard). A ROMAN MYSTERY.
Third Edition. Cr. 8vo. 6s.
THE PASSPORT. *Fourth Ed. Cr. 8vo. 6s.*
Baring-Gould (S.). ARMINELL. *Fifth
Edition. Cr. 8vo. 6s.*
URITH. *Fifth Edition. Cr. 8vo. 6s.*
IN THE ROAR OF THE SEA. *Seventh
Edition. Cr. 8vo. 6s.*
CHEAP JACK ZITA. *Fourth Edition.
Cr. 8vo. 6s.*
MARGERY OF QUETHER. *Third
Edition. Cr. 8vo. 6s.*
THE QUEEN OF LOVE. *Fifth Edition.
Cr. 8vo. 6s.*
JACQUETTA. *Third Edition. Cr. 8vo. 6s.*
KITTY ALONE. *Fifth Edition. Cr. 8vo. 6s.*
NOÉMI. Illustrated. *Fourth Edition. Cr.
8vo. 6s.*
THE BROOM-SQUIRE. Illustrated.
Fifth Edition. Cr. 8vo. 6s.

DARTMOOR IDYLLS. *Cr. 8vo. 6s.*
THE PENNYCOMEQUICKS. *Third
Edition. Cr. 8vo. 6s.*
GUAVAS THE TINNER. Illustrated.
Second Edition. Cr. 8vo. 6s.
BLADYS. Illustrated. *Second Edition.
Cr. 8vo. 6s.*
PABO THE PRIEST. *Cr. 8vo. 6s.*
WINEFRED. Illustrated. *Second Edition.
Cr. 8vo. 6s.*
ROYAL GEORGIE. Illustrated. *Cr. 8vo. 6s.*
MISS QUILLET. Illustrated. *Cr. 8vo. 6s.*
CHRIS OF ALL SORTS. *Cr. 8vo. 6s.*
IN DEWISLAND. *Second Edition. Cr.
8vo. 6s.*
LITTLE TU'PENNY. *A New Edition. 6d.*
See also Strand Novels and Books for
Boys and Girls.
Barlow (Jane). THE LAND OF THE
SHAMROCK. *Cr. 8vo. 6s.* See also
Strand Novels.
Barr (Robert). IN THE MIDST OF
ALARMS. *Third Edition. Cr. 8vo. 6s.*
THE MUTABLE MANY. *Third Edition.
Cr. 8vo. 6s.*
THE COUNTESS TEKLA. *Third Edition.
Cr. 8vo. 6s.*
THE LADY ELECTRA. *Second Edition.
Cr. 8vo. 6s.*
THE TEMPESTUOUS PETTICOAT.
Illustrated. *Third Edition. Cr. 8vo. 6s.*
See also Strand Novels and S. Crane.
Begbie (Harold). THE ADVENTURES
OF SIR JOHN SPARROW. *Cr. 8vo. 6s.*
Belloc (Hilaire). EMMANUEL BURDEN,
MERCHANT. With 36 Illustrations by
G. K. CHESTERTON. *Second Edition.
Cr. 8vo. 6s.*

Benson (E. F.) DODO. *Fourth Edition.*
Cr. 8vo. 6s. See also Strand Novels.
Benson (Margaret). SUBJECT TO
VANITY. *Cr. 8vo. 3s. 6d.*
Bourne (Harold C.). See V. Langbridge.
Burton (J. Bloundelle). THE YEAR
ONE : A Page of the French Revolution.
Illustrated. *Cr. 8vo. 6s.*
THE FATE OF VALSEC. *Cr. 8vo. 6s.*
A BRANDED NAME. *Cr. 8vo. 6s.*
See also Strand Novels.
Capes (Bernard), Author of 'The Lake of
Wine.' THE EXTRAORDINARY CON-
FESSIONS OF DIANA PLEASE. *Third
Edition. Cr. 8vo. 6s.*
A JAY OF ITALY. *Fourth Ed. Cr. 8vo. 6s.*
LOAVES AND FISHES. *Second Edition.
Cr. 8vo. 6s.*
Chesney (Weatherby). THE TRAGEDY
OF THE GREAT EMERALD. *Cr.
8vo. 6s.*
THE MYSTERY OF A BUNGALOW.
Second Edition. Cr. 8vo. 6s.
See also Strand Novels.
Clifford (Hugh). A FREE LANCE OF
TO-DAY. *Cr. 8vo. 6s.*
Clifford (Mrs. W. K.). See Strand Novels
and Books for Boys and Girls.
Cobb (Thomas). A CHANGE OF FACE.
Cr. 8vo. 6s.
Corelli (Marie). A ROMANCE OF TWO
WORLDS. *Twenty-Sixth Edition. Cr.
8vo. 6s.*
VENDETTA. *Twenty-Third Edition. Cr.
8vo. 6s.*
THELMA. *Thirty-Fourth Edition. Cr.
8vo. 6s.*
ARDATH : THE STORY OF A DEAD
SELF. *Sixteenth Edition. Cr. 8vo. 6s.*
THE SOUL OF LILITH. *Thirteenth Edi-
tion. Cr. 8vo. 6s.*
WORMWOOD. *Fourteenth Ed. Cr. 8vo. 6s.*
BARABBAS : A DREAM OF THE
WORLD'S TRAGEDY. *Forty-first Edi-
tion. Cr. 8vo. 6s.*
THE SORROWS OF SATAN. *Fiftieth
Edition. Cr. 8vo. 6s.*
THE MASTER CHRISTIAN. *167th
Thousand. Cr. 8vo. 6s.*
TEMPORAL POWER : A STUDY IN
SUPREMACY. *150th Thousand. Cr.
8vo. 6s.*
GOD'S GOOD MAN : A SIMPLE LOVE
STORY. *137th Thousand. Cr. 8vo. 6s.*
THE MIGHTY ATOM. *A New Edition.
Cr. 8vo. 6s.*
BOY. *A New Edition. Cr. 8vo. 6s.*
JANE. *A New Edition. Cr. 8vo. 6s.*
Crockett (S. R.), Author of 'The Raiders,'
etc. LOCHINVAR. Illustrated. *Third
Edition. Cr. 8vo. 6s.*
THE STANDARD BEARER. *Cr. 8vo. 6s.*
Croker (B. M.). THE OLD CANTON-
MENT. *Cr. 8vo. 6s.*
JOHANNA. *Second Edition. Cr. 8vo. 6s.*

THE HAPPY VALLEY. *Third Edition.
Cr. 8vo. 6s.*
A NINE DAYS' WONDER. *Third
Edition. Cr. 8vo. 6s.*
PEGGY OF THE BARTONS. *Sixth
Edition. Cr. 8vo. 6s.*
ANGEL. *Fourth Edition. Cr. 8vo. 6s.*
A STATE SECRET. *Third Edition. Cr.
8vo. 3s. 6d.*
Dawson (Francis W.). THE SCAR.
Second Edition. Cr. 8vo. 6s.
Dawson (A. J.). DANIEL WHYTE.
Cr. 8vo. 3s. 6d.
Doyle (A. Conan), Author of 'Sherlock
Holmes,' 'The White Company,' etc.
ROUND THE RED LAMP. *Ninth
Edition. Cr. 8vo. 6s.*
Duncan (Sara Jeannette) (Mrs. Everard
Cotes). THOSE DELIGHTFUL
AMERICANS. Illustrated. *Third Edition.
Cr. 8vo. 6s.* See also Strand Novels.
Findlater (J. H.). THE GREEN GRAVES
OF BALGOWRIE. *Fifth Edition.
Cr. 8vo. 6s.*
See also Strand Novels.
Findlater (Mary). A NARROW WAY.
Third Edition. Cr. 8vo.. 6s.
THE ROSE OF JOY. *Third Edition.
Cr. 8vo. 6s.*
See also Strand Novels.
Fitzpatrick (K.) THE WEANS AT
ROWALLAN. Illustrated. *Second Edi-
tion. Cr. 8vo. 6s.*
Fitzstephen (Gerald). MORE KIN
THAN KIND. *Cr. 8vo. 6s.*
Fletcher (J. S.). LUCIAN THE
DREAMER. *Cr. 8vo. 6s.*
Fraser (Mrs. Hugh), Author of 'The Stolen
Emperor.' THE SLAKING OF THE
SWORD. *Cr. 8vo. 6s.*
THE SHADOW OF THE LORD. *Cr.
8vo. 6s.*
Fuller-Maitland (Mrs.), Author of 'The
Day Book of Bethia Hardacre.' BLANCHE
ESMEAD. *Second Edition. Cr. 8vo. 6s.*
Gerard (Dorothea), Author of 'Lady Baby.'
THE CONQUEST OF LONDON.
Second Edition. Cr. 8vo. 6s.
HOLY MATRIMONY. *Second Edition.
Cr. 8vo. 6s.*
MADE OF MONEY. *Cr. 8vo. 6s.*
THE BRIDGE OF LIFE. *Cr. 8vo. 6s.*
THE IMPROBABLE IDYL. *Third
Edition. Cr. 8vo. 6s.*
See also Strand Novels.
Gerard (Emily). THE HERONS'
TOWER. *Cr. 8vo. 6s.*
Gissing (George), Author of 'Demos,' 'In
the Year of Jubilee,' etc. THE TOWN
TRAVELLER. *Second Ed. Cr. 8vo. 6s.*
THE CROWN OF LIFE. *Cr. 8vo. 6s.*
Gleig (Charles). BUNTER'S CRUISE.
Illustrated. *Cr. 8vo. 3s. 6d.*
Harraden (Beatrice). IN VARYING
MOODS. *Fourteenth Edition. Cr. 8vo. 6s.*

THE SCHOLAR'S DAUGHTER. *Fourth Edition. Cr. 8vo. 6s.*
HILDA STRAFFORD. *Cr. 8vo. 6s.*
Harrod (F.) (Frances Forbes Robertson). THE TAMING OF THE BRUTE. *Cr. 8vo. 6s.*
Herbertson (Agnes G.). PATIENCE DEAN. *Cr. 8vo. 6s.*
Hichens (Robert). THE PROPHET OF BERKELEY SQUARE. *Second Edition. Cr. 8vo. 6s.*
TONGUES OF CONSCIENCE. *Second Edition. Cr. 8vo. 6s.*
FELIX. *Fifth Edition. Cr. 8vo. 6s.*
THE WOMAN WITH THE FAN. *Sixth Edition. Cr. 8vo. 6s.*
BYEWAYS. *Cr. 8vo. 3s. 6d.*
THE GARDEN OF ALLAH. *Thirteenth Edition. Cr. 8vo. 6s.*
THE BLACK SPANIEL. *Cr. 8vo. 6s.*
Hobbes (John Oliver), Author of ' Robert Orange.' THE SERIOUS WOOING. *Cr. 8vo. 6s.*
Hope (Anthony). THE GOD IN THE CAR. *Tenth Edition. Cr. 8vo. 6s.*
A CHANGE OF AIR. *Sixth Edition. Cr. 8vo. 6s.*
A MAN OF MARK. *Fifth Edition. Cr. 8vo. 6s.*
THE CHRONICLES OF COUNT ANTONIO. *Sixth Edition. Cr. 8vo. 6s.*
PHROSO. Illustrated by H. R. Millar. *Sixth Edition. Cr. 8vo. 6s.*
SIMON DALE. Illustrated. *Seventh Edition. Cr. 8vo. 6s.*
THE KING'S MIRROR. *Fourth Edition. Cr. 8vo. 6s.*
QUISANTE. *Fourth Edition. Cr. 8vo. 6s.*
THE DOLLY DIALOGUES. *Cr. 8vo. 6s.*
A SERVANT OF THE PUBLIC. Illustrated. *Fourth Edition. Cr. 8vo. 6s.*
Hope (Graham), Author of ' A Cardinal and his Conscience,' etc., etc. THE LADY OF LYTE. *Second Ed. Cr. 8vo. 6s.*
Hough (Emerson). THE MISSISSIPPI BUBBLE. Illustrated. *Cr. 8vo. 6s.*
Housman (Clemence). THE LIFE OF SIR AGLOVALE DE GALIS. *Cr. 8vo. 6s.*
Hyne (C. J. Cutcliffe), Author of ' Captain Kettle.' MR. HORROCKS, PURSER. *Third Edition. Cr. 8vo. 6s.*
Jacobs (W. W.). MANY CARGOES. *Twenty-Eighth Edition. Cr. 8vo. 3s. 6d.*
SEA URCHINS. *Twelfth Edition.. Cr. 8vo. 3s. 6d.*
A MASTER OF CRAFT. Illustrated. *Seventh Edition. Cr. 8vo. 3s. 6d.*
LIGHT FREIGHTS. Illustrated. *Fifth Edition. Cr. 8vo. 3s. 6d.*
James (Henry). THE SOFT SIDE. *Second Edition. Cr. 8vo. 6s.*
THE BETTER SORT. *Cr. 8vo. 6s.*
THE AMBASSADORS. *Second Edition. Cr. 8vo. 6s.*

THE GOLDEN BOWL. *Third Edition. Cr. 8vo. 6s.*
Janson (Gustaf). ABRAHAM'S SACRIFICE. *Cr. 8vo. 6s.*
Keays (H. A. Mitchell). HE THAT EATETH BREAD WITH ME. *Cr. 8vo. 6s.*
Langbridge (V.) and **Bourne (C. Harold.).** THE VALLEY OF INHERITANCE. *Cr. 8vo. 6s.*
Lawless (Hon. Emily). WITH ESSEX IN IRELAND. *Cr. 8vo. 6s.*
See also Strand Novels.
Lawson (Harry), Author of 'When the Billy Boils.' CHILDREN OF THE BUSH. *Cr. 8vo. 6s.*
Le Queux (W.). THE HUNCHBACK OF WESTMINSTER. *Third Edition. Cr. 8vo. 6s.*
THE CLOSED BOOK. *Third Edition. Cr. 8vo. 6s.*
THE VALLEY OF THE SHADOW. Illustrated. *Third Edition. Cr. 8vo. 6s.*
BEHIND THE THRONE. *Third Edition. Cr. 8vo. 6s.*
Levett-Yeats (S.). ORRAIN. *Second Edition. Cr. 8vo. 6s.*
Long (J. Luther), Co-Author of 'The Darling of the Gods.' MADAME BUTTERFLY. *Cr. 8vo. 3s. 6d.*
SIXTY JANE. *Cr. 8vo. 6s.*
Lowis (Cecil). THE MACHINATIONS OF THE MYO-OK. *Cr. 8vo. 6s.*
Lyall (Edna). DERRICK VAUGHAN, NOVELIST. *42nd Thousand. Cr. 8vo. 3s. 6d.*
M'Carthy (Justin H.), Author of ' If I were King.' THE LADY OF LOYALTY HOUSE. Illustrated. *Third Edition. Cr. 8vo. 6s.*
THE DRYAD. *Second Edition. Cr. 8vo. 6s.*
Macdonald (Ronald). THE SEA MAID. *Second Edition. Cr. 8vo. 6s.*
Macnaughtan (S.). THE FORTUNE OF CHRISTINA MACNAB. *Third Edition. Cr. 8vo. 6s.*
Malet (Lucas). COLONEL ENDERBY'S WIFE. *Fourth Edition. Cr. 8vo. 6s.*
A COUNSEL OF PERFECTION. *New Edition. Cr. 8vo. 6s.*
THE WAGES OF SIN. *Fourteenth Edition. Cr. 8vo. 6s.*
THE CARISSIMA. *Fourth Edition. Cr. 8vo. 6s.*
THE GATELESS BARRIER. *Fourth Edition. Cr. 8vo. 6s.*
THE HISTORY OF SIR RICHARD CALMADY. *Seventh Edition. Cr. 8vo. 6s.*
See also Books for Boys and Girls.
Mann (Mrs. M. E.). OLIVIA'S SUMMER. *Second Edition. Cr. 8vo. 6s.*
A LOST ESTATE. *A New Edition. Cr. 8vo. 6s.*
THE PARISH OF HILBY. *A New Edition. Cr. 8vo. 6s.*

THE PARISH NURSE. *Fourth Edition.* *Cr. 8vo. 6s.*
GRAN'MA'S JANE. *Cr. 8vo. 6s.*
MRS. PETER HOWARD. *Cr. 8vo. 6s.*
A WINTER'S TALE. *A New Edition.* *Cr. 8vo. 6s.*
ONE ANOTHER'S BURDENS. *A New Edition. Cr. 8vo. 6s.*
ROSE AT HONEYPOT. *Third Ed. Cr. 8vo. 6s.* See also Books for Boys and Girls.
Marriott (Charles), Author of 'The Column.' GENEVRA. *Second Edition. Cr. 8vo. 6s.*
Marsh (Richard). THE TWICKENHAM PEERAGE. *Second Edition. Cr. 8vo. 6s.*
A DUEL. *Cr. 8vo. 6s.*
THE MARQUIS OF PUTNEY. *Second Edition. Cr. 8vo. 6s.*
See also Strand Novels.
Mason (A. E. W.), Author of 'The Four Feathers,' etc. CLEMENTINA. Illustrated. *Second Edition. Cr. 8vo. 6s.*
Mathers (Helen), Author of 'Comin' thro' the Rye.' HONEY. *Fourth Edition. Cr. 8vo. 6s.*
GRIFF OF GRIFFITHSCOURT. *Cr. 8vo. 6s.*
THE FERRYMAN. *Second Edition. Cr. 8vo. 6s.*
Maxwell (W. B.), Author of 'The Ragged Messenger.' VIVIEN. *Eighth Edition. Cr. 8vo. 6s.*
THE RAGGED MESSENGER. *Third Edition. Cr. 8vo. 6s.*
FABULOUS FANCIES. *Cr. 8vo. 6s.*
Meade (L. T.). DRIFT. *Second Edition. Cr. 8vo. 6s.*
RESURGAM. *Cr. 8vo. 6s.*
VICTORY. *Cr. 8vo. 6s.*
See also Books for Girls and Boys.
Meredith (Ellis). HEART OF MY HEART. *Cr. 8vo. 6s.*
'Miss Molly' (The Author of). THE GREAT RECONCILER. *Cr. 8vo. 6s.*
Mitford (Bertram). THE SIGN OF THE SPIDER. Illustrated. *Sixth Edition. Cr. 8vo. 3s. 6d.*
IN THE WHIRL OF THE RISING. *Third Edition. Cr. 8vo. 6s.*
THE RED DERELICT. *Second Edition. Cr. 8vo. 6s.*
Montresor (F. F.), Author of 'Into the Highways and Hedges.' THE ALIEN. *Third Edition. Cr. 8vo. 6s.*
Morrison (Arthur). TALES OF MEAN STREETS. *Sixth Edition. Cr. 8vo. 6s.*
A CHILD OF THE JAGO. *Fourth Edition. Cr. 8vo. 6s.*
TO LONDON TOWN. *Second Edition. Cr. 8vo. 6s.*
CUNNING MURRELL. *Cr. 8vo. 6s.*
THE HOLE IN THE WALL. *Fourth Edition. Cr. 8vo. 6s.*
DIVERS VANITIES. *Cr. 8vo. 6s.*

Nesbit (E.). (Mrs. E. Bland). THE RED HOUSE. Illustrated. *Fourth Edition. Cr. 8vo. 6s.*
See also Strand Novels.
Norris (W. E.). THE CREDIT OF THE COUNTY. Illustrated. *Second Edition. Cr. 8vo. 6s.*
THE EMBARRASSING ORPHAN. *Cr. 8vo. 6s.*
NIGEL'S VOCATION. *Cr. 8vo. 6s.*
BARHAM OF BELTANA. *Second Edition. Cr. 8vo. 6s.*
See also Strand Novels.
Ollivant (Alfred). OWD BOB, THE GREY DOG OF KENMUIR. *Eighth Edition. Cr. 8vo. 6s.*
Oppenheim (E. Phillips). MASTER OF MEN. *Third Edition. Cr. 8vo. 6s.*
Oxenham (John), Author of 'Barbe of Grand Bayou.' A WEAVER OF WEBS. *Second Edition. Cr. 8vo. 6s.*
THE GATE OF THE DESERT. *Fourth Edition. Cr. 8vo. 6s.*
Pain (Barry). THREE FANTASIES. *Cr. 8vo. 1s.*
LINDLEY KAYS. *Third Edition. Cr. 8vo. 6s.*
Parker (Gilbert). PIERRE AND HIS PEOPLE. *Sixth Edition.*
MRS. FALCHION. *Fifth Edition. Cr. 8vo. 6s.*
THE TRANSLATION OF A SAVAGE. *Second Edition. Cr. 8vo. 6s.*
THE TRAIL OF THE SWORD. Illustrated. *Ninth Edition. Cr. 8vo. 6s.*
WHEN VALMOND CAME TO PONTIAC: The Story of a Lost Napoleon. *Fifth Edition. Cr. 8vo. 6s.*
AN ADVENTURER OF THE NORTH: The Last Adventures of 'Pretty Pierre.' *Third Edition. Cr. 8vo. 6s.*
THE SEATS OF THE MIGHTY. Illustrated. *Fourteenth Edition. Cr. 8vo. 6s.*
THE BATTLE OF THE STRONG: a Romance of Two Kingdoms. Illustrated. *Fifth Edition. Cr. 8vo. 6s.*
THE POMP OF THE LAVILETTES. *Second Edition. Cr. 8vo. 3s. 6d.*
Pemberton (Max). THE FOOTSTEPS OF A THRONE. Illustrated. *Third Edition. Cr. 8vo. 6s.*
I CROWN THEE KING. With Illustrations by Frank Dadd and A. Forrestier. *Cr. 8vo. 6s.*
Phillpotts (Eden). LYING PROPHETS. *Cr. 8vo. 6s.*
CHILDREN OF THE MIST. *Fifth Edition. Cr. 8vo. 6s.*
THE HUMAN BOY. With a Frontispiece. *Fourth Edition. Cr. 8vo. 6s.*
SONS OF THE MORNING. *Second Edition. Cr. 8vo. 6s.*

THE RIVER. *Third Edition. Cr. 8vo. 6s.*
THE AMERICAN PRISONER. *Third Edition. Cr. 8vo. 6s.*
THE SECRET WOMAN. *Fourth Edition. Cr. 8vo. 6s.*
KNOCK AT A VENTURE. With a Frontispiece. *Third Edition. Cr. 8vo. 6s.*
THE PORTREEVE. *Fourth Edition. Cr. 8vo. 6s.*
See also Strand Novels.
Pickthall (Marmaduke). SAÏD THE FISHERMAN. *Fifth Edition. Cr. 8vo. 6s.*
BRENDLE. *Second Edition. Cr. 8vo. 6s.*
'Q,' Author of 'Dead Man's Rock.' THE WHITE WOLF. *Second Edition. Cr. 8vo. 6s.*
THE MAYOR OF TROY. *Fourth Edition. Cr. 8vo. 6s.*
Rhys (Grace). THE WOOING OF SHEILA. *Second Edition. Cr. 8vo. 6s.*
THE PRINCE OF LISNOVER. *Cr. 8vo. 6s.*
Rhys (Grace) and Another. THE DIVERTED VILLAGE. Illustrated by DOROTHY GWYN JEFFREYS. *Cr. 8vo. 6s.*
Ridge (W. Pett). LOST PROPERTY. *Second Edition. Cr. 8vo. 6s.*
ERB. *Second Edition. Cr. 8vo. 6s.*
A SON OF THE STATE. *Second Edition. Cr. 8vo. 3s. 6d.*
A BREAKER OF LAWS. *A New Edition. Cr. 8vo. 3s. 6d.*
MRS. GALER'S BUSINESS. Illustrated. *Second Edition. Cr. 8vo. 6s.*
SECRETARY TO BAYNE, M.P. *Cr. 8vo. 3s. 6d.*
Ritchie (Mrs. David G.). THE TRUTHFUL LIAR. *Cr. 8vo. 6s.*
Roberts (C. G. D.). THE HEART OF THE ANCIENT WOOD. *Cr. 8vo. 3s. 6d.*
Russell (W. Clark). MY DANISH SWEETHEART. Illustrated. *Fifth Edition. Cr. 8vo. 6s.*
HIS ISLAND PRINCESS. Illustrated. *Second Edition. Cr. 6vo. 6s.*
ABANDONED. *Cr. 8vo. 6s.*
See also Books for Boys and Girls.
Sergeant (Adeline). ANTHEA'S WAY. *Cr. 8vo. 6s.*
THE PROGRESS OF RACHAEL. *Cr. 8vo. 6s.*
THE MYSTERY OF THE MOAT. *Second Edition. Cr. 8vo. 6s.*
MRS. LYGON'S HUSBAND. *Cr. 8vo. 6s.*
THE COMING OF THE RANDOLPHS. *Cr. 8vo. 6s.*
See also Strand Novels.
Shannon. (W.F.) THE MESS DECK. *Cr. 8vo. 3s. 6d.*
See also Strand Novels.

Sonnischsen (Albert). DEEP-SEA VAGABONDS. *Cr. 8vo. 6s.*
Thompson (Vance). SPINNERS OF LIFE. *Cr. 8vo. 6s.*
Urquhart (M.), A TRAGEDY IN COMMONPLACE. *Second Ed. Cr. 8vo. 6s.*
Waineman (Paul). BY A FINNISH LAKE. *Cr. 8vo. 6s.*
THE SONG OF THE FOREST. *Cr. 8vo. 6s.* See also Strand Novels.
Waltz (E. C.). THE ANCIENT LANDMARK: A Kentucky Romance. *Cr. 8vo. 6s.*
Watson (H. B. Marriott). ALARUMS AND EXCURSIONS. *Cr. 8vo. 6s.*
CAPTAIN FORTUNE. *Third Edition. Cr. 8vo. 6s.*
TWISTED EGLANTINE. With 8 Illustrations by FRANK CRAIG. *Third Edition. Cr. 8vo. 6s.*
THE HIGH TOBY. With a Frontispiece. *Third Edition. Cr. 8vo. 6s.*
See also Strand Novels.
Wells (H. G.). THE SEA LADY. *Cr. 8vo. 6s.*
Weyman (Stanley), Author of 'A Gentleman of France.' UNDER THE RED ROBE. With Illustrations by R. C. WOODVILLE. *Twentieth Edition. Cr. 8vo. 6s.*
White (Stewart E.), Author of 'The Blazed Trail.' CONJUROR'S HOUSE. A Romance of the Free Trail. *Second Edition. Cr. 8vo. 6s.*
White (Percy). THE SYSTEM. *Third Edition. Cr. 8vo. 6s.*
THE PATIENT MAN. *Second Edition. Cr. 8vo. 6s.*
Williamson (Mrs. C. N.), Author of 'The Barnstormers.' THE ADVENTURE OF PRINCESS SYLVIA. *Second Edition. Cr. 8vo. 3s. 6d.*
THE WOMAN WHO DARED. *Cr. 8vo. 6s.*
THE SEA COULD TELL. *Second Edition. Cr. 8vo. 6s.*
THE CASTLE OF THE SHADOWS. *Third Edition. Cr. 8vo. 6s.*
PAPA. *Cr. 8vo. 6s.*
LADY BETTY ACROSS THE WATER. *Third Edition. Cr. 8vo. 6s.*
Williamson (C. N. and A. M.). THE LIGHTNING CONDUCTOR: Being the Romance of a Motor Car. Illustrated. *Fourteenth Edition. Cr. 8vo. 6s.*
THE PRINCESS PASSES. Illustrated. *Seventh Edition. Cr. 8vo. 6s.*
MY FRIEND THE CHAUFFEUR. With 16 Illustrations. *Seventh Edition. Cr. 8vo. 6s.*
Wyllarde (Dolf), Author of 'Uriah the Hittite.' THE PATHWAY OF THE PIONEER. *Fourth Edition. Cr. 8vo. 6s.*

Methuen's Shilling Novels

Cr. 8vo. Cloth, 1s. net.

ENCOURAGED by the great and steady sale of their Sixpenny Novels, Messrs. Methuen have determined to issue a new series of fiction at a low price under the title of 'THE SHILLING NOVELS.' These books are well printed and well bound in *cloth*, and the excellence of their quality may be gauged from the names of those authors who contribute the early volumes of the series.

Messrs. Methuen would point out that the books are as good and as long as a six shilling novel, that they are bound in cloth and not in paper, and that their price is One Shilling *net*. They feel sure that the public will appreciate such good and cheap literature, and the books can be seen at all good booksellers.

The first volumes are—

Balfour (Andrew). VENGEANCE IS MINE.
TO ARMS.
Baring-Gould (S.). MRS. CURGENVEN OF CURGENVEN.
DOMITIA.
THE FROBISHERS.
Barlow (Jane), Author of 'Irish Idylls. FROM THE EAST UNTO THE WEST.
A CREEL OF IRISH STORIES.
THE FOUNDING OF FORTUNES.
Barr (Robert). THE VICTORS.
Bartram (George). THIRTEEN EVENINGS.
Benson (E. F.), Author of 'Dodo.' THE CAPSINA.
Bowles (G. Stewart). A STRETCH OFF THE LAND.
Brooke (Emma). THE POET'S CHILD.
Bullock (Shan F.). THE BARRYS.
THE CHARMER.
THE SQUIREEN.
THE RED LEAGUERS.
Burton (J. Bloundelle). ACROSS THE SALT SEAS.
THE CLASH OF ARMS.
DENOUNCED.
FORTUNE'S MY FOE.
Capes (Bernard). AT A WINTER'S FIRE.
Chesney (Weatherby). THE BAPTIST RING.
THE BRANDED PRINCE.
THE FOUNDERED GALLEON.
JOHN TOPP.
Clifford (Mrs. W. K.). A FLASH OF SUMMER.
Collingwood (Harry). THE DOCTOR OF THE 'JULIET.'
Cornford (L. Cope). SONS OF ADVERSITY.
Crane (Stephen). WOUNDS IN THE RAIN.
Denny (C. E.). THE ROMANCE OF UPFOLD MANOR.
Dickson (Harris). THE BLACK WOLF'S BREED.
Dickinson (Evelyn). THE SIN OF ANGELS.

Duncan (Sara J.). *THE POOL IN THE DESERT.
A VOYAGE OF CONSOLATION.
Embree (C. F.). A HEART OF FLAME.
Fenn (G. Manville). AN ELECTRIC SPARK.
Findlater (Jane H.). A DAUGHTER OF STRIFE.
Findlater (Mary). OVER THE HILLS.
Forrest (R. E.). THE SWORD OF AZRAEL.
Francis (M. E.). MISS ERIN.
Gallon (Tom). RICKERBY'S FOLLY.
Gerard (Dorothea). THINGS THAT HAVE HAPPENED.
Gilchrist (R. Murray). WILLOWBRAKE.
Glanville (Ernest). THE DESPATCH RIDER.
THE LOST REGIMENT.
THE KLOOF BRIDE.
THE INCA'S TREASURE.
Gordon (Julien). MRS. CLYDE.
WORLD'S PEOPLE.
Goss (C. F.). THE REDEMPTION OF DAVID CORSON.
Gray (E. M'Queen). MY STEWARDSHIP.
Hales (A. G.). JAIR THE APOSTATE.
Hamilton (Lord Ernest). MARY HAMILTON.
Harrison (Mrs. Burton). A PRINCESS OF THE HILLS. Illustrated.
Hooper (I.). THE SINGER OF MARLY.
Hough (Emerson). THE MISSISSIPPI BUBBLE.
'Iota' (Mrs. Caffyn). ANNE MAULEVERER.
Jepson (Edgar). KEEPERS OF THE PEOPLE.
Kelly (Florence Finch). WITH HOOPS OF STEEL.
Lawless (Hon. Emily). MAELCHO.
Linden (Annie). A WOMAN OF SENTIMENT.
Lorimer (Norma). JOSIAH'S WIFE.
Lush (Charles K.). THE AUTOCRATS.
Macdonell (Anne). THE STORY OF TERESA.
Macgrath (Harold). THE PUPPET CROWN.

Mackie (Pauline Bradford). THE VOICE IN THE DESERT.
Marsh (Richard). THE SEEN AND THE UNSEEN.
GARNERED.
A METAMORPHOSIS.
MARVELS AND MYSTERIES.
BOTH SIDES OF THE VEIL.
Mayall (J. W.). THE CYNIC AND THE SYREN.
Monkhouse (Allan). LOVE IN A LIFE.
Moore (Arthur). THE KNIGHT PUNCTILIOUS.
Nesbit (Mrs. Bland). THE LITERARY SENSE.
Norris (W. E.). AN OCTAVE.
Oliphant (Mrs.). THE LADY'S WALK.
SIR ROBERT'S FORTUNE.
THE TWO MARY'S.
Penny (Mrs. Frank). A MIXED MARAGE.
Phillpotts (Eden). THE STRIKING HOURS.
FANCY FREE.
Pryce (Richard). TIME AND THE WOMAN.
Randall (J.). AUNT BETHIA'S BUTTON.
Raymond (Walter). FORTUNE'S DARLING.
Rayner (Olive Pratt). ROSALBA.
Rhys (Grace). THE DIVERTED VILLAGE.

Rickert (Edith). OUT OF THE CYPRESS SWAMP.
Roberton (M. H.). A GALLANT QUAKER.
Saunders (Marshall). ROSE A CHARLITTE.
Sergeant (Adeline). ACCUSED AND ACCUSER.
BARBARA'S MONEY.
THE ENTHUSIAST.
A GREAT LADY.
THE LOVE THAT OVERCAME.
THE MASTER OF BEECHWOOD.
UNDER SUSPICION.
THE YELLOW DIAMOND.
Shannon (W. F.). JIM TWELVES.
Strain (E. H.). ELMSLIE'S DRAG NET.
Stringer (Arthur). THE SILVER POPPY.
Stuart (Esmè). CHRISTALLA.
Sutherland (Duchess of). ONE HOUR AND THE NEXT.
Swan (Annie). LOVE GROWN COLD.
Swift (Benjamin). SORDON.
Tanqueray (Mrs. B. M.). THE ROYAL QUAKER.
Trafford-Taunton (Mrs. E. W.). SILENT DOMINION.
Upward (Allen). ATHELSTANE FORD.
Waineman (Paul). A HEROINE FROM FINLAND.
Watson (H. B. Marriott). THE SKIRTS OF HAPPY CHANCE.
'Zack.' TALES OF DUNSTABLE WEIR.

Books for Boys and Girls

Illustrated.   Crown 8vo.   3s. 6d.

THE GETTING WELL OF DOROTHY. By Mrs. W. K. Clifford. *Second Edition.*
THE ICELANDER'S SWORD. By S. Baring-Gould.
ONLY A GUARD-ROOM DOG. By Edith E. Cuthell.
THE DOCTOR OF THE JULIET. By Harry Collingwood.
LITTLE PETER. By Lucas Malet. *Second Edition.*
MASTER ROCKAFELLAR'S VOYAGE. By W. Clark Russell.

THE SECRET OF MADAME DE MONLUC. By the Author of "Mdlle. Mori."
SYD BELTON: Or, the Boy who would not go to Sea. By G. Manville Fenn.
THE RED GRANGE. By Mrs. Molesworth.
A GIRL OF THE PEOPLE. By L. T. Meade. *Second Edition.*
HEPSY GIPSY. By L. T. Meade. 2s. 6d.
THE HONOURABLE MISS. By L. T. Meade. *Second Edition.*
THERE WAS ONCE A PRINCE. By Mrs. M. E. Mann.
WHEN ARNOLD COMES HOME. By Mrs. M. E. Mann.

The Novels of Alexandre Dumas

Price 6d.   Double Volumes, 1s.

THE THREE MUSKETEERS. With a long Introduction by Andrew Lang. Double volume.
THE PRINCE OF THIEVES. *Second Edition.*
ROBIN HOOD. A Sequel to the above.
THE CORSICAN BROTHERS.
GEORGES.

CROP-EARED JACQUOT; JANE; Etc.
TWENTY YEARS AFTER. Double volume.
AMAURY.
THE CASTLE OF EPPSTEIN.
THE SNOWBALL, and SULTANETTA.
CECILE; OR, THE WEDDING GOWN.
ACTÉ.

THE BLACK TULIP.
THE VICOMTE DE BRAGELONNE.
    Part I. Louise de la Vallière. Double
    Volume.
    Part II. The Man in the Iron Mask.
    Double Volume.
THE CONVICT'S SON.
THE WOLF-LEADER.
NANON; OR, THE WOMEN' WAR. Double
    volume.
PAULINE; MURAT; AND PASCAL BRUNO.
THE ADVENTURES OF CAPTAIN PAMPHILE.
FERNANDE.
GABRIEL LAMBERT.
CATHERINE BLUM.
THE CHEVALIER D'HARMENTAL. Double
    volume.
SYLVANDIRE.
THE FENCING MASTER.
THE REMINISCENCES OF ANTONY.
CONSCIENCE.
PERE LA RUINE.
*HENRI OF NAVARRE. The second part of
    Queen Margot.
THE GREAT MASSACRE. The first part of
    Queen Margot.
THE WILD DUCK SHOOTER.

Illustrated Edition.

Demy 8vo. Cloth.

THE THREE MUSKETEERS. Illustrated in
Colour by Frank Adams. 2s. 6d.

THE PRINCE OF THIEVES. Illustrated in
Colour by Frank Adams. 2s.
ROBIN HOOD THE OUTLAW. Illustrated in
Colour by Frank Adams. 2s.
THE CORSICAN BROTHERS. Illustrated in
Colour by A. M. M'Lellan. 1s. 6d.
THE WOLF-LEADER. Illustrated in Colour
by Frank Adams. 1s. 6d.
GEORGES. Illustrated in Colour by Munro Orr.
2s.
TWENTY YEARS AFTER. Illustrated in Colour
by Frank Adams. 3s.
AMAURY. Illustrated in Colour by Gordon
Browne. 2s.
THE SNOWBALL, and SULTANETTA. Illus-
trated in Colour by Frank Adams. 2s.
THE VICOMTE DE BRAGELONNE. Illustrated in
Colour by Frank Adams.
    Part I. Louise de la Vallière. 3s.
    Part II. The Man in the Iron Mask. 3s.
CROP-EARED JACQUOT; JANE; Etc. Illus-
trated in Colour by Gordon Browne. 2s.
THE CASTLE OF EPPSTEIN. Illustrated in
Colour by Stewart Orr. 1s. 6d.
ACTÉ. Illustrated in Colour by Gordon
Browne. 1s. 6d.
CECILE; OR, THE WEDDING GOWN. Illus-
trated in Colour by D. Murray Smith.
1s. 6d.
THE ADVENTURES OF CAPTAIN PAMPHILE.
Illustrated in Colour by Frank Adams.
1s. 6d.

Methuen's Sixpenny Books

Austen (Jane). PRIDE AND PRE-
JUDICE.
Bagot (Richard). A ROMAN MYSTERY.
Balfour (Andrew). BY STROKE OF
SWORD.
Baring-Gould (S.). FURZE BLOOM.
CHEAP JACK ZITA.
KITTY ALONE.
URITH.
THE BROOM SQUIRE.
IN THE ROAR OF THE SEA.
NOÉMI.
A BOOK OF FAIRY TALES. Illustrated.
LITTLE TUPENNY.
THE FROBISHERS.
Barr (Robert). JENNIE BAXTER,
JOURNALIST.
IN THE MIDST OF ALARMS.
THE COUNTESS TEKLA.
THE MUTABLE MANY.
Benson (E. F.). DODO.
Brontë (Charlotte). SHIRLEY.
Brownell (C. L.). THE HEART OF
JAPAN.

Burton (J. Bloundelle). ACROSS THE
SALT SEAS.
Caffyn (Mrs)., ('Iota'). ANNE MAULE-
VERER.
*Capes (Bernard). THE LAKE OF
WINE.
Clifford (Mrs. W. K.). A FLASH OF
SUMMER.
MRS. KEITH'S CRIME.
Connell (F. Norreys). THE NIGGER
KNIGHTS.
Corbett (Julian). A BUSINESS IN
GREAT WATERS.
Croker (Mrs. B. M.). PEGGY OF THE
BARTONS.
A STATE SECRET.
ANGEL.
JOHANNA.
Dante (Alighieri). THE VISION OF
DANTE (CARY).
Doyle (A. Conan). ROUND THE RED
LAMP.
Duncan (Sara Jeannette). A VOYAGE
OF CONSOLATION.
THOSE DELIGHTFUL AMERICANS.

Eliot (George). THE MILL ON THE FLOSS.
Findlater (Jane H.). THE GREEN GRAVES OF BALGOWRIE.
Gallon (Tom). RICKERBY'S FOLLY.
Gaskell (Mrs.). CRANFORD.
MARY BARTON.
NORTH AND SOUTH.
Gerard (Dorothea). HOLY MATRI-MONY.
THE CONQUEST OF LONDON.
MADE OF MONEY.
Gissing (George). THE TOWN TRAVEL-LER.
THE CROWN OF LIFE.
Glanville (Ernest). THE INCA'S TREASURE.
THE KLOOF BRIDE.
Gleig (Charles). BUNTER'S CRUISE.
Grimm (The Brothers). GRIMM'S FAIRY TALES. Illustrated.
Hope (Anthony). A MAN OF MARK.
A CHANGE OF AIR.
THE CHRONICLES OF COUNT ANTONIO.
PHROSO.
THE DOLLY DIALOGUES.
Hornung (E. W.). DEAD MEN TELL NO TALES.
Ingraham (J. H.). THE THRONE OF DAVID.
Le Queux (W.). THE HUNCHBACK OF WESTMINSTER.
Levett-Yeats (S. K.). THE TRAITOR'S WAY.
Linton (E. Lynn). THE TRUE HIS-TORY OF JOSHUA DAVIDSON.
Lyall (Edna). DERRICK VAUGHAN.
Malet (Lucas). THE CARISSIMA.
A COUNSEL OF PERFECTION.
Mann (Mrs. M. E.). MRS. PETER HOWARD.
A LOST ESTATE.
THE CEDAR STAR.
Marchmont (A. W.). MISER HOAD-LEY'S SECRET.
A MOMENT'S ERROR.
Marryat (Captain). PETER SIMPLE.
JACOB FAITHFUL.
Marsh (Richard). THE TWICKENHAM PEERAGE.
THE GODDESS.
THE JOSS.
Mason (A. E. W.). CLEMENTINA.
Mathers (Helen). HONEY.
GRIFF OF GRIFFITHSCOURT.

SAM'S SWEETHEART.
Meade (Mrs. L. T.). DRIFT.
Mitford (Bertram). THE SIGN OF THE SPIDER.
Montresor (F. F.). THE ALIEN.
Moore (Arthur). THE GAY DECEIVERS.
Morrison (Arthur). THE HOLE IN THE WALL.
Nesbit (E.). THE RED HOUSE.
Norris (W. E.). HIS GRACE.
GILES INGILBY.
THE CREDIT OF THE COUNTY.
LORD LEONARD.
MATTHEW AUSTIN.
CLARISSA FURIOSA.
Oliphant (Mrs.). THE LADY'S WALK.
SIR ROBERT'S FORTUNE.
THE PRODIGALS.
Oppenheim (E. Phillips). MASTER OF MEN.
Parker (Gilbert). THE POMP OF THE LAVILETTES.
WHEN VALMOND CAME TO PONTIAC.
THE TRAIL OF THE SWORD.
Pemberton (Max). THE FOOTSTEPS OF A THRONE.
I CROWN THEE KING.
Phillpotts (Eden). THE HUMAN BOY.
CHILDREN OF THE MIST.
Ridge (W. Pett). A SON OF THE STATE.
LOST PROPERTY.
GEORGE AND THE GENERAL.
Russell (W. Clark). A MARRIAGE AT SEA.
ABANDONED.
MY DANISH SWEETHEART.
Sergeant (Adeline). THE MASTER OF BEECHWOOD.
BARBARA'S MONEY.
THE YELLOW DIAMOND.
Surtees (R. S.). HANDLEY CROSS. Illustrated.
MR. SPONGE'S SPORTING TOUR. Illustrated.
ASK MAMMA. Illustrated.
Valentine (Major E. S.). VELDT AND LAAGER.
Walford (Mrs. L. B.). MR. SMITH.
THE BABY'S GRANDMOTHER.
Wallace (General Lew). BEN-HUR.
THE FAIR GOD.
Watson (H. B. Marriot). THE ADVEN-TURERS.
Weekes (A. B.). PRISONERS OF WAR.
Wells (H. G.). THE STOLEN BACILLUS.
White (Percy). A PASSIONATE PILGRIM.